Ottoman Medicine

Ottoman Medicine

Healing and Medical Institutions, 1500–1700

MIRI SHEFER-MOSSENSOHN

SUNY
PRESS

Cover art entitled "The Story of the Toothache Tree." In Turkestan there is a certain tree which cures toothaches. The wood of the tree is burnt and the ashes rubbed on the painful tooth. The smoke from the wood is also effective. In the picture, one youth with a swollen face holds his head over the smoke of fire made of the Toothache Tree, while another youth stands nearby. "Wonders of Art and Nature," manuscript held at the British Library, Harl. 5500, f.75v, reproduced by permission of the British Library.

Published by State University of New York Press, Albany

Printed in the United States of America

For information, contact State University of New York Press, Albany, NY
www.sunypress.edu

Production by Diane Ganeles
Marketing by Michael Campochiaro

Library of Congress Cataloging-in-Publication Data

Shefer-Mossensohn, Miri, 1971–
Ottoman medicine : healing and medical institutions, 1500–1700 / Miri Shefer-Mossensohn.
p. cm.
Includes bibliographical references and index.
ISBN 978-1-4384-2529-0 (hardcover : alk. paper)
ISBN 978-1-4384-2530-6 (pbk. : alk. paper)
1. Medicine—Turkey—History. 2. Medical care—Turkey—History.
I. Title.

RA537.M67 2009
610.9561—dc22 2008024275

10 9 8 7 6 5 4 3 2 1

To I. with endless love and gratitude

Contents

Illustrations

Preface

This is a book on sickness and health and how one dealt with it as a patient, a healer, and health administrator in the Ottoman Middle East in the early modern period. In some cases the story had a happy ending; in so many other instances, suffering, misery, and finally death were involved. This is of course not one the most cheerful topics one could choose as a focus to a scientific enquiry. I have chosen it nevertheless, as health and sickness and finally death are an inherent part of life. This may be not terribly optimistic, but it has the merit of being realistic. Moreover, they are intimately connected to so many other aspects of life—intellectual debates, social interactions, religious beliefs, economic processes, and political order—and as a result they are very promising as a venue for delving into past societies.

The multifaceted of medicine turned this project into a double journey. It started as a foray into history, and I hope to bring to life in these pages a rich picture of the lives of people in the early modern Middle East. It was also a personal one. As I proceeded with this study I had to redefine my assumptions of what health and medicine were, not only for people of a distant time and place, but also for me and the society in which I live.

This book is about contemporary social consciousness and awareness, as the history of medicine is not of historical value only. In this case the past is very much relevant to our own modern society. It is also connected with the current public debate worldwide about the role that the medical establishment and the scientific community should play in a modern society, and how they should respond to the social and natural environment, especially when the cost of medical treatment is higher than ever. This debate is related also the current crisis within orthodox medicine. More people choose alternative medicines rather than orthodox medicine and technology and question their moral basis. Academic studies add to the critical discourse of what is "good" or "modern" about contemporary health care institutions by going back to historical examples, Western and non-Western alike. This in turn should help society educate better medical personnel (whatever "better" is). By making the medical system better not only the lives of the sick and feeble are better, but the world becomes better, more just.

This work has two layers. The first layer is the story of Middle Eastern medicine(s) and medical institutions: what types of medicine(s) existed in the Middle East, who were its founders were, who worked in it, who the patients were, and where it was located. The second and more important layer deals with Middle Eastern society and culture from a medical point of view. The chapters in this book are devoted to subjects like prevention and curative therapeutics; holism, nature and ecology; charity, entitlement, and group identity; health and social hierarchy; dialogues between medicine and religious belief; and medicine, power and social order.

I accumulated quite a debt to so many people, and am glad I am able to at least partially repay it by presenting them with this book; I would like to acknowledge their support here.

The project originated as a doctoral dissertation. Later on it went through a series of transformations, and (I hope)—improvements. However, I still owe a debt to my teachers at Tel Aviv University: my doctoral advisor, Professor Amy Singer; Professor Ehud Toledano, who did not carry any official roles but was and still is a constant source of support and inspiration; and Professor David J. Wasserstein, now of Vanderbilt University, who tutored a young research assistant. In London, I owe Professor Lawrence I. Conrad (now of Hamburg) much gratitude for hosting me for three months while carrying out my project at the wonderful facilities of the Wellcome Institute for the History of Medicine. In Istanbul Professor Nil Sarı of the Department of History of Medicine at the Cerrahpaşa Faculty of Medicine in Istanbul was gracious enough to take real interest in the research of someone who at the time was still a novice in Ottoman medicine and Ottoman sources. In Cambridge it was Dr. Kate Fleet, the head of the Skilliter Centre for Ottoman Studies at Newnham College, who was a wonderful hostess. I was affiliated with the Centre for a term and benefited greatly from the vast Ottoman literature (primary and secondary) there. With Dr. Leigh N. B. Chipman of Ben Gurion University, a friend and colleague, I share interest in Muslim medicine. I thank her for all her help with editing the text.

The names of museums, libraries, and archives bring to mind faces and names of people I enjoyed working with and to whose help

I am immensely grateful. In Istanbul I worked in the Başbakanlık Osmanlı Arşivi (the Archives of the Ottoman Prime Ministry), the Topkapı Sarayı Müzesi Arşivi and Kütüphanesi (the Archives and Library of Topkapi Palace), and the Süleymaniye Library; in Ankara at the Vakıflar Genel Müdürlüğü Arşivi (the Archives of the General Directorate for Charitable Institutions); in London at the British Library and the Wellcome Institute for the History of Medicine Library; in Cambridge at the Cambridge University Library; and in Princeton at the Firestone Library. The hospitality of librarians who supplied me with good advice with regard to the collections at their charge (and not to mention other types of help in the form of endless cups of hot tea and good conversation) helped me to move forward.

At the State University of New York Press, I would like to thank Dr. Michael Rinella, Diane Ganeles, and Wyatt Benner for their expert guidance in producing this book.

My thanks are also to the anonymous readers for the Press. Their endorsement and constructive criticism are very much appreciated. Finally, Tomer Miron, Liran Yadgar, Barak Rubinstein, and Ido Ben-Ami, my former and current research assistants, helped me in various ways in preparing this manuscript.

I am happy to acknowledge the generous financial support from various institutions and grants that made the research and writing it up possible: the Israel Science Foundation (grant number 535/04), the Dan David Prize Scholarship in History, the Skilliter Centre for Ottoman Studies Research Grant, the Friends of the Library Fellowship at Princeton University Library, the Rothschild Fellowship, and a Research Scholarship from the Turkish Ministry of National Education (Milli Eğitim Bakanlığı), and the Department of Middle Eastern and African History at Tel-Aviv University.

Finally, I would like to mention my family: my parents, brother, and in-laws, and especially my husband (to whom I dedicate this book) and two daughters, who were born into this project and grew with it. We all know how much I owe you. At this point I also remember my late grandfather, who would have been happy and proud to see his granddaughter writing a book.

As the book was copyedited, my father, Dr. Michael Shefer, passed away. I wish he could have seen the book.

Note on Transliteration

The problem of transliteration in Ottoman studies is complicated because of the very broad geographical, cultural, and lingual scope of the subject matter. Spreading over three continents for six hundred years, the Ottoman Empire was inhabited by members of many linguistic groups living alongside each other, including—in addition to users of Turkic dialects—users of Serbo-Croat, Berber, Hebrew, Arabic, Persian, Kurdish, and many more. Moreover, Ottoman society and culture enabled—indeed, encouraged—routine crossing of lingual and cultural boundaries. The result was an extraordiary cultural mixture and diversity. To deal with it, any single system of transliteration is found lacking either grammatically, phonetically, or aesthetically. Hence I adopted a compromise that allowed me to achieve consistency as much as possible while emphasizing the theme of cultural diversity with regard to Ottoman medical realities of the early modern period and accurately reflecting the languages of the sources used here, which are mainly Ottoman Turkish and Arabic. In addition, I tried to simplify forms as much as possible to make the text accessible to medical historians who are nonspecialists in Middle Eastern studies.

Throughout the book I make the case of the high level of Ottomanness of medicine in the Middle East of the sixteenth and seventeenth centuries. With the Ottoman context in mind I find it appropriate to write most terms and names of places and individuals in Ottoman-Turkish forms. For the sake of simplicity, I rendered such terms and names in a modern Turkish form rather than following formal transliteration tables of Ottoman-Turkish. In modern Turkish, *c* is pronounced as *j* is in English, *ç* as *ch*, *ğ* is unvocalized and lengthens the preceding vowel; *ı* (undotted i) sounds like *u* in the word *turn*; and *ş* is pronounced like *sh*.

At the same time I give ample room to provincial-cultural variations, recognizing the Arab character of the Ottoman-Arab provinces.

Therefore, in cases where the context is Arabic-speaking I have used Arabic forms.

This dual system of transliterations allows me to make a distinction, for example, between a *cerrah*, a surgeon in a Turkish speaking site, and his colleague in an Arabic environment, who is a *jarrāḥ*. I write about *darüşşifa*s and *medrese*s, and refer to such physicians as Emir Çelebi. Although he worked many years in a Cairo hospital, Emir Çelebi owed his fame in the seventeenth-century Ottoman court to a medical treatise written in Ottoman-Turkish. However, I discuss also Ottoman physicians like the sixteenth-century physician, Dā'ūd al-Anṭākī, who operated from Antakya in an Arabic-speaking environment, and Ṣālih b. Naṣrallah Ibn Sallūm, the seventeenth century physician from Aleppo who rose to be the imperial head physician but still wrote only in Arabic.

INTRODUCTION

The Marriage of Medicine and Society

Susan Sontag once wrote that we all hold dual citizenship, in the kingdom of the well and in the kingdom of the ill. Sooner or later we are obliged, at least for a spell, to be citizens of that other place.[1] Although illness is so common, it is far from being taken in stride. Rather it was—and still is—regarded as a dramatic and surprising event. Yet there is hardly anything surprising about it. Human life was, and still is, riddled with illness and death. Illness is one of the more regular events in our lives, one that happens to all of us over and over again. Still, each time illness happens, it catches us by surprise. Moreover, illness arouses passionate feelings. Some illnesses are regarded as horrid for the individual in question and his or her surrounding family. Some diseases are romanticized (like the case of TB). Other illnesses are used by some as metaphors for ill deeds and ill nature in the suffering individual or the community at large. The origins of disease are mysterious (like leprosy in the Middle Ages or HIV in our own society). Illness needed explanation. At the basis of everyday realities stand health and illness. These, among other factors (financial, etc.), determine the ability of a person to lead the life of his or her choice. Health and illness affect not just the length of life but its quality. Hence the importance of medicine that should—at least ideally—transfer people from the realm of disease to the realm of health.

This book is about health as much as it is about illness. Not only does each mirror the other, they exist only in relation to each other. Medicine in the early modern Middle East was not only for the ill; it concerned itself primarily with the healthy. Medicine defined what health and illness were, and suggested means to safeguard the former. Moreover, medicine and illness are not simply the backdrop to other historical processes. Illness is more than a minor nuisance that happens to people while they live their lives. Rather, it is a major factor in their lives and how they think of it. Illness is not a marginal and deviant occurrence.

The central theme of this book is that medicine is a human experience and as such is embedded in society and culture. Attitudes prevailing in the early modern Ottoman society concerning health and illness did not exist in isolation from the general social and cultural consensus. Hence, medicine discussed here comprises the realm of knowledge and social applications embedded in a specific historical setting, rather than discussed as a universal reality. The historical setting here is the Ottoman Empire of the fifteenth to seventeenth centuries. The center of attention is the core area of the Ottoman world—that is, the Balkans and Anatolia as far as the Sivas-Kayseri area,[2] with occasional reference to the Arab provinces. Although it is possible to see medicine as an ahistorical clinical reality and to focus on nosologies and treatments, here medicine is presented as the socially and culturally constructed and organized responses of individuals, social networks, and professional communities to health and illness. It is society and culture that endow human medical experience with meaning and that shape various aspects of "reality."[3] Here we shall see how Ottomans in the early modern period made sense of their medical realities; we shall see how medical realities and knowledge of medicine were reflected in the minds of Ottomans, who then articulated their perceptions and in so doing shaped the nature of that "reality."

The study follows the many interactions between medicine (namely, theories and practices), and society (that is, the people who carry those theories and practices—the ill, the practitioners, the healthy). Illness and health do not "belong" to the patients or their doctors but are much wider phenomena embedded in very many layers of social and medical concepts, activities, arrangements, and relationships. There is a constant dialogue in these matters between society and individuals, and this dialogue eventually molds such concepts. Health and illness are social and public events, not only an individual experience and reality.

The basic argument of this book is that the ways in which we conceive health and illness, and organize medical care, reflect the society in which we live. Our understanding of medical concepts and institutions as cultural and social constructs enables us to understand the social organization and cultural values that mold them. Hence constructing the medical-health system of the early modern Middle East tells us who these individuals and their communities were, and what their goals and social values were. To understand a human society one needs to decode the ways in which the society perceived health and illness. I suggest, therefore, that etiologies, therapeutic techniques, and institutions related to medicine, like hospitals and endowments, are a suitable framework for disentangling the complex and elusive life of men and women in the premodern Middle East. Medicine here is a prism through which we can reconstruct social and cultural realities, and we do not stay within the supposedly strict realm of medicine.

These contexts of medicine result in the presentation of an alternative picture of medicine in the Middle East, one that is less heroic or dramatic but perhaps more real. The binary image so far existing in the literature, either heroic (scientific discoveries, progress) or abysmal (redundant, declining medicine) is replaced by a more nuanced one. Here medicine is linked to other fields of knowledge and social activity shared by medical men, men of letters, men of religious scholarship, and laymen and laywomen. The links between medicine and the rest of early modern Ottoman intellectual and social life were many and close. Medicine was a subject of high intellectual status and at the same time also a popular, oral, and empiric activity. Such medicine is largely terra incognita, both for historians of the Middle East and for historians of medicine.

The (In)Visible Middle Eastern Ill in the Scholarship

The history of medicine was centered for a long period on physicians, their interests, and their worldview of what medicine and health constituted. This was a medicine "from the inside" as many historians of medicine used to come from various medical fields, like physicians, nurses, public health officers, or medical administrators. It was an "internalist" intellectual history of medicine that focused on recorded achievements. It was the story of exceptional individuals and their triumphs. The first signs of change were seen in the middle of the twentieth century with George Rosen and some others and gained acceptance later in the 1970s and 1980s.[4] The changes originated in the expropriation of history of medicine by a new generation of historians with new research interests (like social, financial, political, and cultural factors affecting medicine). These new historians wrote the history of medicine "from the outside," introducing new research methodologies borrowed from the social sciences. The result is an interdisciplinary field inviting scholars to consider medicine as a social category. This "social history of medicine" includes such topics as the sociology of the medical profession, medicine and popular culture, and public health. Two primary goals of most work in the social history of medicine appear to be first the delineation of the profiles of complete local or regional medical communities—that is, of all those who practiced healing of any kind, however varied their level of academic preparation, wealth, status, or full-time commitment to the healing arts—and second, the exploration of the experience of ill health and its treatment across the broadest possible social spectrum.[5]

One of the outcomes of this new discipline is the positioning of the patient as the focus of study. In a seminal article on the methodology of medical history, the late Roy Porter called the physician-centered account a major distortion of history. He urged the scholarly community to replace it with one that considers how ordinary people have actually regarded health and illness, and managed their encounter with medical personnel.[6] Porter's plea to map the experiences of the ill has been heard, and in the last twenty years our body of knowledge of lay perceptions of medicine has grown considerably.

While Roy Porter advocated history of medicine from below, another research path highlighted societal power over the ill individuals via the power of medical knowledge. This theory is associated, of course, with Michel Foucault. He outlined "the great confinement" from the Middle Ages onward. This process of segregation of anyone who was perceived as not able to or as not wanting to conform to everyday routines reached its height in the eighteenth century. It was rationalized by contemporaries as a means to protect the interests of two social groups that conspired together: the aristocratic elite and the rising bourgeoisie.[7] This is *mentalités* history, on the borders between history (here: of medicine), psychology, and social science, at the juncture of the individual and the collective. This elusive French term refers to mind-sets, social attitudes, and the forms through which they are conveyed. These may include language (oral and body) and rituals, among other things. This type of history focuses on decoding the manner in which historical circumstances were portrayed and presented in contemporary sources. Its interest is in image and representation rather than in compiling data.[8]

There is a fly, however, in this intellectual ointment. The Middle Eastern ill and illness are (still) missing from the pages of history, as work on social history of medicine is clearly Western-oriented. Many historians of medicine did not include Muslim aspects in their discussion and thus produced Eurocentric narratives. An example is Guenter Risse's masterful exposition of the history of hospitals. Risse traces the evolution from antiquity to contemporary hospitals by favoring the Christian and Anglo-Saxon worlds. It starts with Asclepius, moves on to Byzantium, and focuses on European history, mainly Western (with one subsection dedicated to Vienna), and culminates in the United States.[9]

We can find a similar situation in the wider field of history for science, where studies influenced by Thomas Kuhn are charting how sciences (in the plural) and their cultures coevolve. Yet even the post-Kuhnian stream of studies that brought in skepticism about the separability of science from society seems parochial if one asks questions outside the European-American medical systems.[10] Indeed, for this very reason some historians have criticized the "tyranny" of Anglo-Saxon models forced upon the history of medical systems in non-Western societies. It was mainly Western medicines that were revisited and reconsidered as multifaceted phenomena.

Likewise, scholars of Muslim medicines too have not concerned themselves with the social practice of Middle Eastern physicians, and their interactions with patients did not interest the scholars. The experience of illness and how medicine was viewed from the angle of the ill were also not commented on. Those few studies which did mention illness and ill people described neglect, stoic attitudes, and even fatalism as characterizing the Muslim Middle East. Medicine in the Muslim Middle East has indeed received considerable attention, yet few have considered it in its social and cultural contexts. Although social history of medicine is a well-established field, for historians of the Middle East it still remains at the periphery of the discipline. While a great deal has been written, very creatively from a methodological point of view, about medicine as a social phenomenon in European and U.S. history, this is a new area of interest for historians of Muslim societies in general and Ottoman society in particular.

History of medicine is a field with a history of its own within Middle Eastern history. The discourse has focused on famous physicians and their great medical discoveries, or, alternatively, the intellectual decline thereof. As Emilie Savage-Smith has observed in a state-of-the-art article, the questions that have customarily been asked of early Islamic science have concerned the reception, transformation, and transmission of earlier scientific ideas. This was the rather traditional text-bound approach to the history of Islamic medicine.[11]

Manfred Ullmann's *Islamic Medicine*, published more than thirty years ago, is symptomatic of the scholarship that reigned supreme for a long time.[12] Under this title Ullmann focused exclusively on only one type of Muslim medicine, presenting it as the only medicine there was, or the only type that counted as "medicine," the others being mere folklore or superstitions. For him, medicine was an intellectual activity, rather than a social phenomenon embedded in a specific culture. And Muslim medicine was presented as an Arabic medicine in the sense it existed (that is, was written) in Arabic. Ullmann studied Arabic manuscripts minutely, since he, like other scholars of his period, among them Max Meyerhof and Joseph Schacht, came from an academic background in Arabic philology.[13] Moreover, Ullmann was very much influenced by the "decline theory." This paradigm maintained that after a golden period under the Abbasid caliphate, continuous decline started in the Muslim world as a whole. It encompassed all aspects of Muslim life, including intellectual and scientific thought. These two factors explain Ullmann's almost total silence on Turkish and Persian medicines. According to Ullmann, after the end of the Islamic (Arabic) golden age in the thirteenth century nothing good or innovative happened in Muslim medicine till the westernization of the nineteenth century. Hence, Ullmann devoted only a small portion of his book to the Ottoman period, and the few Ottoman physicians who are mentioned are only those who wrote in Arabic and were accessible to him.

Only in the beginning of 2007, almost thirty years later, were we presented with an updated replacement to Ullmann's monograph in the form of *Medieval Islamic Medicine*, which was included in the New Edinburgh Islamic Surveys.[14] The different title is telling. Peter E. Pormann and Emilie Savage-Smith declare the mandate they took upon themselves: they surveyed medicine in a specific historical reality, that of medieval Muslim societies. Intentionally they left out later Muslim medical systems, like the Ottoman. However, they end their excellent survey with a chapter entitled "Afterlife" where they discuss in brief various trends in Muslim medicine in the Middle East, Persia, and India from the early modern period till today.

A rare example of scholarly work focused on Persian medicine is the that of Cyril Elgood, who published several monographs on premodern Persian medicine using Persian sources.[15] However, other than the choice of a different geographical scope, Elgood's work represents the same scholarly fashion as Ullman's. In terms of methodology, both were text-bound and interested only in learned (that is, written) medical traditions. They belonged to the same historiographical generation.

Meanwhile, from the 1930s onward, many studies on Turkish medicine have been published, but in Turkish (the authors were Turks), which made them inaccessible to most Western and Middle

Eastern readers. These scholars, such as Osman Şevki Uludağ, Mehmet Cevdet, Adnan Abdülhak Adıvar, Ahmet Süheyl Ünver, and Bedi N. Şehsuvaroğlu did focus on medicine in later periods in the premodern Muslim world, including the Ottoman period.[16]

Despite these noted differences, the two groups of scholars were partners in a similar discourse on the history of medicine in a Muslim society. First, both groups wrote a "Whiggish" history, looking for heroes, success stories, and scientific progress. They were fascinated by what Charles E. Rosenberg described as "a past that could be constructed as progressing toward an enlightened and ethical present. The intellectual significance of individuals and events was seen in terms of their relationship to the development of a contemporary understanding of the human body and not to the particular historical context in which those individuals worked and thought."[17] Second, if one group focused on medicine in Arabic to the exclusion of other types of medical activity, the other's focus was mainly Turkish. Furthermore, both groups concentrated on "learned medicine." They downplayed the importance of other types of medicine, so-called popular medicine, and thus not "scientific" and important. Their studies too were text-based and tried to discern "what happened" rather than why history unfolded in certain ways or medicine's relation to other processes in society (economic, social, cultural, or intellectual). They did not pay attention to medical clinical reality and those who shared in its practice, healers and patients alike.

All was not static, however. There were intellectual changes in the 1970s, when historians of the Middle East started to write about medical education and professionalism, hospitals, plagues, and westernization and modernization. Some of these studies were prepared by scholars like Franz Rosenthal, an Arabist. Rosenthal previously had worked on the concept of knowledge in medieval Arabic Muslim society and the classical heritage in Islam. Now his work included studies on gambling, hashish, and other narcotics, and on the medical profession, although still within the context of "high" and learned medicine.[18]

It is especially in the past quarter of a century that there has been a new wave of studies on medicine in the field of Islamic studies. In part these studies were inspired by the new trends in history of medicine in general, within which social aspects have gained momentum in the last thirty years. These studies showed that a body of evidence pertaining to the experience of illness in the historical Middle East still exists. If the ill and disabled were left in history's shadow, it was because they were hidden from scholars' sight, rather than due to contemporaries' lack of interest. Let me select three names to illustrate the considerable distance the field has gone, and that there is still a long way to go. The attention of most historians of Islamic science was and still is directed toward Arabic sources. The vast quantity of Turkish and Persian manuscript and archival sources still interest only a few scholars.[19]

One of the first "encouraging trends," as Savage-Smith termed them in the late 1980s, is the research of Michael W. Dols, who wrote several pioneering works on various aspects of plagues, leprosy, hospitals, and madness in the medieval Muslim Middle East. He lays the groundwork for understanding the physical realities as well as the social and cultural aspects of illness and disability.[20] Lawrence I. Conrad has been carrying the torch since Dols's untimely death with regard to studying plagues in the early Muslim Middle East (as well as other topics related to the history of medicine).[21]

A second name is Khaled Fahmy. Fahmy considered modernization and state building in late nineteenth-century Egypt, mainly under British rule, through the prism of medicine and medical institutions. His main interest lay with medicine and power, whether between the state and its organs and the population, or between genders.[22] It is interesting to note that the geographical area of North Africa and Egypt has been privileged more than other regions of the Middle East to be the focus of studies on the history of medical professionalism and public health in the late eighteenth and early nineteenth centuries.[23]

While illness in either the medieval or modern periods has started to be addressed, the examples above demonstrate there is still a lacuna in the scholarship with regard to the early modern period. In most of the publications the ill do not occupy a central spot. Instead, the studies focus on demography and internal and international politics rather than on the realities of individual ill people.[24] Certain remnants from previous trends in scholarship still linger.

The majority of the work on this period is still conducted in Turkey, by Turkish scholars, in the Turkish language. A minority (although a growing one) publishes also in English or German,[25] but with few exceptions they too do not seek audiences outside Turkish academic journals. More importantly, to a large extent work on Ottoman medicine is still a "history of heroes." Ekmeleddin İhsanoğlu, without whose publications any survey of studies of Ottoman science cannot be complete, and the third name to be mentioned here, referred to this point. In the preface of his collection of articles published by Ashgate in the Variorum Collected Studies Series İhsanoğlu presented his research program. He explained that while studying the history of Ottoman science it is imperative to consider nonscientific activities, like political, economic, and social factors, as well.[26] Despite this declaration in İhsanoğlu's own work, descriptive narratives of physicians and the contents of their manuscripts are the usual context. The few ill people who do appear are discussed under the heading of "famous illnesses of famous people," which is yet another version of the history of "big names."

The present book tries to contribute to filling up some of the gaps in our knowledge and understanding of Muslim medicines in past Muslim societies by focusing on two major areas so far neglected in Middle Eastern history: Ottoman medicines and the experiences of illness. It is done by offering a work of fusion. In addition to social history of medicine brought into a Middle Eastern context, there are other fields of research from history and social sciences pertaining to medicine and illness that are absorbed into this book. They help to ask and attempt to answer basic questions about what illness was as a human experience. The result, it is hoped, is a thick description of this phenomenon in the early modern Middle East. In focusing on the early modern Middle East, this study adds to the growing literature on medicine and society in non-Western societies. Moreover, in this way cross-fertilization is achieved: This work considers research issues raised by historians and anthropologists of Western societies, adjusts these topics to the Ottoman case, and tries to discuss them in a context that can enrich works on Western medicine as well.

Recent evolutions within history, for example, have had an influence on this study. The first is "disability history," which in its present form was launched in the middle of the 1980s. Disability was added to historical inquiries as an analytical category of society on a par with key terms like "gender," "race," and "class." It thus adds another theoretical tool to exploring the "Other." As in the case of social history of medicine, physical impairment is considered here as (only) a part of a multifaceted reality of abnormality that also includes social and cultural power relations that may yield oppression and inequality.[27] Disability studies focus on the interaction between individuals and their society.

The second evolution within recent history unfolds a story of interaction with the organic world. This is "environmental history"—that is, the story of humanity as a participant in local, regional, and worldwide ecosystems. In the words of Emmanuel Le Roy Ladurie, the field embraces climate, epidemics, natural calamities, population explosion, urbanization, industrial overconsumption, and pollution.[28]

The present work does not make nature and the environment its focus, but reflects on the fact that early modern Middle Easterners were aware of the environmental consequences of their behavior. Moreover, the category of "nature" adds an important dimension to medicine and health; the context of ecology with its physical and moral dimensions. It highlights the fact these are also, to a degree, ecologically circumscribed.

The dynamics in the realm of history did not occur in isolation from changes within anthropology, including its exciting and promising subdisciplines of medical anthropology.[29] The goal of medical anthropology is the comprehensive description and interpretation of the interrelationships between human behavior, past and present, and health and disease. Another aim is the improvement of human health levels through greater understanding of health behavior in directions believed to promote better health. The field has a wide range of interests, some of which are close to biology (human development, genetics, etc.). Other of its interests are closer to sociology and culture. These involve "ethnomedicine," medical personnel and their professional preparation, illness behavior, the doctor-patient relationship, and the dynamics of the introduction of Western medical services into traditional societies. The field bears a Geertzian influence in considering medicine as a public cultural phenomenon rich with symbols and values.

It is, however, the understanding of medicine as a composite system, made of subsystems and multiple institutions, beliefs, and practices, that most influenced the present book. At the same time, beneath the surface of luxuriant variety, several unifying principles and mechanisms operated to bring systematic organization to the seemingly random action (here Claude Lévi-Strauss and structuralism contributed to medical anthropology). We shall see that the Ottoman Empire produced a variety of medical systems rather than one, universal and uniform. Yet they interacted in a way that proved that there was one "medical space" in which they all participated.

Medical anthropology formulates several universals, some of which echo findings from social history of medicine. These are that medical systems are integral parts of cultures; that illness is culturally defined; that all medical systems have both preventive and curative sides; and that medical systems have multiple functions, in addition to caring for a patient, among them enacting social roles and norms or offering devices to control behavior. Although the infrastructures that make up a medical system are accepted as very powerful and can shape human action, medical anthropology leaves room also for the doer, presenting the actor's point of view. Illness is also what people make within the constraints of the system they operate in; they are active persons who shape their reality and are not mere passive recipients.[30]

The Aims and Scope of the Book

The ill and their illness in the Muslim Middle East were missing from historical narratives but certainly not from historical realities. A society never stops being interested in medicine and health, and never neglects trying to improve them. This is after all a very basic human need, both mentally and physically. It was certainly so in the early modern Middle East, where life was riddled with health hazards and death lurked at every corner, with life expectancy at around the age of forty. Such is the hunger for preserving health and curing illness as commodities that there has nearly always been a buyers' market for them. However, buyers, suppliers, and, indeed, markets have varied enormously, not only over time but also within a country in any one period, with different groups and classes of patients patronizing different types of medical practitioners.[31] The present book shows that the Ottoman understanding of health and usage of medicine were much more complex than previously envisioned.

This volume does not claim to deal with every aspect of health, disease, and medicine in the early modern Ottoman Middle East. Although readers will find here a wide-ranging study of some aspects of medicine in the Ottoman Middle East, the book in no way pretends to present the definitive history of Ottoman health care. This has yet to be written. Such an attempt at comprehensive coverage would have led to too much diffuseness in a volume of the present length or to an unacceptably long monograph. Consequently, I have preferred to include detailed studies of certain important issues pertaining to health and disease and agencies of health care and leave other important but so far neglected questions to future investigations.

Thus, one task this book takes on is to chart the gaps in our knowledge and understanding with regard to Ottoman medicine and health. Many aspects have not been written about because this cannot yet be done. Sources are still to be located, studied, and deciphered. Methodological problems are to be solved, mainly the tangled and not always obvious relationship between the sources pertaining to health care (medical, legal, financial and literary) and historical medical reality.

Intentionally I chose to follow a topical framework rather than a geographical or chronological one. The benefit of this approach is that it scans a wide spectrum of discussion on medical topics. The four chapters and conclusion portray Ottoman health care in a way that weaves together social, cultural, and political dimensions into a coherent picture of a complex, multifaceted system. As an aid to facilitate orientation with the main Ottoman medical institutions, I include a list of the main hospitals discussed here as an appendix.

Each of the four numbered chapters of this book deals with different aspects of health beliefs and health maintenance and preventive practices that existed in the early modern Middle East. The chapters discuss various sectors in society that were involved in medicine, among them are professional healers, patients, health administrators, and philanthropists. They explore issues of power, knowledge, personal and social norms, and social structures and networks related to medicine and health. The chapters explain how both the personal and the communal affect the perception, experience, and expression of health and illness and how care is delivered. They illustrate how elite and nonelite Ottomans talked about medicine and health and how they lived it. Two realities unfold here: a discursive one that exists in the realm of language and thought, alongside a social reality of how people experienced medicine and health in concrete life experiences.

The first two chapters discuss treatment as intervention, whether symbolic or instrumental, and show etiquette, treatment style, and therapeutic objectives. The chapters show that practitioner and patient shared in the responsibility for the treatment: decisions about its nature and course and its ultimate success are determined by both. The medical reality of the early modern Ottoman world was that of medical ideas and skills widely disseminated in the community and not segregated in the profession. Laymen could understand as well as manipulate many medical ideas, and the result was a shared medical language for both healers and patients.

The first chapter, "Medical Pluralism, Prevention, and Cure," presents the medical settings: what types of medicine existed in the early modern Ottoman Empire and the Middle East. The Ottoman medical system was based on several traditions—Galenic humoralism, folkloristic medicine, and religious medicine. Like in our modern medical system (which features the existence of "alternative" medicine), various traditions complemented one another and competed with one another for hegemony (and finances) within the medical system. The discussion revolves around medical theories and actual therapeutics, and tries to get as close as possible to the patient's bed: how were patients really treated at home and in the hospitals? Clinical reality can be elusive, as medical practice was not necessarily identical to the medical theory discussed in learned treatises. The chapter highlights two characteristics of Ottoman medicine. The first: in contrast to our modern medicine, Ottoman medicines emphasized preventive measures rather than curative, "heroic," and invasive procedures. The second characteristic is that medical options were tied to social and economic realities. Medicine was a means for social demarcation and in turn helped to reinforce those status distinctions.

Chapter 2, " 'In health and in sickness': The Integrative Body," continues to discuss the interaction between medical theory and clinical reality, but here the emphasis is on the integrative dimensions of Ottoman medicines. The chapter argues that all the traditions that make up the Middle Eastern medical system shared an integralistic approach to healing. All recognized that the emotional, spiritual, physical, and ecological elements of each person comprise a system, although the exact definition of each component and the relative balance between them varied from one medical tradition to another. This was on the theoretical level. On the practical level, the chapter demonstrates how all medical traditions attempted to treat the whole person, concentrating on the cause of the illness as well as symptoms. The chapter stresses four examples where such philosophical, psychological, and theological attitudes were most apparent: the use of all the human senses in the healing process; the intentional use of belief in various forms (belief in oneself, in one's healer, or in God) to promote health; the importance of water for the constant upkeep of hygiene and for therapy; and finally, Ottoman perceptions of health and illness as much more than physical conditions. This chapter helps us to understand the distinction between health and well-being, as the latter was not the medical absence of illness but also the ability to live a full social life. This last section in the second chapter serves as a summation to the first two chapters. It explains why although Ottomans ascribed much importance to preventive medicine, as explained in the first chapter, there were nevertheless many curative measures. Indeed, there were multiple means to treat all kinds of aches and ailments. This feature of Ottoman medicine goes hand in hand with the great significance Ottomans attached to health and the major political, social, cultural, financial, and religious consequences of ill health in that society.

This book is also about how that society organized health care and its institutions. This is the subject of the third chapter, " 'Feed the hungry, visit the sick, and set those who suffer free': Medical Benevolence and Social Order," which discusses how charity was a basic financial and legal mechanism for medical aid in general and for hospital management in particular. The chapter considers the two sides of charity, the partners to the "gift exchange": those who offer it (e.g., the founders of hospitals) and the consumers (e.g., the patients in the hospitals). The discussion reveals that benevolent donors had concrete materialistic and political aims in this world, in addition to gaining merit for pious deeds in the world to come. More importantly, by discussing medical philanthropy we can discern two related social process. One was the means by which medical charity expressed and controlled Ottomans' conceptions of belonging to their society during the early modern period. Those who were entitled to medical services were so entitled because they were members of Ottoman society. An interrelated aspect of this issue was the means by which medical aid reveals the identity of marginal groups in Ottoman-Muslim society. While clearly there was a process of marginalization in action in pre-modern Ottoman society, this was not a society that was quick to exclude minority groups from within the larger community. The second process was using medical charity for social order by controlling people's behavior, through moral and professional codes, financial resources, and a sense of obligation. In other words, medical charity is presented here as a means to bring about social cohesiveness.

Chapter 4, "Spaces of Disease, Disease in Space," examines the physical setting of hospitals in the Ottoman Empire in the early modern period. I present this physical setting by investigating the location and structure of hospitals in the Ottoman realm as a whole and within the urban space in particular. My aim is not to focus on the architectural aspects of these buildings as such. Following Charles E. Rosenberg's *The Care of Strangers* on the rise of the American hospital system,[32] I use hospitals as a means to learn about social and cultural assumptions that are otherwise not easily visible; since they govern hospital life, they are revealed. I discuss the perceptions of these buildings by contemporary Ottomans as a reflection of the competing etiologic theories (miasma, celestial causes, contagion, and jinns) that were at work in the Ottoman society. Their existence explains the diverse (and sometimes opposing) Muslim medical and religious attitudes toward diseases, like the plague, as some stayed put and some ran away. Ottoman hospitals were an epitome of one medical tradition, humoralism, and thus an epitome of the ecological concepts embodied in this medical tradition.

The final pages of the book are dedicated to two questions that are hinted at in previous chapters. First, how far and in what ways was the Ottoman medical system indeed "Ottoman"? Second, was this medical system at all successful in Ottoman eyes? By reconsidering issues analyzed in the previous chapters, the discussion here confronts the question of the extent to which medicine is a universal and cosmopolitan entity, or else is embedded in specific social and cultural contexts.

Several themes weave the chapters together. One is the discussion of multiple and contradictory/conflicting morals and worldviews. Ottoman medicine was a blend of customs, ideas, and realities aiming to solve a constant human problem—illness and death. Individuals and communities decided for themselves issues like right and wrong, true or false. Ottomans selected their own medical paths to follow as occasion arose (and it always did). The story throughout the book is one of constant interpretations and contested ideas and ideals. Society juggled different medical beliefs and customs, and different medical professionals competed among themselves and with the widespread tradition of self-treatment. We learn of the harmonious but sometimes tense or ambiguous and overlapping relationship between traditional and customary medical and health practices and innovations, between public and private considerations, between the individual and his worlds, between individual needs and societal ones. The narrative explores the process of the failed attempts to establish one medical system as canonic and defuses dichotomies like high/learned/elite versus low/oral/popular in the medical realm. It is a story of the dynamics of dissemination and transmission of medical knowledge. The relationship between producers, transmitters, and consumers of that knowledge changed, yet all played active roles in the realm of medicine, albeit different ones.

Balance (Arabic, *mīzān*), too, serves as a theme throughout the book. The chapters bring forth various balances pertaining to the human being; some are "real," physical, while others are symbolic. The opening two chapters present balances within the human being. The first chapter discusses various working explanations existing in Ottoman medicine concerning the physical balance in the body. These explanations were different interpretations of what Greek Galenic medicine termed "humors," the four basic "fluids" of the body (blood, phlegm, black bile, and yellow bile), corresponding to the four elements in nature (air, water, earth, and fire). The second chapter tackles the balance Ottomans sought to establish within the body between body and soul, between the material and the spiritual. There is a pattern of the integrative, or holistic, in Ottoman medicine. The following two chapters leave the body and seek to position man in balance with his social and physical surroundings. The third chapter discusses the balance between the individual and society via the obligation to give and the need to receive. The chapter explores various needs of society and how the elite controlled it by balancing the offerings of medical charity between as many groups as possible. The fourth chapter picks up the ecological balance: the fact that man had to be one with his surrounding nonhuman world. This theoretical moral concept had physical implications in the situating of hospitals within the urban space and in the organization of their inner space, such as the inclusion of walls and gardens as an integral part of the hospital.

The last two numbered chapters are connected in discussing the community and its borders, in the social context (chapter 3) and in the physical meaning of quarantines and hospitals' walls (chapter 4). Medical charity, with its choice of entitled beneficiaries and the implementation of etiological theories in the realm of public health, reveals what Muslim Ottomans understood to be their community, who was part of it, who was regarded as being on the fringes, and who belonged at all. Illness was one of the indicators of the "other" in early modern society; yet it was not a final marker. Even while ill and admitted into hospitals, people were not cut off from society. Hospitals were situated in most cases in very central places in the urban space. Once illness (including lunacy) was removed, the ad hoc marginalization stopped and people were reintegrated into society.

The book discusses inter alia various aspects of medical professionalism. It is brought up in the first chapter while discussing surgery. The Ottoman period saw growing professionalism within medicine. The institutionalization of surgery as a discipline of its own, for example, was one aspect of this process. Medicine is discovered to be a body of knowledge and a profession that arouses opposing emotions. As discussed in the third chapter in the context of physicians working pro bono as a form of medical charity, there was a debate about the nature of occupation: was it indeed a noble calling, a field of knowledge (*ilm*), or a craft (*sina'a*)? The conclusion sums up by saying that medicine as a body of knowledge was respected, even admired; but the profession elicited some disparagement. Medical healers were idolized in some sources as having special knowledge and capabilities for the good of people, but in many others they were the target of jests and were accused of charlatanism, miserliness, and foolishness. Physicians were feared because of their ability to harm people, whether intentionally (they were able to do so with their gifts of special knowledge and capabilities) or unintentionally, as a result of an error. Yet physicians were sued for their failures. This shows that they did not induce that much fear in their patients.

The treatment of this subject here only scratches the surface and will be scrutinized in another study, but we can safely say that whatever the precise reaction medicine and medical professionals caused, one thing did not happen: they were not ignored, nor taken for granted, nor met with indifference.

In preparing this work, several problems had to be solved. One was the need to place limits on a topic that entices its students to deviate to other relevant subjects. As Mary Lindemann observed,[33] the history of medicine and society is especially notorious for presenting such a challenge. There are numerous routes through which one may trace the concepts and organization of health and illness in a given society. The solution was a combination of selections followed rigorously, yet within these selections I allowed myself to be tempted to broaden the discussion.

A choice was made of (only) one route to follow, and this is the interplay between knowledge and practice. Knowledge and practice shape each other; moreover, much of what we know about an object can be attained through the practices surrounding it. Each chapter deals with these two aspects of medicine, their complex relationship with each other, and their relationships with society. Yet this theme was a springboard to discussions of several basic principles that govern human lives and how abstract concepts about life and death, health and illness, entitlement and obligation, nature and the environment, are put into social praxis. Hence the various chapters deal with medical, legal, and literary discussions and clinical realities and their social meanings (chapter 1), holistic therapeutics and concepts of health (chapter 2), medical welfare and philanthropy as connected to social discipline (chapter 3), and, lastly, medical institutions and urban space and nature (chapter 4).

Another means of focusing the discussion was to prefer the urban segment of society. The geographical scope of the book is the central urban centers in the Ottoman Empire, and it does not comment on the medical realities of the rural parts of the empire. This is not to say that the peasants lacked medical attention. Rather, medical aid in the countryside was organized in a different way, and as a result is excluded from this work. As the rural area encompassed the majority of the empire in terms of geography and population, this book should be followed by a sequel.

In my case, I believe the focus here has several merits. First, the urban centers were the seats of Ottoman power. The state was more salient in the cities. The empire maintained a system of several urban centers. The Ottoman capital moved from Bursa, the first capital in the fourteenth century, to Edirne in the 1360s and finally to Istanbul after the conquest of Constantinople in 1453. Even after the official move, the previous capitals retained some power and imperial symbolism. Sultans invested in magnificent complexes of buildings in Bursa and Edirne many years after they officially sat in another capital. Several seventeenth-century sultans moved their royal court to Edirne for several months each year. The Ottoman ideology was further disseminated through a network of provincial centers in western and central Anatolia that hosted princes' courts. Until the days of Süleyman I in the sixteenth century, teenage Ottoman princes were sent off to such towns to mature and acquire hands-on experience in administration and politics (another object was to distance a potential heir to the sultanate from the center and reduce his political threat to the reigning sultan, till his death). In these urban centers the Ottoman state and Ottoman elite were visible and active, and so it was also in the medical realm.

Another reason to choose this specific geographical area is related to the first one. As these centers were the seats of power, they were better documented. The central administration was naturally interested in regulating these places politically, socially, and financially. The Ottoman elite lived here, and here it patronized cultural and intellectual activity. It was in the centers that manuscripts on every subject imaginable were produced, works related to medicine included. The same scholars also documented the activities of an elite that was involved in medicine as patients and as patrons of medical charity. The centers drew many travelers, both locals and Europeans. They were diplomats, merchants, and adventurers. Some of them were interested in medicine, botany, and nature. They all wrote later about their experiences and impressions of medicine and health in the Ottoman Empire.

The subject of the book and its focuses determined the sources, and this was the second problem that had to be solved in preparing this work. Because this is the first foray into the social history of Ottoman medicine, the sources for this kind of research had first to be found and evaluated. As the point of departure is the center of the empire, I located the sources representing the viewpoints of the three capitals. In addition to the geographical aspect of this selection, these sources are the product of a certain social group—namely, the political, social, and military elite of the Ottoman Empire. The sources range from the foundation deeds of the hospitals, the annual reports of the pious foundations (*muhasebe defterleri*), decrees of the sultans (sing. *ferman*), to medical treatises, travel literature, and biographical dictionaries. There is a variety of written sources—archival, literary, and medical—as well as pictorial miniatures in manuscripts depicting medical scenes. The more diverse the sources, the more complex the picture we can construct out of them, and therefore gain closer access to the realities of the premodern era.

Our understanding of what constitutes "health" and "illness" is ever changing. Here we focus on the early modern period. Focusing on the early modern period is not an arbitrary choice. I borrow this periodization from European history, although it is not a natural outgrowth of Middle Eastern realities. Moreover, it is an artificial term in the European context, too. However, "early modern" recognizes the beginning of a new period and world in the fifteenth century, a period and world different from the previous one, that of the Middle Ages.

In Europe "early modern" is the period of the humanists and Renaissance, a profound intellectual change intertwined with deep changes in society and economy, including religious ideas and institutions, politics, the state, and warfare. This was the age of technological and scientific discoveries and advances like the printing press or sea voyages. The modern experience of Europe and the end of the old ways starts in the late eighteenth century with the fall of the ancien régime and industrial society replacing an agrarian one. Medicine was linked to all these changes and was thus affected too.[34]

For the Middle East with regard to medicine I define "early modern" as the fifteenth through the seventeenth centuries. I argue that Middle Eastern medicine changed profoundly during this period. Intellectually, professionally, and administratively it is a period that should be studied on its own merit. Moreover, the fifteenth century through the seventeenth century was a period that became a formative link between medieval medicine and the modern medical system in the Middle East. It was a period when Ottoman medicines went through systemization, organization, and professionalization on a scale not experienced before. Throughout the book various aspects of this process will be discussed. The conclusion will argue that these changes in the realm of medicine are not separable from the wider process of Ottomanization that various institutions went through during the fifteenth to seventeenth centuries, changes that set the stage for the modern medical systems of the future.

I have in mind hospitals, a prominent medical institution, and the Ottoman Empire, the important political entity in the region in that period, as a dual yardstick. After a period of an almost complete halt in the foundation of large-scale hospitals in the later Middle Ages (from the Zangids onward only a few new big hospitals were erected), the

Ottomans renewed with gusto the tradition of imperially patronized hospitals and were associated with hospital foundation from the late fourteenth century. Whereas hospitals were founded in major cities all over the Ottoman Empire in the fifteenth and seventeenth centuries, this activity came to a halt in the eighteenth century. When it was resumed at the end of the end of the eighteenth century, again the hospitals were founded with elite and even imperial backing, but they were of a different type. New hospitals in the eighteenth and nineteenth centuries were established against the background of reforms based on Western models of modern society, culture, and state. These reforms touched upon medicine and hospital management as well as upon so much else. The medicine practiced in the new westernized hospitals was not humoralism, the medical theory studied and practiced for hundreds of years by Muslim and Ottoman doctors within and outside hospitals as learned medicine. Instead, patients were now treated according to a new conceptualization of medicine, illness, and health that emphasized biology and pathology over the holistic and human approach of previous centuries. The conceptual changes affected the location of new hospitals, too. New hospitals were no longer part of the charitable complexes system—that is, imperial complexes composed of mosques, soup kitchens, and several other dependent charitable institutions.[35] The post-1700 medical realities and changes lie therefore outside the scope of this work.

The early modern period was a period of change in Ottoman medicine. At the same time, there was also continuation. Hospitals serve again an example. On the one hand, they were physically bigger than the pre-Ottoman Muslim hospitals. They employed a larger staff that displayed wider medical capabilities and a higher level of medical professionalism. Yet the medical, administrative, and architectural basis for this new hospital was clearly that of previous centuries. The Ottomans, as in other aspects of their culture, drew on previous traditions and made them their own.

CHAPTER 1

Medical Pluralism, Prevention, and Cure

Medicine in the Muslim Middle East in the early modern period, like other traditional medical systems (for example, the Chinese one),[1] was composed of several subsystems, each promoting a unique etiology and practice, and each enjoying a different legitimacy. This was only to be expected in the Ottoman Empire, the most important political unit in the Middle East from 1300 till World War One; it was vast enough to contain different geographical zones and climates, and diverse cultural heritages. Yet these medical subsystems were not independent of each other. None enjoyed complete hegemony or was regarded by all as superior to others, absolutely true, and exceptionally efficient. Instead of replacing each other, the different medical systems complemented one another. It was a situation of "not only/but also," in contrast to the dichotomy of "either/or." In the Ottoman context, that means that humoralism inherited from antiquity, folklore based on custom, and religious medicines were all solidly present in the medical scene.[2]

The relationship of competition between and completion of these three medical theories and practices is one theme in this chapter. Another type of relation explored here is the still evasive one between medical theory and clinical reality. Cristina Álvarez-Millán showed quite conclusively for the Arab-Muslim Middle Ages the existence of a gap between the learned and written tradition and the clinical one, sometimes in the practice of the same physician. On top of this, in Muslim societies there was no scientific and literary tradition of discussing medical clinical experience. As Lawrence I. Conrad claimed, medical writing is sometimes also a literary activity with social and cultural goals; clinical and pedagogical instruction was not necessarily one of them.[3] Sometimes technology precedes the theoretical understanding of why a certain procedure/medicine/medical device works.

In other cases, the knowledge of what should be done and why is present before there are the means to apply it. And sometimes medical practices from different theoretical systems are lumped together. Naturally, practice was not independent of or divorced from theoretical discourse, but intertwined with it.

Following Peregrine Horden, I take the evidence as revealing contemporary medical and social concerns. The fact that manuscripts seem to rely heavily on one another, and sometimes blatantly copy from one another without acknowledging their intellectual debt, means we cannot hope to extract from them proper statistics of the ailments of that era. However, although we lack as yet a complete list of important diseases, an Ottoman nosography, we do posses textual representations thereof. Far from being the full reality of pathology, then, it does reflect at least some of the health concerns of that society.[4]

Two characteristics of Ottoman medicine reveal themselves as salient. First, Ottomans ascribed much importance to preventive medicine (*himaya*), though at the same time there were also many curative measures, and indeed there were multiple (and competing) means in the medical scene to treat all kinds of aches and ailments. Second, medical therapeutics had pronounced and far-reaching social aspects. Being embedded in the hierarchical Ottoman society, the realm of medicine too acknowledged social and financial differences. Ottoman medicines offered multiple methods for getting better and keeping one's health; not unlike today, they were not available to all. To many Ottomans, social and economic realities narrowed their medical options. Medicine was also a means for social demarcation and in turn helped to reinforce those status distinctions.

Ottoman Medical Etiologies

Ottoman medicine and therapeutics are best understood as a system, inasmuch as they encompassed all of the health-promoting beliefs and actions, scientific knowledge, and skills of the members of the group that subscribed to the system.[5] Seeing it as a system allows us to visualize Ottoman medicine as a superstructure, constructed of smaller building blocks of medical ideas and practices. This is to be expected in an empire as vast as the Ottoman, subject as it was to several climates and environments, and enriched by numerous cultural and scientific influences. The three building blocks, folkloristic popular medicine, religious medicine ("Prophetic medicine"), and mechanistic medicine based on humoralism had their own body of medical knowledge, unique disease theory, and characteristic therapeutic techniques. Each boasted a different set of credentials.

Popular medicine was sanctioned by custom, by a wide consensus from below, not by any religious, judicial or scientific authority. In the Ottoman empire, this medical folklore was in itself of many varieties, partly because of the Ottoman past, partly because of the Ottoman present. The Ottomans inherited shamanistic medical traditions from central Asia that Turkish tribes immigrating to the Middle East and Asia Minor brought with them. The Ottomans blended their Turkish past with other traditions that they encountered in their expansions, ranging from Hellenic Anatolia and the Christian Balkans to the local folklore in the Arab provinces. All these pasts functioned in a concrete present. The Ottoman Empire was made of several climate zones, each with its unique medical problems and flora and fauna from which medication was prepared. The medical illnesses riddling a port city like Tunis in North Africa and the medical steps to combat them were hardly the same as those of Baghdad in Iraq on the shores of the Tigris River, or Sofia in the European hinterland.

Mechanistic medicine, based on humoralism inherited from Greek antiquity, is another medical tradition present in the Ottoman medical system. This tradition asserted its legitimacy by drawing on the scientific treatises of the sages of antiquity, the patronage of a Muslim urban elite, and the dominant role it played in the intellectual and literary discourses of famous medical figures. This medicine based itself on the physical and philosophical metatheory of the four elements. The human body was understood to correspond with this theory, as it is a microcosm of nature. The body consists therefore of four humors, or fluids, the physiological building blocks of the body: blood (air), phlegm (water), black bile (earth), and yellow bile (fire). In the case of illness, which is a state of imbalance in the body, it was up to the humoralist physician to diagnose which of the four humors was in excess or deficient. The physician then proceeded to recommend a course of treatment, counteracting the offending humor by means of an opposite regimen. Excess in black bile, for example, known to be cold and dry, necessitates adding warmth and moisture artificially.[6]

Humoralism presented itself primarily as a preventive system. Ideally, a patient consulted a doctor while healthy in order to ward off Illness. The humoral doctor was supposed to identify the particular humoral balance that made a specific individual healthy and instruct him or her how to maintain it. However, maintaining the appropriate balance was far from easy, as it was based on the integration of so many variables (the theme of integralism is the subject of the next chapter). The physician had to advise the patient about the lifestyle in the broadest sense that matched his or her balance. Physicians were to consider all aspects of life—that is, everything from choosing a climate and topography to live in, to deciding on a profession (in the case of men), to organizing hours of rest and activity during the day, to fixing a suitable food regimen, and much more. All these different aspects were part of the broad concept of "diet." "Diet" comes from Greek, where *diata* means "regimen for life" rather than our narrower modern understanding of the food regimen, usually in the context of restriction of food in order to lose weight. In the humoral context, "diet" refers to the *sex res non-naturales*, the six nonnaturals, which include light and air, food and drink, work and rest, sleep and waking, excretions and secretions (which include also baths and sexual intercourse), and finally dispositions and states of the soul. (The naturals are temperament, the humors, the faculties, and the *pneuma*, spirit.) Diet is thus "the manner by which a man through his daily activity found himself in a lively and permanent relation with his surrounding world."[7] The six nonnaturals are a link with the body's vital processes. The six nonnaturals should be used quantitatively and qualitatively in the proper place and time and in the correct order. The "naturals" will thus be conserved in good condition and guarantee health.[8]

In Ottoman society, as well as in other early or premodern societies (Christian and Muslim alike), humoralism filled the niche of "learned medicine" of its time. It enjoyed supremacy in urban communities, in the sultanic palaces, and among the wider Ottoman elite. Chronicles and biographical dictionaries, two literary by-products of this social group, described ailments and explained death as stemming from changes in the humoral balance. This was also the medical system practiced in Ottoman hospitals.

Muslim religious medicine, the third medical tradition present in the Ottoman medical system, was similar in its contents to both popular and humoral medicines, but its legitimacy lay elsewhere. Instead of relying on custom or learned treatises, Muslim believers accept religious medicine as originating from (and therefore sanctioned by) the sayings of the Prophet Muhammad. One aspect of Muhammad's prophetic charisma and a source for divine blessing is the healing powers attributed to him. Although too few to constitute a complete medical system, the sayings in which Muhammad gave his (positive or negative) opinion on medical practices were the basis upon which Muslim scholars built from the ninth century onward. Hence this type of medicine is aptly known as "Prophetic medicine" (*al-ṭibb al-nabawī* in Arabic or *tibb-i nebevi* in Ottoman Turkish). Translations of Arabic treatises on the subject into Ottoman Turkish, in addition to the composition of original works in Turkish, attest to the popularity of this branch of religious knowledge among Ottoman Muslims.[9]

Popular medicine was transmitted orally, whereas humoralism and Prophetic medicine were both grounded in written traditions. Moreover, humoralism and Prophetic medicine each had a unique written literary genre. Popular medicine emphasized techniques and results, not bookish learning and the accumulation of knowledge.

In addition to the different modes of legitimacy and theoretical and practical concepts of disease and health, each system had its own corps of specialist healers. The Ottomans might have been familiar with an example set in the *Ḳutadġu Biliġ* (Knowledge That Brings Happiness), a political essay that, in an Islamic setting, describes an ideal monarchy. It was the first long narrative poem in Turkic literature, as well as the oldest monument of Turkic-Islamic literature, and come from another Turkish-Muslim state of the eleventh century in central Asia, the Karakhanid realm. The author of the *Ḳutadġu Biliġ* differentiated between physicians (*hekim*), who cure with medications, and healers (*esfuncu*), whose expertise lay in healing illnesses (mainly mental) caused by demons and spirits (*jinns*).[10]

Muslim humoralism is theologically neutral in its attitude toward health and medicine (its adversaries in medieval Europe claimed it was even atheist and retained its pagan roots; some modern scholars describe it as rational and secular). Its physiological etiology did not judge the patients' religious devotion or blame their misfortune on their sinfulness and infidelity.[11] Prophetic medicine, on the other hand, did have a pronounced ethical and theological worldview because of the ever-present monotheistic dilemma of divine justice. Suffering was promoted in intellectual circles as a purifying element, and therefore positive and desirable. Suffering was celebrated as a religious virtue, and illness was perceived as martyrdom, awarding the ill person with holiness and piety, and thus hastening his or her entrance into paradise. An example to this is the Prophetic saying "A believer will suffer no illness without God expiating his sins."[12]

Despite all the differences, these three systems—folkloristic medicine, Prophetic medicine, and humoralism—were not autonomous or separate. People tended to adhere to only one of these three medical systems, but Ottoman medical subsystems could not afford to be exclusive. Moreover, in reality both healers and patients fused medical ideas and practices, sometimes without consciously knowing this. Such was the case when the source for a specific piece of knowledge or procedure was rooted in learned written medicine but after several generations diffused orally to popular medicine, its "high" origin long forgotten.[13] The three systems were not perceived as incompatible alternatives. Patients crossed from one sector to another in their search for proper—that is, effective—treatment.[14]

This reality brought about brutal competition among healers. If different types of healers offered the patients—their clients—more or less the same therapeutics, and none could boast superior success rates, healers could not single themselves out and justify the high level of financial rewards they expected. Humoral doctors, for example, could not necessarily demand (and get) the financial premium they believed befitted their long process of training and their theoretical knowledge. They wished to strengthen their position as carriers of classical (and superior) tradition, in contrast to the "charlatans" who could offer no more than harmful superstitions. Their guildlike organizations in the bigger cities were used, among other things, to bring pressure on the Ottoman authorities to remove their competitors. Humoral physicians could not (or refused to) recognize the medical logic behind their competitors' practice, especially when the similarities were great. They claimed, for instance, that these medical procedures were beneficial to the patient only when *they* were the ones implementing them.[15]

Three examples will suffice to illustrate the considerable overlap, even ambiguity, in knowledge and technology. The first is phlebotomy, a therapeutic technique used by all three medical systems. Phlebotomy was one of the most frequently used therapeutic and prophylactic treatments for many centuries in the Middle East, as well as in Europe. Humoralism adopted bloodletting as a means to relieve the body from surplus humors that upset the balance in the body (and hence corrupted it). Manuals guided the doctor in words, and sometimes also in pictures, as to when to draw blood, how much to draw, and what body part to draw from. The decision depended on the patient's age and constitution, the season of the year, the weather, and the time of day.[16] Phlebotomy was popular also in folkloristic medicine, sometimes to the extent that people practiced it on themselves. Certainly, phlebotomy was used also when people were not ill as a preventive measure to keep one's health. Even the Prophet Muhammad is reported to have allowed it, whereas other popular forms of treatment, like cauterization, were forbidden.[17]

The dialogue between the three subsystems was not restricted to the therapeutic side of medicine. One evidence is that they all would touch the patient as a diagnostic tool to grasp his or her inner pathological problems. Another is that they shared sources for knowledge or "truth"; all would draw on authorities and theories usually connected with rival systems.

Direct physical contact between physician and patient, even their being in the same room together, was not trivial (in contrast to today, when we expect to be touched by the doctor when he or she examines us, and regard it a basic condition of sound medical practice). Medieval biographical dictionaries celebrate the supernatural abilities of some famous physicians, who correctly diagnosed a medical problem of someone not in their immediate presence. We can find fantastic anecdotes about doctors commenting to their companions upon seeing someone on the street in passing that the person in question was sure to die in the next day or two; and lo and behold—that is exactly what happened! Moving from literary embellishments to humoral medical writings, we can find that in addition to pulse reading, there were other highly respected and much practiced diagnostic methods, like scrutinizing urine (uroscopy), which could of course be done when not in the presence of the patient. Therefore, it is worth noting that both humoralism and Prophetic medicine assigned importance to the doctor's touching the patient. A humoralist doctor would feel the pulse at the wrist (Chinese medicine, of course, emphasizes pulse taking, too). According to Prophetic sayings, Muhammad laid his hands on the body of ill persons to discern what ailed them. Various versions pinpoint different body parts, either the forehead or the upper chest between the nipples.[18] The body part designated for touching may be different, but the reasons behind diagnosis by touch were similar. Medical authors did not refer to reasons other than the medical/physical, but there is a psychological meaning as well, of which they may have not been consciously aware. Touching established an intimate physical connection between doctor and patient. From the latter's point of view, the healer assumed responsibility for the situation at the moment of touching, and the healing process started.

Maybe most surprising is to find medical writers quoting the "great names" associated with rival medical theories as authorities. It is not at all trivial to read Muslim scholars who, while discussing Prophetic medicine, connect medicine with the divine relying on Galen, the Greek pagan, as a source for unearthing the mysteries of health and disease. Pagan Galenism (and the figure of Galen himself) indeed underwent a process of depaganization in order to be adopted by a monotheistic Muslim society.[19] But this is a basic characteristic of Prophetic medicine. It did not mean to discard humoral Galenism as such; far from it. Authors on religious medicine even accepted pre-Muslim authorities in addition to more obvious Muslim ones, like Ibn Sina and others.

They did, however, position them—Muslim and non-Muslims alike—as authorities inferior to the divine legitimacy of Prophetic medicine. It was a confrontation of authorities, not of contents.

A good example is Jalāl al-Dīn al-Suyūṭī (d. 1505), the famous Egyptian scholar, one of the most famous figures in premodern Islamic history. Al-Suyūṭī enjoyed a great reputation as a scholar, and an aura of godliness surrounded him even during his lifetime. According to the medieval Egyptian chronicler Ibn Iyās (d. 1524), on his death al-Suyūṭī's standing reached its zenith: his clothes were bought as if they were relics![20] A versatile writer, known usually for his religious scholarly work (mostly hadith, the sayings of the Prophet, and Qur'anic studies), he was active also in the field of medicine. His treatise *Al-manhaj al-sawī wal-manhal al-rawī fī al-ṭibb al-nabawī* (The Proper Road and the Thirst-quenching Spring of Prophetic Medicine), is—as its title indicates—a discussion of medicine as formed by, and legitimized by, the sayings of the Prophet Muhammad.[21] This treatise and others by al-Suyūṭī enjoyed a wide reputation. Before he reached the age of thirty, his works were sought after in the Middle East and later in the entire Muslim world; they circulated from India to North Africa. In the framework of our discussion here, it should be noted that two manuscripts of *Al-manhaj al-sawī* were kept at the libraries of Topkapı, the Ottoman imperial palace.[22] Al-Suyūṭī's text, which is devoted to Muslim Prophetic medicine, reminds the reader very much of Greek Galenic theory. His treatise on Prophetic medicine takes the *form* of a Galenic book. It starts with medical theory and then goes on to discuss principles of treatment based on this theory. The *contents* of the text are influenced by Galenism. The constitution of man is explained by al-Suyūṭī as being made up of the four elements, and he included putrefied air (miasma), food and drink, and physical and emotional factors on his list of causes of disease. These are the accepted etiological agents in the humoral tradition. At the same time, al-Suyūṭī composed this medical treatise as a Muslim scholar, not a Galenic humoral physician. Al-Suyūṭī begins his work with an exposition of the four humors as a report in the first person by God describing his creation of the world and humanity. In other works he discusses his belief in the curative powers of words (whether written, recited, or worn) from the Qur'an or God's names. He also acknowledged the evil eye and the jinn as etiological agents. Al-Suyūṭī fused medicine with faith, God, and worship, and placed humoralism in a divinely ordained world.

Al-Suyūṭī is by no means unique, although some writers on Prophetic medicine composed their treatises to resemble religious texts, relying more exclusively in contents and format on the sayings of the Prophet Muhammad without attempting to assume a medical or scientific aura. Al-Suyūṭī's work is an example of a mature stage in the development of Prophetic medicine from the late Mamluk period. It came into being when Muslim scholars did not stop at collecting medical-related sayings related to the Prophet Muhammad, or as they had in earlier stages. Rather, they went on to compose comprehensive medical works, based on hadith but explained in the light of Galenic medicine. The scholars' aim was not to build a new Muslim medical system, confronting the existing systems, from non-Islamic origins. Instead, they wished to legitimize medicine in the eyes of Muslim scholars, making it relevant to a Muslim world view centered on complete faith in God. Medicine—in effect repeating humoralism in its physiology and etiology—was portrayed as an integral part of a devout Muslim lifestyle, and was even a religious obligation according to some legal scholars.[23]

On the other side of the spectrum of medical writing, humoral writers themselves supplied religious authority to their Galenic arguments. Take Zeyn al-Din al-Abidin b. Halil as an example. He devoted his work in Ottoman turkish on diet entitled *Shifa'-ı al-feva'id* (The Advantages of Health) to Murad IV (reigned 1623–40). The treatise outlines different types of dishes and beverages according to their humoral attributes (cold, warm, moist, and dry). The author explains how these attributes, combined with different cooking methods and the exact timing of a dish during a meal affect one's inner balance. Zeyn al-Din al-Abidin grouped his discussions into seventeen headings ranging from water for drinking to pulse, meat, poultry, desert and mountain game, and sea and lake fish, and he finishes with fresh and dry fruit. Humoralism is the basis for the work, and Galen is often quoted. At the same time Zeyn al-Din al-Abidin brings forward Muslim prophets like Joseph and Solomon, in addition to Muhammad himself, as medical authorities.[24]

Therapeutics: The Clinical Reality

It is not an easy task to reconstruct the process of healing, despite the fact that there seem to be a lot of sources on Ottoman medicine. The relationship between medical practice and medical theory is always very intricate and hard to pinpoint. Therapeutics, of any kind, can be (and many a time are) noticeably different from the notions outlined in learned medical treatises. Yet because of the gap between the two forms of medicine, we cannot assume that we know the ways the two corresponded with each other. The problem of evidence arises. Medical theory is accessible for historical inquiry—it is for all to see, discussed in learned treatises, many of which have survived to this day. Clinical reality is concealed, and only hinted at.

Pluralism characterized the Ottoman medical system on the intellectual level. But what was the clinical reality? Was it the same in the so-called private sector and the hospitals? And did social and financial factors affect the treatment? What follows is an attempt to reconstruct Ottoman therapeutics inside and outside its hospitals to learn not only what doctors claimed to be the most suitable and effective remedy for a certain disease, but what their actual clinical recommendation was. We shall follow the hierarchy that the learned medicine specified—diet, followed by medication, and, only when all else failed, surgery. Although other orders are justified, I have chosen the humoralistic hierarchy as a starting point to give the discussion some order, because despite competing etiologies and practices, it enjoyed elite patronage and hegemonic status in elite circles. One characteristic is clear: Ottomans were not averse to taking medicine.[25]

"An apple a day keeps the doctor away": Medical Dietary

Traditionally, consuming rich and balanced food was extolled as a habit leading to good health. Anthropological literature reminds us that all human societies regarded a controlled diet as a central element in illness-preventive measures and medical treatment (in addition to being related to other nonmedical domains in personal and communal life, like religion, magic, social demarcation, and personal identity). Therapeutic abilities are assigned to certain foodstuffs or dishes. Some of them include local ingredients; others include rare items that are not usually present in the kitchen for regular meals.[26] This was certainly true of the Ottomans, who linked food with potential health benefits.

The Ottomans drew on several sources of inspiration to link food and health. It was a common thread in Turkish lore in central Asia, as can be learnt from the *Ḳutadġu Biliġ*. This eleventh-century treatise discusses in detail the connections between food, nutrition, and health. It discusses the positive and negative attributes of certain vegetables and fruits and the recommended way to prepare them as a dish. It specifies, for example, the various good effects apples have on the human body and how it makes the heart and stomach stronger and healthier.[27]

Food was a vital therapeutic tool in one medical theory and practice common among Ottomans in the early modern period. In the humoralistic system, the recommended course of treatment was usually by diet; as a means of counteracting the offending humor with an opposite regimen. Food and beverages were the first course of action, to be followed (only if they failed) by more invasive and violent measures. Humoralism promoted a hierarchy of treatments, from dietetics to medications and surgery.

Food and beverages acted also as an insurance against illness, not only as curative agents. Ottomans believed that a strict regimen could guard one's body and soul against illness. Ottoman humoralism was very much a preventive system, in contrast to our modern medicine, which likes to think of itself as heroically curative. The words of an eleventh-century Chinese physician who also belonged to a preventive system that developed dietary medicine are applicable to the Ottoman understanding of the importance of a nutritional regimen. According to him, "[E]xperts at curing diseases are inferior to specialists who warn against diseases. Experts in the use of medicines are inferior to those who recommend proper diet."[28] However, regimen is much more than a careful diet: it is a lifestyle. Humoralism is an integralistic approach to health and the human body and adjusting one's diet to one's physical and mental attributes is just one component. Theoretically, following a regimen carefully should shield a person from any illness.

European travelers commented on the elaborate Ottoman elite cuisine culture in the early modern period and the varied foodstuffs available.[29] Here we are concerned with the medical considerations shaping Ottoman cuisine, rather than gastronomical preferences. However, differentiation between gastronomy and the pharmaceutical is not clear. It is impossible at times to decide whether a specific item was edible or medicinal, or perhaps it served both purposes (some condiments could add yet another use—devotional—when they were applied to give a good smell to a holy site or an object).[30]

Palace culture appreciated the medical aspects of food. Many physicians in the imperial court were interested in dietetic medicine. In 1575 several treatises on medical culinary matters were loaned from the inner library at the palace (*iç hazine*) to the imperial head physician (*hekimbaşı*), who wanted to study them. Five years later they were still out, now given to the next head physician.[31] New treatises on medical dietetics were composed at the imperial court, like Zeyn al-Din al-Abidin's *The Advantages of Health.* This treatise still exists in multiple copies in various libraries in Turkey and around the world. It was printed in Cairo in 1872 together with another work by the same author on tea and pepper—all this attests to the author's prestige. Zeyn al-Din al-Abidin outlines different types of dishes and beverages according to their humoral attributes. The author explains how these attributes, combined with different cooking methods and the timing of a dish during a meal, affect one's inner balance.

We are still guessing to what extent such medical-culinary treatises or recipe collections influenced actual cooking at the palace. So many cooks in this period could not have read such learned didactic works, anyway.[32] However, the purchases for the imperial kitchens or hospitals' larders hint at possible medical influences shaping gastronomic decisions. As Michael Rogers, who studied sixteenth-century Istanbul palaces, commented, it seems as if the spices for the imperial kitchens were ordered by an accomplished druggist with a pharmacopoeia in mind. Although many kinds of spices or seasonings are of culinary importance, the full lists make it probable that their primary importance was medical, not gastronomic.[33]

Despite detailed lists of foodstuffs purchased for several hospitals, we do not know what hospital patients ate or took as medication. The lists of purchases for the hospital warehouses include items for both the kitchen and the pharmacy, but do not distinguish which is which. This is the case in four budget reports from the late fifteenth century of the imperial complexes of Sultan Mehmet II Fatih (reigned 1444–46, 1451–81) and Beyazid II (reigned 1481–1512) (other budget reports do not elaborate on hospital expenses).[34] For instance, the purchases included opium, but Anatolian cuisine makes extensive use of poppy and opium for human beings as well veterinary purposes. Several popular sweet pastes included poppy seeds and were believed to have nutritional values as well as having proven abilities to cure.

If the case of poppy and opium is not clear-cut, what can we say about foodstuffs like oil and honey, or a beverages like coffee? All were believed to serve both for gastronomic purposes and as medications. In September 1689 the governor (*nazir*) of a Meccan hospital dispatched a letter to the imperial palace where the benevolent founder, Gülnüş Sultan, lived. He described the supplies needed at the hospital. With regard to olive oil he remarked that the cooks at the nearby soup kitchen use it, and so do the physicians and surgeons at the hospital; as a result he must purchase oil in greater quantities and the expense account increases.[35]

The gastronomic (and social aspects thereof) had medical consequences. Each meal in the imperial palace was conducted as a ceremony that included a strict code of behavior and comprised lavish dishes consumed in leisure made of meat, fish, rice, sweets, water, and şerbets. Another aspect of the ceremony was social stratification by food: there was a clear distinction according to hierarchy in the meals offered to palace officials and guests; the most senior of them (and the sultan at the very top) were served especially lavish and extravagant dishes: food was a social signifier.[36] The lowest servants, however, ate dishes that alleviated their hunger but had poor nutritional value, like bread and porridge.[37]

The clients of charitable soup kitchens, or imarets, fared better than some servants in elite palaces. Soup kitchens operated according to strict stipulations determining who was given what and when, trying to prevent giving to the "wrong" people or not giving to the "right" ones. On one hand, food quantities in many imarets were measured because of budget limitations. On the other hand, the offerings seemed on the whole more balanced and nutritious. As the kitchen based itself mainly on products available on the local markets, it could offer fresh items. Typical dishes included cereals, fresh fruit, and vegetables changing with the seasons. In some cases it included also meat.[38]

The example of meat well illustrates that the vast variety of foodstuffs one was supposed to consume in order to create a balanced diet in order to keep healthy or to combat illness was available for daily consumption only at the kitchens of the Ottoman elite and for the elite. Meat in various forms was regularly discussed in both Ottoman medical and culinary treatises. Zeyn al-Din al-Abidin, for instance, grouped his discussions under several headings, ranging from water for drinking to sea and lake fish, and finishing with fresh and dry fruit. His discussion of food in a medical-dietetic context is subdivided further into meat, poultry, and desert and mountain game. Indeed, various kinds of meat and fowl were discussed in detail by many Ottoman medical writers who commented on the many types known to them: not just the common chicken but also duck, goose, pigeon, and quail. Almost all the parts of these birds were used: their flesh, gall, fat, brain, heart, and even dung were used for some medico-gastronomic purposes. The flesh was usually seen as being an aphrodisiac and having a fattening and activating effect on the body.[39]

Most Ottomans below the upper echelon did not consume meat regularly. We know this from the diet of soldiers on the march in the early modern period and the many recipes of dishes offered in the soup kitchens.[40] It is true that by some, meat was regarded a basic element in one's diet. This is apparently what a Jerusalemite judge (*kadi*) had in mind when he stipulated a divorced wife should receive alimony and orphans should be allotted money from the inheritance at an amount sufficient to afford a daily diet of meat, oil, and bread. Yet Jerusalemites consumed less than one-third or even one-quarter of the amount of mutton and beef of the average Istanbuli.[41]

At the same time, the impression of George Sandys, an early seventeenth-century English traveler in the Ottoman Empire, was that the population in the capital did not consume that much meat. According to him, if Istanbulis ate meat at all, it was usually mutton, but more regularly they fed on fish, rice (*pilav*), and eggs. Those who could not afford even these products lived on fruit, roots, and various plants. Onion, garlic, porridge, flour, and honey were popular foodstuffs.[42] Hans von Hradiczin Dernschwam, an ex-trader who visited the Ottoman Empire in the 1550s with the Habsburg embassy, related how Ottomans preferred mutton to any other meat, and it was served in various forms frequently, maybe in nearly every meal for those who could afford it. The poorer people lived mostly on much cheaper foodstuffs, like green vegetables, beans, and lentils.[43] In reality, consumption of meat became a symbol of social and economic status, a matter of fashion as well as of availability.[44] If the doctor then stipulated a dish with meat, could the patient follow that order?

Ginger and Viper Flesh: The Ordinary and the Bizarre in Middle Eastern Pharmacology

Medication, like medical dietary, served both preventive and curative aspects of medical treatment. And medication, like diet, was a social symbol, as those of means could afford medication prepared of rarer and more expensive ingredients (although the outcome was not necessarily more effective medically). The affluent patients in the imperial palace, for example, received medication prepared from drugs like opium or hashish, pulverized gems (colored and clear), and precious metals. This possibility did not exist for the patients in the hospitals: such materials were certainly not on the lists of products bought for hospitals. On the open market such ingredients were available only for those who could buy it at full price. This was the case of some specific medications that improved the quality of life, but because they were not emergency medicines many had to deny themselves their use. That applied to things like aphrodisiacs, hair products preventing balding, or drugs for strengthening memory.

The gap in the medical options open to various Ottomans was due to financial realities. There is of course the fact that few people could have afforded the more unusual or imported (and therefore expensive) ingredients, like gold dust and other precious stones, rare flowers, fruit, or animals. An extreme example is theriac (a word loaned from Greek), the famous cure-all antidote that reached Muslims from antiquity. Theriacs existed in many versions. They had various purposes, but the more famous were intended as antidotes for poisons. Theriacs were among the most complex of Muslim pharmaceutical forms, as they contained huge number of ingredients. The most important (and the most unusual) of these were vipers' flesh and snakes' venom. The process of manufacturing was complex and time-consuming.[45]

In addition to financial realities shaping medical options, there existed an ethical-medical discourse on adapting medical treatment to poor patients. The moral and theoretical standpoints were discussed at length by various physicians in their treatises. This discourse concerned itself not only with the obvious financial constraints that demanded the doctor adapt his course of treatment to less expensive options, but also with social hierarchy. Here the discussants—all of whom were members of the elite—thought of social differentiation and demarcation. The elite is expected by its own members as well as by the nonelite to follow a refined lifestyle (this is a privilege as well as an obligation—noblesse oblige); this applies also to their medical options. Physicians to the elite should offer their high-ranking patients courses of treatment suitable to their social standing. This had consequences on the patient-doctor relationship and diagnostic procedures (e.g., whether a male-physician was allowed to treat his female patient directly), and also affected the actual treatment. These privileged patients received delicate, nice-smelling, and tasty medication that suited their noble sensitivities. Poor patients, in contrast, had to be satisfied with simple and coarse medication.[46]

Middle Eastern pharmacology in the early modern period continued previous medieval Arabic pharmacies. The continuation is evident in two aspects. First: most drugs used were of plant origin, hence the uncertainty in certain cases whether the recipes are for condiments, for foods, or for medications. This was the theoretical reality, as evident from the pharmacological compendia of the time. Thanks to the survival of dozens of medical recipes from the imperial Ottoman palace, we have some clues to clinical reality (although we do not know necessarily whether these prescriptions were actually prepared; and if they were, whether they were taken; and if taken, whether the patient followed the dosage and usage instructions).[47] The range of products used by pharmacists was very wide. It included oils, fats, and dairy products (olive oil, butter, milk, and cheese products); pulses (like lentils, chickpeas, peas, and beans);

herbs, seeds, and nuts (cumin, coriander, mustard, cress, pistachio, and sesame were quite popular); sweets like honey, jujubes, peaches, plums, and dates; cooked foods; alcoholic drinks (wine and various beers); cosmetics (henna and hair dyes); and precious perfumes. Such commodities were stored in various vessels, boxes, and baskets made of glass, wood, or metal.[48]

Second, early modern pharmacy continued previous forms of pharmacological literature. The literary models that existed in the Ottoman Empire evolved over hundreds of years. The Ottomans inherited these genres while adapting them. For example, many Ottoman physicians now composed pharmaceutical manuals in Ottoman-Turkish, not in Arabic. But like before, the various works were organized internally in a manner suitable for their use, whether as a quick reference for the doctor or pharmacist, for learned and thorough discussion or for a lexical interest. Some formed part of a larger medical encyclopedia, where one part was devoted to pharmaceuticals, and were not independent works. Each drug was analyzed according to its humoral characteristics and how it affected the body—that is, whether it cooled, dried, heated, or wetted the body (not that there was necessarily unanimity among scholars about the typology of drugs).

Medical formularies (Arabic, *aqrābādhīn*) are one of the oldest forms of Arabic pharmacological literature. These included prescriptions for various types of compound drugs ordered according to pharmaceutical forms, like kneaded preparations, electuaries, pills, aperients, pastilles, powders, syrups, lohochs and robs, gargles, collyria, suppositories, pessaries, cataplasms, oils and lotions, and dentifrices, pomades, and poultices. Another type was books on toxicology that discussed poisons that killed by sight, sound, odor, and contact. Dictionaries of synonyms were lists of simples, usually in alphabetic order, whose main aim was to help the reader identify the drug in other languages. Synoptic texts supplied summaries in the form of tables for quick usage. Lists of *materia medica* addressed therapeutic considerations, giving the opinions of various writers on the description and preparation of simples. Some works focused on substitute drugs: many simples were impossible to procure or too expensive outside major cities, so the compounder had to know of a suitable substitute. (In addition, many frauds were practiced, so the customer also had to be aware of possible substitutes.) Yet another type of pharmaceutical work concentrated on medical specialties, such as treatment of eye ailments, with minute description of the appropriate drugs, their preparation, and their pharmacological properties.[49]

The literary reality is a mirror of the pharmaceutical reality, which recognized a surprisingly wide range of forms in the early modern period. Analytical study of several prescriptions written down in the imperial palace illustrates that most prescriptions were *mürekebbat*, compound medicine (polypharmacy). Formulations included several plants and the preparation included several stages, like powdering in a mortar, mixing, sieving, boiling, kneading, and evaporation. This is in contrast to a simpler pharmacy in which formulations were based on single plants (Ottoman Turkish *müfredat*), which apparently was the more prevalent one in regular apothecary shops.[50]

Beside very modern methods like sprays, the Ottomans prepared most forms familiar to the modern patient, such as infusions, decoctions, pomades, pilules, syrups, pastilles, powders, emulsions, suppositories, and clysters (rectal or urethral). Medications were eaten, drunk, or swallowed—that is, taken by mouth. There was also nasal medicine: fumes were inhaled and powders snuffed, sometimes with a blower used to open the nostrils. Baths, too, were used, so the patient would inhale the fumes from the drug more easily (the entire body was not necessarily immersed in the drug). Other medications were not ingested but rubbed on the outside, as in the case of ointments.

Two things may be said for all pharmaceutical forms. First, the task of preparing a drug was hard work physically. Hence, one of the professional criteria in Ottoman imperial hospitals with reference to pharmacists who specialized in drug pounding (*edviye-i kub* or *daqq-i edviye*) was their physical suitability for the job. They were supposed to be big and strong men, exactly like the hospitals' guards-cum-doormen.[51]

Second, since drug assay of botanicals was (and still is) difficult, the amount of the active principle was uncertain even though the dosage remained constant. Chemistry and other sciences were not sufficiently developed to yield the proper information demanded of them. Authors of pharmacology texts were not unaware of this issue and tried to give precise instructions for the correct time to gather certain plants and even for hunting snakes for theriac in order to control the percentage of the active substances within a drug.[52]

Two forms seem to have been especially popular among Ottomans, and they are mentioned in scientific and nonscientific works alike. One was syrup (*shurba* or *sharab* in Arabic or *şerbet* in Ottoman-Turkish); the other was doughy paste (Ottoman *ma'cun*).[53] Many other forms of prescriptions existed, but they were less popular. Or to put it more correctly: they were less known outside medical circles, hence they were not referred to in literary sources.

Syrups were based on juices concentrated to a certain viscosity so that when two fingers were dipped into the juice, it behaved as a semisolid when the digits were opened. Very often sugar and honey were added together or separately as thickeners and sweeteners. Rob (*rubb*) was a special type of syrup. Often it was the concentrated juice of the raisin, but most of the time, by extension, the word was applied to all fruits and plants, juices of which were purified and concentrated over a fire or in the sun. Julep (literally, "rosewater," from *gulāb* in Persian) was a light syrup. Syrups were a regular part of meals in the Ottoman palace, where a lot of water and juices were drunk. It could be that some or most of these fruit-based beverages did not carry particular therapeutic attributes; they were prepared by the kitchens, not at the palace pharmacy. The terminology is confusing, since the same terminology was used in kitchens and in pharmacies.

Confections too were very popular among Ottomans. The medieval Arabic literature differentiated between bitter and sweet tastes, and good or bad odors, but it seems most Ottoman pastes, especially the more famous ones, were sweetened and smelled good (those made to act as purgatives could be bitter). *Ma'cun*s existed in many versions and were popular among Ottomans from all classes of society. They were prepared for court consumption and were part of popular festivals. They included sugar and/or raisins, honey, almonds, and various aromatics, like cinnamon. In fact, they became almost something of a sweet to be consumed in nonmedical settings as a festive dish on important occasions. This was the case of the *mesir*, a local confection of the city of Manisa, which the hospital in town specialized in. It was believed to be a powerful *ma'cun*, as befits the medical abilities of its creator, an eminent physician in Manisa, Merkez Muslih al-Din Efendi (died 1551–52), the founder of the hospital for the imperial family and its first governor. But this *ma'cun* gained its fame at least partly due to its being a secret recipe, the mystique adding to its fame. Prepared especially for the annual festival of the Persian New Year (*nevruz*), it was so important in the social life of the community that its manner of distribution was regulated by the local judge. The urban elite (persons associated with the Ottoman bureaucracy) were to get it first and then, only if something was left, the poor were entitled to their share. Despite the secrecy surrounding this particular confection, the list of ingredients made its way into the court archive. The prescription comprised no less than forty different ingredients, among them red and black pepper, ginger, coriander, coconut, aniseed, saffron, cinnamon, mustard, nigella, cardamom, indigo plant, cumin, vanilla, orange peel, and sugar.[54]

Honey appears in very many recipes and in very many pharmacological forms. Why was honey used? Honey was widespread partly because it was rather cheap. It was one of the basic products of the premodern Middle East. But honey became a popular substance because in addition to its nourishing value it could be used for preparing and administering various remedies. The more religiously inclined found reassurance in the sayings of the Prophet, who acknowledges honey as having healing qualities. The "scientific" minds could find in pharmacological works discussions of honey as an important ingredient in a complex drug. It prevents whatever it is mixed with from changing and deteriorating; it is nutritious and adds a pleasant smell and taste to what could otherwise be disagreeable; and it also strengthens the various materials mixed together.[55]

Narcotics were a special case of medication. For centuries hashish and opium (*afyun*) were prominent among the drugs used by Muslims medically and also socially for recreational reasons, or even as agents to maintain health.[56] Opium is singled out here because it was especially accepted as a healing substance among Ottomans. However, the distinction between opium and hashish and numerous other narcotics is sometimes not at all clear in the sources. Not only is the terminology confusing, but there were recipes mixing several drugs to the point it is hard to decide which is the most potent and effective, or establish the exact species and plant parts used.[57] Some sources lump the terms together. There were contemporary observers who sometimes referred to opium, hashish, coffee, and tobacco together, or expressed similar feelings toward them (in favor or against). Other sources developed specific debates concerning each topic; certainly the religious scholars and the authorities dealt with wine, tobacco, opium, and coffee in diverse ways.[58] Despite the differences, the consumption of all substances was considered at the very least as having the potential to deteriorate into vice.

Opium appeared, and in large quantities, on the lists of products purchased for the imperial kitchens. Opium served as a laxative, and purgatives were quite common in the pharmacological repertoire of the palace. It was used also in other forms for patients in Topkapı.[59] But opium was not the prerogative of the upper echelon. It was used by Ottomans from all walks of society as a cure to all aches and pains. Poppy and opium (consumed as oil and syrup for drinking) were taken by many for toothaches, headaches, or coughs.

Opium was bought for the hospital of Mehmet II in the fifteenth century. Yet the shopping list of the Edirne hospital did not include it. Opium served as the basis for various painkillers for stomachaches, toothaches, and a long list of other ailments. Several medical treatises refer to opium to as an anesthetic, a medication suitable (in different dosages, of course), for children and grown-up people alike. It was quite common to use it as a pacifier for cranky infants. Opium soothed children suffering from various aches (for ear infections, drops of opium mixed with warm milk were dripped into the ear). Usually it was taken by the mouth as a powder, pill, or fluid, but there were other methods: sniffing opium, for instance, was recommended as a medication for certain eye problems.[60] Opium was used as a cure for seasickness, as the French traveler Thevenot discovered, not too happily. He was on a boat on his way to Rhodes and was highly nauseated. His companion pitied him and gave him something to eat, promising it would ease his suffering, which indeed it did. Thevenot asked for a second helping but then discovered it was an opiate. He was annoyed with his friend for giving him a drug without consulting him first. Thevenot claimed he did not want to poison himself.[61]

The demand for opium was quite high. The markets had to supply the needs of the medical establishment as well as social activities and the kitchens. Ottoman cuisine, especially in the Aegean regions, made routine use of poppy for gastro-medical purposes. But opium was easy to find. Opium could be bought as a regular commodity in the common market, like the central "Egyptian Market" in Istanbul (*mısır çarşısı*) that specialized (and still does) in condiments and herbal medical substances.[62] European observers attest there was no shortage. The cultivation of opium was prevalent in central and southeastern Anatolia, with poppy apparently indigenous to the area since the Hittites (the second millennium BCE). Kayseri, Niğde, and Antakya were noted as centers of opium agriculture in the early modern period. Opium was one of the important products in the Anatolian intercity trade, and was sent to further destinations in camel caravans.[63] Opium was a global commodity, and Anatolia was the major European supplier in the early modern period. It was considered of good quality (certainly better than Indian opium) and contained more morphine.[64]

Opium was a medication, and at the same time also recognized as a source of medical problems. Treatment with opium is what brought one Jewish physician into power because his ability to alleviate his patient's aches, but the same opium treatment also brought him down, when he was accused of using the opium to hurt the patient intentionally.

Moses Hamon, a member of a prominent Jewish family originally from Granada, Spain, who immigrated to the Ottoman lands in the 1490s, treated the gout (*nikris*) problem of Süleyman I (reigned

1520–66) by massaging the aching leg with an opium-based ointment. It was a controversial treatment, and this was the reason given by Nev'izade Ata'i, a prominent Ottoman poet of the early seventeenth century and one of Hamon's biographers, for his disrupted career at court. Other versions of the incident—for example, those relying on contemporary Jewish sources—stress the political struggle at court and anti-Jewish sentiments. Moses was backed by the powerful triumvirate of Hurrem Sultan, Süleyman's favorite concubine and then wife; her daughter Mihrimah, and her son-in-law, Rüstem Paşa, who later rose to become the grand vizier. Hamon's career matched the rise and fall of his patrons. Here, however, we are interested in the link Ata'i makes between treatment with opium and the end of Hamon's career. Ata'i continued a sixteenth-century collection of biographies of Ottoman religious scholars, or ulema, and dervishes. He referred also to Hamon in a nonsympathetic manner. He deliberately corrupted his name, calling him Haman, recalling the biblical figure who appears in the Qur'an as Pharaoh's sinful vizier. Ata'i discussed (very favorably) Hamon's rival at court, Şeyh Qayṣūnīzāde Mahmud, a scion of an esteemed family of Egyptian Muslim physicians who served the Mamluk sultans in Egypt. After the Ottoman conquest at the beginning of the sixteenth century, they were transferred to Istanbul, where they served the Ottomans. Qayṣūnīzāde led a faction of Muslim doctors within the imperial medical corps who opposed Hamon on religious, medical, and political grounds. A medical-professional competition was combined with political struggles within the palace. Qayṣūnīzāde and his supporters used Hamon's particular treatment of Süleyman to accuse him of malpractice, hinting at an intentional attempt on the ruler's life. Their argument in the public disputation between them was based on the fact that the ointment was not known to other physicians and thus suspected of harming the sultan. Qayṣūnīzāde suggested that the opiate gave the patient a temporary sensation of relief while in fact causing long-term and serious damage. Note that Qayṣūnīzāde did not take issue with treatment with opium as such, only this particular usage of it. The struggle between the two doctors ended with Qayṣūnīzāde's triumph: he received the prerogative of treating the sultan and, indeed, succeeded in curing him quickly. Qayṣūnīzāde replaced Hamon as personal physician to the sultan after the former was removed from office. Moses Hamon died shortly afterward of humiliation and a broken heart.[65]

Opium was used as a means of control. It was used to control the wild insane (they were drugged and quieted), but addiction to narcotics was one of the known sources for insanity, as in the case of Ibn Munqār, a seventeenth-century scholar born in Damascus who came to Istanbul. His biography echoes the typical story of the innocent country boy who could not resist the sinful temptations of the cosmopolitan capital. Yet he is also shown to be an educated young man who could not have been that naive. Ibn Munqār was the son of a learned Damascene scholar from a prominent family in that town. His father did well in the imperial religious institution and was appointed to a judgeship in Istanbul. The son followed in his father's footsteps and gained much fame even as a very young man, due to his erudition in several fields of religious knowledge; his expertise in Arabic poetry was also soon recognized. When he traveled to Istanbul upon his father's demise to claim his inheritance, he easily gained access to the highest religious circles and was made assistant to an important scholar in the capital. He adopted the lifestyle of his new social circle, including consuming opium at social events. The biographer claims it was the opium that threw him out of balance, to the point that he had to be hospitalized. Later on, several acquaintances from Damascus accompanied him back to his hometown, where he was put in a house set up especially for him, and was under constant supervision. When his illness worsened he was even chained to the walls. A former colleague lamented at his young life wasted away because of opium.[66]

Ibn Munqār's tragic story hints at yet another medical problem associated with opium: it was feared to be addictive. Contemporary medical works offered "proven" receipts for warding off the addiction in the first place, or at least easing the process of kicking the habit. One was a formula for a laxative of opium, pepper, ginger, cinnamon, and honey, which one had to take in smaller and smaller dosages till the body was used to no drug at all. The inclusion of opium in small dosages may have eased the shock for the body and prevented withdrawal symptoms.[67]

Opium's addictive quality was one of the main reasons narcotics caught the attention of the authorities. Consumption of both opium and hashish (tobacco was added from the seventeenth century onward) was part of a Muslim man's lifestyle in certain social circles. In certain social circles the use of psychoactive drugs developed into a "narcotic culture," as the use of narcotics was so widespread and was accompanied by a certain code of behavior and social norms. European observers commented that it was not uncommon to see Ottoman bureaucrats, even religious scholars, consume opium in cafés in Istanbul after working for hours, in order to sharpen their tongues and improve their mood.[68] It was suggested that a drug culture was even more prevalent in Anatolia than in other places, like Europe, because opium had been cultivated there for centuries.[69] The mid-sixteenth-century German merchant Hans Dernschwam opined that in the Ottoman core areas opium and cannabis had no rival in the form of alcohol (at least in public), as in Europe.[70] Opium made its way into the plays of the popular Turkish shadow theater, Karagöz (named after one of the heroes). This important factor in public entertainment in Ottoman Anatolia included key figures who were heavy smokers of drugs or tobacco. Karagöz himself, a down-to-earth, witty man, had a small bag attached to his belt for carrying tobacco. His costar, Hajivat, a friend and foe, a target for many of Karagöz's practical jokes and even occasional blows, was an educated and gentle man who smoked opium.[71] But what was portrayed as an affable quality in popular entertainment was viewed by the political and religious authorities quite differently.

The Ottoman authorities tried—unsuccessfully—to stop the use of narcotics and their abuse. It was neither the first time authorities in the Muslim Middle East intervened in such matters, nor that such a step failed. The legal, moral, and medical debate around smoking, as part of the wider discussion on vice (like prostitution and consumption of prohibited substances), went on for centuries. This debate included also a political aspect, when the authorities took a stand in the name of law and order.[72]

In 1670–71 Mehmet IV (reigned 1648–87) issued a decree ordering the destruction of all taverns in the vast Ottoman Empire. He wanted to prevent the drinking of alcohol and the smoking of tobacco and opium.[73] Several years previously, he caught an officer in his summer camp in Edirne smoking tranquilly in his tent, a man-servant massaging his legs. The furious sultan imposed severe punishment on the offender: unless he ransomed himself he would be executed. The courtier lost most of his fortune to smoke.[74] Mehmet IV followed in his grandfather's footsteps. Murad IV is very famous for a similar decree concerning tobacco. Murad made a name for himself as someone who abhorred the substance, and contemporaries likened him to James I of England, also a sworn enemy of tobacco. Murad IV forbade smoking under the death penalty if disobeyed. He had traders in tobacco caught and amputated their legs in the public square.[75] The decrees relied at times on precedents set by Süleyman I, who had issued several resolutions on abolishing coffeehouses and wineshops.[76] In September 1725 Ahmet III (reigned 1703–30) issued a sultanic decree (*ferman*) concerning the smoking of hashish. The habit was denounced in religious and political terms as an act of heresy (*ilhad, zandaqa*), an unwelcome invention (*bid'a*), and rebellion (*siyanet*). This particular decree was addressed to the heads of the judicial and military institutions in Edirne, instructing them to warn the people of Edirne not to engage in trade in hashish, let alone consume it. The objective was to remove hashish totally from the local markets. He who was caught buying, selling, or smoking hashish was to be punished severely, and his name sent to the capital. The central administration may have wanted to have the names at its disposal to allow follow-up. It may have been used also as a further threat to the offenders, or maybe a reminder to the Ottoman officials that the central government expected to see action and results.[77] As the repetitive acts reveal, the authorities did not succeed in repressing the consumption of narcotics, and their efforts were not necessarily constant or consistent.

Addiction to opium—any addiction—was not approved of in Ottoman society. In his repeated intake of the drug the addict increases amounts in order to retain the feeling of satisfaction. Continued use of the drug results in a physical or psychological dependence and an urgent compulsion to get it.[78] Since an addicted person cannot behave in the controlled and rational manner expected from an adult, addiction could cause one to behave in an unmanly and un-Muslim manner. But the elite expected its members to have dignity and refinement. This is why Mustafa Ali (died 1600), an Ottoman bureaucrat and historian, objected to unrestrained behavior during drinking parties. Guests who drank too much, ate too much, talked in a confused way, or fell asleep could spoil a party for the other participants. Spoiling a party (because one was out of control), he explained, was very bad manners.[79]

At the very least, the addicts were made fun of. Evliya Çelebi (c. 1611–85), the renowned Ottoman traveler, literatus and courtier, dedicated a section on famous lunatics of his time in the "book" devoted to Istanbul, the first in his vast account of his travels. Evliya loved Istanbul, the city of his birth, and knew it intimately, including many local madmen who became part of the landmarks. Evliya related a story about one of them, a neighborhood lunatic who was addicted to sniffing tobacco. The local boys routinely played pranks on him, such as selling him sand instead of tobacco. As Evliya wittily put it, the madman occasionally puffed away one hundred silver coins of worthless sand.[80]

While this causes embarrassment to the individual and his family, the authorities were not interested in the likes of Evliya's hero, who was not harmful, except to himself. Rather, the authorities were concerned that under a condition of hazy consciousness and altered mood, one might act unpredictably in a harmful manner, whether physically or verbally. European observers claimed that under the influence of opium Muslim Ottomans could beat up Jews and Christians that they came across. According to Nicholas de Nicolay, who resided in Istanbul between 1551 and 1552 as part of the French embassy, the worst were the soldiers.[81]

The interest of the authorities in narcotics rose not out of health considerations but out of political ones, although medical aspects of use (and abuse) of opium and other narcotics were discussed. Drugs were tolerated, but the authorities feared that narcotics and the drug culture around it, like madness, might upset the public order.[82]

Nonaddicts who consumed drugs socially were also suspect, as far as the political and religious authorities were concerned. Gatherings in public places were politically, socially, and religiously suspect. The Bohemian and loose conduct associated with such activities was the reason for this suspicion. How else could one describe the kind of literary meetings that took place in cafés or taverns (*meyhane*s), where men and women mingled and music was played?

This was certainly what the historian and bureaucrat Ibrahim Peçevi (1574–ca. 1649–50) thought. His reasons for abhorring coffee and tobacco are telling. Peçevi mentioned the nauseating smell. Ascribing much importance to personal cleanliness and appearance, he complained the smoke soiled his clothes, turban, and beard. Coffee and tobacco were said to have ill effects on the brain; moreover, the consumption of both, with the related lifestyle, led to wasting of too much time and money on mere entertainment, meaningless pleasure, and immoral frivolities.[83]

The illegal aspect of opium consumption angered the religious scholars. Peçevi explained that numerous ulema made great efforts to forbid the consumption of coffee, tobacco, and opium. They explained why it was unlawful, but all three substances became very popular. One of the ulema doing so was Ebu Su'ud Efendi (1490–1574), the influential head mufti under Suleyman I and his successor Selim II (reigned 1566–74) during the sixteenth century. He issued numerous legal decisions (*fetva*s) where he criticized the habit. He compared it to consuming alcohol and drunkenness, which are strictly forbidden in the Qur'an.[84]

Surgery?

In humoral theory surgery was the last option a physician should consider. Learned medical treatises reveal this hierarchy: surgery is discussed in these books, but it is clear it was a minor weapon in the humoral medical arsenal. This type of treatment offered the healer limited options: it was mainly a curative measure, although some intrusive procedures were used as preventives. Surgeons bore the professional title of *jarrāḥ* (Arabic) or *cerrah* (Ottoman Turkish) to distinguish them from physician (*tabīb/tabip* or *ḥakīm/hekim*). Surgery was thus recognized as a medical field in its own right—a social and medical indication of its independent status. But this differentiation made it possible to place surgeons in a slot below physicians in the professional hierarchy. Salaries paid to medical personnel in Ottoman hospitals reveal that surgeons were always paid considerably less than physicians.

The clinical reality, however, was much more complex. A certain degree of medical professionalization did exist, and according to it surgery was less appreciated than "natural" medicine, but the borders of the disciplines were still vague. Actual practices combined various fields of expertise: sometimes physicians carried out chirurgical operations, and it is not clear whether a surgeon's practice was restricted to operations only. Indeed, surgery was carried out in nonhumoral medical contexts as well. Folk or religious medical practitioners conducted operations too. Moreover, even humoral practitioners carried out various surgical operations on a daily basis and considered them routine. This explains evidence found in archaeological excavations from medieval Muslim settlements where various surgical and dental instruments, like cauteries, trocars, extractors, suture instruments, scalpels, pincers, pinchers, forceps, and scissors have been found.[85]

We know today that the established wisdom of an earlier generation of scholars who maintained that surgery was forbidden for Muslims due to legal and theological sentiments is obsolete. Anatomy was studied and surgery was certainly practiced. But what was done and to what extent? We know that anatomy and surgery were discussed in learned medical treatises, but the writings of so many famous physicians were riddled with myth when reporting (boasting?) about surgery. In these cases there was a considerable gap between what is described as established knowledge and clinical realities.[86]

We cannot ignore the objective problems facing surgery and dissection in the early modern Middle East (some of which were present also in medieval Europe; others were unique to the geographical area and culture of the Middle East). The warm weather throughout most of the region is one problem. That could have made an intensive study of corpses as part of the study course of a medical student very difficult to pursue. If that was a student's background, what could he practice well as a professional? There was also the patients' understandable fear, since in many cases major surgery was fatal. At the time, sanitization and pasteurization were not thought of, and were not a legal obligation for medical doctors. But even if the surgery was not fatal, it was certainly painful and difficult to endure, as this was also the period before the age of painkillers and anesthesia as routine procedures in intrusive operations. So even if the physicians had the know-how, where would they gain the experience? They might have had no opportunity to try it out—their patients would not agree to undergo that process. But more broadly, the attitude toward surgery was ambiguous. While there was no strict ban and it existed as an option to be discussed, it was not wholeheartedly embraced.

Knowledge of anatomy was an integral part of medical sciences in Ottoman society. As in other branches of medicine, anatomy was based on Galenic writings. By the early modern period *tashrīḥ* (the technical term for anatomy) came to denote in the Muslim medical context a description of the human body, as well as its empirical application in the form of dissection. Thus, we can find descriptions of the bones, muscles, nerves, arteries, veins, and the compound organs, which included the eye, the liver, the heart, and the brain.[87]

Many Ottomans lauded the study of anatomy. Hajji Khalifa, the seventeenth-century scholar and a scribe in the financial bureau of the army known as Katip Çelebi, included "tashrīḥ" in his gigantic bibliographic encyclopedia in Arabic, *Kashf al-ẓunūn 'an asāmī al-kutub wal-funūn* (Uncovering of Ideas: On the Titles and the Names of the Sciences). His editorial decision attests that anatomy was a respected field of knowledge in the early modern Middle East. He praised the subject: "He who does not know astronomy and anatomy is lacking in his knowledge of God." Here Hajji Khalifa repeats sentiments that many writers before him had expressed: that the study of anatomy is a means to demonstrate the greatness of God's perfect design. Anatomy here is the textual description of the systems in the body and their functions, rather than the actual dissection of bodies in order to determine these systems and functions.[88]

Surgery was considered an integral part of medical sciences studied by many, Anatomy was part of the course in the Süleymaniye medical school in Istanbul, and attending such classes was at times a condition for appointment as surgeons at the palace medical corps.[89] However, the anatomical and surgical manuals produced in the Ottoman Empire are few. Although most standard medical compendia discussed the bodily systems as well, this was clearly not their focus. The number of works specializing in anatomy and surgery was tiny.

One rare example to Ottoman chirurgical tracts is the seventeenth-century writer Şams al-Din Itaki's *Tashrih-i abdan ve tarjuman-i kabala-yi falasufan* (The Anatomy of the Body Parts and Expounding the Role of the Philosophers), of which seven manuscripts are in existence. Şams al-Din Itaki was born in Shirvan. He had to leave his hometown on the Ottoman-Safavid border after losing his family in the course of the wars between the two empires in the 1620s. He moved to Istanbul and introduced himself to court by dedicating his treatise to Murad IV through Topal Recep Paşa, who acted as vizier for a short while in 1632. This places the writing of the treatise around 1630. The vizier liked his work and bestowed upon him the prestigious position of keeper of the Holy Mosque in Mecca.

Itaki based himself in part on Ibn Sina's *Qānūn*. Following Ibn Sina's classification, Itaki too separated the organs into two groups: simple organs that are of the same structure (blood, bone and muscle) and complex ones (like the systems of respiration and digestion). At the same time Itaki diverged from Ibn Sina. On some points Itaki gave different information or a different explanation. This was the case, for example, in Itaki's discussion of the nerve system or the embryo. Another departure from Ibn Sina was due to Itaki's adoption of Ibn al-Nafīs's summary and criticism of Ibn Sina, in his *Sharḥ tashrīḥ al-qānūn* from the thirteenth century, although he did not necessarily grasp the full significance of the difference (Ibn al-Nafīs, for example, corrected Galen and Ibn Sina in his theory of the pulmonary circulation of the blood, anticipating William Harvey).[90]

Following his Arabic sources, Itaki usually used Arabic terms, but he added their Turkish equivalent, and in some rare cases mentions also the Persian terminology. In this regard Itāki's work was an important stage in the evolution of technical-medical terminology in the Ottoman-Turkish language.

Itaki's work is noted because of his use of several illustrations in his discussion of various body parts. As in previous works in the Muslim world, we find discussed the human skeleton, muscles, veins and arteries, nerves, and the growth of the fetus. Here Itaki mingles two separate traditions. On the one hand, he followed the tradition starting with *Tashrih-i mansuri*, a fourteenth-century anatomy work in Persian by Mansur b. Muhammad b. Ahmad b. Yusuf b. Ilyas dedicated to the ruler of Fars and Timur's grandson. This is the first work known to include anatomical illustrations in the Muslim world. Itaki, like Ibn Ilyas, uses whole figures in order to portray various "systems" (nerves, muscles, blood vessels, etc.), depicting them in a distinctive squatting posture. Itaki also reproduces Ibn Ilyas's woman figure to portray the growth of the fetus. This particular illustration is Ibn Ilyas's innovation, as the other illustrations were apparently influenced by earlier Latin medical diagrams, although it is not known how.

On the other hand, Itaki was influenced by Andreas Vesalius (1514–64) and his *De Humani Corporis Fabrica* (The Structure of the Human Body), printed in Basel in 1543. Vesalius used the help of an artist, Jan van Kalker, to produce the woodcut illustrations for his anatomical text and atlas (hence anatomical information was displayed by means of the classical statuelike figures, familiar to artists). Itaki used this model for his illustrations of eye muscles, brain, skull, bones of hands and feet, and the vertebral column. From Juan de Valverde, a Spaniard anatomist, Itaki copied a female figure displaying her reproductive organs, which appeared in the 1556 *Historia de la Composicion del Cuerpo Humano* (The Account of the Composition of the Human Body).[91]

This blending of two anatomical traditions is also a blending of two distinct artistic tastes and fashions. The Muslim illustrations are flat, two-dimensional, schematic, and impressionistic renderings of human beings. It seems Itaki drew the illustrations himself, rather than used an accomplished artist. We may associate these artistic-scientific trends with the religious instruction that led to a cultural tendency of refraining from the figurative or realistic expression of humans, lest it be suspected as the creation of idols; as it is said in the Qur'an: "Set not up with God another god."[92] This rule was kept strictly in mosques, which are adorned only with colors and architectural, geometrical, and epigraphic elements. There are no pictures of humans or animals. Outside of mosques human figures were portrayed, even as illustrations for religious texts, but in a decidedly nonrealistic manner. In Europe, however, starting with Leonardo da Vinci (1452–1519) for artistic purposes and then Andreas Vesalius for medical-scientific purposes, 3-D images of human body parts and anatomical systems were produced, and the artists tried to imitate reality as much as possible. They present an important stage in the scientific revolution in Europe during the Renaissance and early modern period. In the Muslim Middle East, in contrast, there was no wish for naturalism, and the result is not realistic or clinically accurate.

Moving from the realm of anatomy, a field of knowledge, to its practice, surgery, we notice that here too there were no explicit legal, religious, or cultural strictures banning human anatomical dissection in particular. Its practice, however, was varied.

An early Ottoman treatise attests to the study of anatomy as preparation for an applicable art, surgery. The fifteenth-century work

Cerahiyyet-ül-Haniyya (The Surgical Operation of the Khan) by Şerefeddin Ali b. al-Haj Elias Sabuncuoğlu from Amasya focuses on surgery and explains procedures and the uses of surgical devices. Like Itaki, Sabuncuoğlu dedicated his work to the reigning sultan, Mehmet II. And like Itaki, Sabuncuoğlu signifies an important step in the evolution of medicine and medical terminology in the Ottoman Empire. He was one of the first in Anatolia to write a scientific treatise in Turkish and thus is part of the larger cultural change of Ottomanization.

Sabuncuoğlu claimed in his various works that he wrote only about clinically proven procedures. In addition to other medical texts, he based himself on the results of his own experiments. In some cases he mentioned that he tried a specific treatment on himself or one of his animals (chickens, for example).[93] This touch of empiricism should not be ignored, but not overemphasized. Sabuncuoğlu was not the only Ottoman physician who boasted the use of empirical evidence. However, the basic tenets of Ottoman medicine were not changed, including the reliance on accepted wisdom from previous generations. Empiricism did not become the central form of medical inquiry in Ottoman learned medicine.

Emir Çelebi, a seventeenth-century physician who worked in the famous Manṣūrī hospital in Cairo and then became imperial head physician to Murad IV, shared Sabuncuoğlu's views. In his medical encyclopedia *Enmüzec-ül-tibb* (Summary of Medicine), composed in 1625, Emir Çelebi claimed his aim was to discuss both medicine as a body of knowledge (*ilm*) and also its application (*amal*) (this is a quite common division of medicine and not the innovation Emir Çelebi implied). He presents himself as an authority on both. Emir Çelebi was against blind borrowing of knowledge from past generations. He suggested that each physician experiment for himself and reach the conclusion of what is correct in medicine. Yet, despite his claims in the introduction of his treatise and his clinical background, the final product follows the familiar textual-theoretical trend. Like other medical encyclopedias, this work is organized alphabetically, and mentions the symptoms and cures for every illness. He relies on the usual suspects like Galen or Ibn Sina and does not seem to refer to his experience as a hospital physician.[94]

Sabuncuoğlu's treatise is basically an Ottoman version of al-Zahrāwī's section on surgery from his vast compendium *Kitāb al-Taṣrīf*. The title hints that it is a self-contained medical manual for medicine; the student needs to look no further to another treatise. Abū al-Qāsim Khalaf ibn 'Abbās al-Zahrāwī, who died in the beginning of the eleventh century (the precise date of his death has been the subject of much speculation), known to the West as "Albucasis," was a Spanish physician from Cordoba. Little is known about him (quite surprisingly, considering his fame and influence). It was said—not by him—that he was a personal physician to Umayyad caliphs ('Abd al-Raḥman III and his son al-Ḥakam II) and the chamberlain Ibn Abī Amīr al-Mansūr. According to one copier of his treatise, al-Zahrāwī was an ascetic, which may explain his modesty in his success. Al-Zahrāwī's book on surgery and surgical devices is in fact only one part, the thirtieth and last chapter, of *Kitāb al-Taṣrīf*, although it is one of the longest. This is probably the earliest work on surgery in Arabic, and certainly the earliest one that contains illustrations of surgical and dental instruments. Al-Zahrāwī claims he wanted to revive this lost art. He tells of four separate incidents he witnessed in which physicians operated on patients with tragic results because of their lack of knowledge in anatomy and training in surgical technique. In this art, errors may lead to death. He discusses cauterization, incisions, puncturing, venesection, cupping, surgery on abscesses, and the withdrawal of arrows from the body and foreign bodies from the ear and nose. He describes many operative procedures and instruments that do not appear in extant classical writings. These may be his own improvements and innovations. Among al-Zahrāwī's possible inventions one should mention his design for a vaginal speculum, the syringe, the use of animal guts as suture materials, and a formula for a kind of plaster casing anticipating the modern plaster cast. This treatise became widely known, learned and copied in the Muslim world, as attested by the many copies spread in libraries all over the Muslim world. Quickly it was also translated into Latin and became a standard text in Europe as well.[95]

Sabuncuoğlu prepared an Ottoman edition of al-Zahrāwī's chapter on surgery in the fifteenth century. But his was not a mere translation. There are some additions, as Sabuncuoğlu prided himself on the devices he invented and produced. Another important change was the addition of many illustrations that show the textual explanation and instructions in pictures. While al-Zahrāwī had included dozens of illustrations of instruments, many more illustrations of supposedly surgical procedures were added to Sabuncuoğlu's text, and several include only utensils.[96]

In Sabuncuoğlu's work the illustrations portray scenes in which physicians treat patients. The physicians in all the miniatures, save a few, are bearded, mustached, older Muslim men. Their social standing is conveyed to the observer by depicting their heads as covered with a turban; and they wear colored and well-sewn clothes (blue, red and green are the prominent colors, but yellow appears as well). The exceptions are female healers (who are also well dressed), who appear in obstetrics-related procedures. Female healers do not appear in all obstetrics-related procedures, and mostly male physicians are depicted as treating gynecological problems in women. The patients include men and women, old and very young. Many of them are portrayed half naked with their backs, buttocks, or genitals exposed. Many miniatures include motifs from nature in the form of flowers, bushes or trees that hint at the scene occurring in a peaceful, calm, and healthy place. The copy of the manuscript kept at the İstanbul Üniversitesi Library includes miniatures that depict more varied and concrete backgrounds for the operations, ranging from open fields and rivers to interiors of homes or hammams (at any rate, doctor's clinics or hospitals do not appear).[97] This picturesque background goes hand in hand with the spirit of the pictures, which is impressionistic rather than realistic. This is not an exact rendering of nature/reality that a medical student can study from. Rather, it is in the two-dimensional, flat, anatomic tradition of Muslim art.

Evliya Çelebi, the renowned Ottoman traveler of the seventeenth century, presents us with literary evidence for the familiarity of Ottomans with surgery. Evliya included a description of several operations he claimed to have witnessed in European hospitals in Vienna and Monastir in the year 1665.[98] Evliya accompanied Kara Mustafa Paşa, who was sent on an embassy from Mehmet IV to the Habsburg king Leopold I (1640–1705) following the Treaty of Vasvár, a truce between the two empires after their war over Transylvania in the 1660s. Ten years later Kara Mustafa Paşa would become the Ottoman grand vizier. Eventually Kara Mustafa Paşa lost favor with the sultan, his political fortunes ebbed, and he was executed in Belgrade in 1683, several months after his military defeat in the siege of Vienna.

Evliya claims that while in Vienna, he met the emperor, who supplied him with a European passport to allow him to continue his excursions in Europe. According to Evliya, he went as far as Spain, the Netherlands, North Germany, and Denmark. This seems highly unlikely. We can attribute this astonishing claim to Evliya's known tendency to exaggerate and embellish reality. Some of his descriptions are surprisingly accurate, although in other cases his information (for example, numbers and quantities) is suspect.

Evliya was not averse to complimenting himself. In the section on surgeries in Vienna he boasts of his worldly experience and vast knowledge, thinly veiled as praise from a supposedly objective third party. During the brain surgery he observed, the chief surgeon at the hospital invited Evliya to come closer and inspect the patient's open skull and his brains. The curious Evliya readily agreed, but covered his mouth and nose with a handkerchief. The physician was puzzled by Evliya's action and asked the reason for that. Evliya answered that he did not want to cough or sneeze by mistake at the open wound. The impressed physician exclaimed "Bravo!" and recommended that Evliya study medicine and science, as clearly he showed aptitude for these subjects. The Viennese physician added it was evident Evliya had learned a lot on his travels.

Evliya, after all, was a storyteller (among other things), and a very accomplished one. His travel stories were a popular and entertaining piece of literature among elite Ottomans (and modern Ottomanists). He included information he believed to be correct, but this included fact as well as fiction, well-evidenced and balanced and reliable information alongside myths, fables, and clichés. Indeed, previous studies of "Evliya-logists" (prominent among them those of Robert Dankoff), have shown how Evliya took over legends and accounts from previous sources and presented then as facts in his (supposedly) first-person narratives. He had the double aim to report and instruct as well as to amuse and divert. As a result, Evliya's autobiographical account should not be taken at face value. The importance of Evliya's account is that it supplies us with patterns of conceptions and attitudes prevailing in Ottoman society. Evliya was a unique individual, yet despite his eccentricities he was a typical Ottoman of his day. He thus provides a view of the Ottoman mind from the inside.[99]

The Ottoman mentality (borrowing Dankoff's phrase) of the seventeenth century—that is, the special Ottoman way of looking at the world, revealed in Evliya's writing—bears of course also on the section that interests us here, the surgeries supposedly watched in Vienna. Should we trust it? Did Evliya really witness these operations? Did such operations, some of them quite unusual, even take place in early modern Vienna? And what does Evliya's interest in such operations tell us about Ottoman attitudes toward medical cutting into the body in the early modern period?

The first event Evliya relates is also the most extraordinary: a sort of brain surgery. It took place in the hospital of St. Stephen's Cathedral (the Stephansdom) on the banks of the Danube, apparently the most important hospital at the time, at least according to Evliya's account. Evliya claimed that the medical staff associated with the institution was especially accomplished, and the hospital could boast royalty among its patients. St. Stephen's Cathedral was the burial place of several members of the Habsburg family from the seventeenth century onward, and royal patronage of such a medical institution seems likely. During the operation the surgeons removed part of the patient's skull at the cap to recover a rifle bullet that had entered the patient's head.[100]

A study of the state of the surgical art and medical devices in contemporary Europe suggests that the descriptions are actually quite factual. By Evliya's time European medicine was starting its revolution and evolution. It was after Paracelsus and his medical chemistry. After Vesalius, surgery and anatomy in Europe were steadily moving away from Galen, al-Zahrāwī, or Ibn Sina. So many of the great artists of the time, including Raphael, Michelangelo, and da Vinci, began to study anatomy closely, realizing that knowledge of the muscles and bones in particular was essential for accurate reproduction of the human form in their paintings and sculptures. For centuries surgeons "saw what they believed," but by the seventeenth century this had been changed to "believed what they saw." This was the age of the surgeon–anatomists. They were well acquainted with the anatomy of the human body, and they advocated and performed their own dissections of humans. An exemplar of the period is Vesalius. Despite many attacks he was ready to point out mistakes in classical writings. His corrected no less than two hundred mistakes in Galen's anatomy. He explained that he relied on direct dissection of humans rather than, like Galen, of animals. Diverging from Galen was not easy. Michael Servetus (1511–53) of Spain claimed blood mixed with air in the lungs passes back into the heart; this was one reason why he was proclaimed a heretic and was burned at the stake. Evliya lived in the period of William Harvey (d. 1657), the Englishman who showed that the circulation of blood was continuous and unidirectional. It was the age of the microscope. Harvey's work was completed by Marcello Malpighi (d. 1694), who showed the capillary vessels for the first time with the help of a microscope. The seventeenth century, Evliya's period, was even a period of several surgical firsts, like the removal of abdominal organs or cutting into the brain.[101]

It is true that Evliya could have obtained most of the information about the operations he describes without leaving his house in Istanbul. As we have seen with Vesalius's influence on Itaki, some of the new ideas and discoveries from Renaissance Europe were making their way slowly to the Ottoman Empire. Evliya could have read about some procedures in Ottoman treatises on the subject, or heard from his many informants, but not of the new techniques Evliya reports. Most scientific changes in Europe occurred far away from the public eye. Although some new knowledge proliferated and reached a broad public, maybe in a simplified or modified format,[102] mostly it was known and of interest to a small group of people: intellectual circles around universities or private societies in some European centers. In order to write in Ottoman Turkish in the middle of the seventeenth century about trepanning (cutting a section out of the skull), one of the operations Evliya described, he had to witness them (or maybe it was someone else who reported back to him).

In any case, Evliya was overwhelmed by the high level of medical practice in Europe. He was puzzled and maybe also shocked by the nature of some of the procedures he saw. Evliya noted particular procedures, the like of which he had not heard of before. He certainly did not condemn the essence of surgical intervention or condemn advances, experiments, and discoveries that are deviations from the accepted wisdom in this art and craft, however bold or even pretentious.

However, Evliya gives the impression that, on the whole, the scientific and clinical tradition he saw was quite familiar to him. The medical-surgical tradition in the Ottoman Empire shared many features with the European clinical reality. Both continued the same medical tradition, that of medieval Islam. Its vast literature was translated into Latin and colloquial Christian languages and thus transferred to Europe. And apparently Renaissance anatomy *reformed* the accepted anatomic wisdom from antiquity rather than rejecting it altogether. Renaissance scholars of anatomy revived knowledge from antiquity and emulated the ancient scholars rather than pursued a new and "modern" research agenda. Even after Vesalius and his contemporaries, European anatomy still reflected the conventional wisdom in the Ottoman Empire. That medical wisdom could have been known to Evliya.[103]

As mentioned, the evidence from many diverse sources suggests that surgery was practiced regularly and was quite common. European travelers attest that they witnessed various surgical procedures, even self-treatment, in public places. Two procedures seem to be mentioned more than others were phlebotomy and cauterization. Bloodletting (*ḥijāma*) was a popular medical practice in the Middle East well into the nineteenth century. The fact that Muhammad the Prophet was known to approve such treatment, and even underwent it himself, gave bloodletting extra legitimation. The humoral reasoning behind it was that the removal of blood should alleviate problems rising from excess or corruption of blood in the body. Before the discovery of the circulation of the blood in the seventeenth century, and even afterward, there was a belief that blood could accumulate and get "spoiled" in the extremities of the body, hence the need to get rid of it (emetics and purgatives were intended to achieve similar aims with other humors). Bloodletting was a routine medical treatment for various aches and pains (head, eyes). It was also used as preventive medicine (at court it became part of the lifestyle), although lone voices were heard that bloodletting might bring more harm to the patient than good.[104]

Bloodletting was practiced using various methods. The one described by Thevenot was "venesection," which involved puncturing a large external vein. Another was to draw blood from an artery, usually in the temples, but venesection was easier to control. Blood flows in the veins at a steady and moderate speed, whereas in arteries it flows in pulses: the heart contracts and thus pushes blood in the body. Two other alternatives for bloodletting were attaching a glass containing hot air and thus creating vacuum on blood vessels ("cupping"), and attaching live leeches to suck out the "bad" blood from the body instead of bleeding it out. Physicians theorized rules concerning specific hours of days, the week, the month, and the season when phlebotomy should be conducted in order to achieve the intended goal.

The French traveler Thevenot, who toured the Ottoman Empire in the 1670s, documented cases he saw of people bleeding themselves. However, the more common occurrence was to hire a professional. This was a routine treatment for aches in all parts of the body, especially the head, and the bloodletter was supposed to bleed the vein in the spot where the pain was felt most. First a turban was tied around the patient's head (hopefully not too tight, lest one choke the patient). Then the bloodletter touched the patient's forehead, looking for the right vein and spot. When those were determined he slashed the skin and opened the vein with a chisel or sharp stick (he described it as "cruel" and fit to slaughter a beast). After shedding a substantial quantity of blood he closed the vein with a piece of cotton or camel droppings.[105]

Phlebotomy made its way into art. An anonymous work from the late sixteenth century on the wonders of art and nature in Ottoman Turkish includes ninety miniatures, one of which features a sadistic bloodcupper who tortured his unsuspecting patient. It tells the story of a Muslim traveler who arrived in India and entered a guesthouse to rest. He concluded a contract with a cupper who happened to be there. By this contract, he was to be cupped in exchange for his turban, seen in the miniature on the floor near the upturned bowl. He did not know that he would be subject to torture by the bloodletter, who is seen cutting his back (see fig. 1).

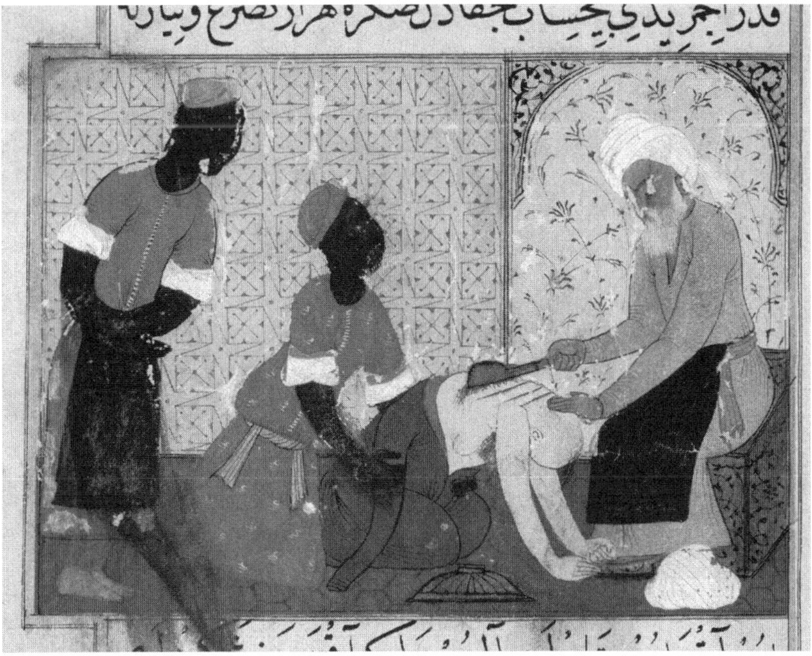

Figure 1. A sadistic bloodcupper tortures his unsuspecting patient. "Wonders of Art and Nature," manuscript held at the British Library, Harl. 5500, f.40r, reproduced by permission of the British Library; Nora M. Titley, *Miniatures from Turkish Manuscripts: A Catalogue and Subject Index of Paintings in the British Library and British Museum* (London: Library, 1981), 30–31.

Cauterization (Ottoman-Turkish *dağ* "branding with a hot iron," or Arabic *'ilāj bi-nār,* "treatment by fire"), was also very popular in the Muslim Middle East for medical (as well as for cosmetic) purposes. It was carried out by placing a white-hot iron on a designated spot on the body, and removing it after a few seconds. The pain could be excruciating, and the sources describe how several big men were drafted in order to hold the patient's limbs down and "glue" him. Cauterization was used as a treatment for a variety of ailments in all body parts, ranging from headaches to fistulas and hemorrhoids. Cauterization treated also nonphysical problems, like forgetfulness (!) or moods (such as melancholy, *maliholiya*). Sabuncuoğlu discussed several such cases throughout his chirurgical manual. Several Prophetic sayings specifically reject cauterizations for human beings and animals. Yet, the fact the Prophet was said to forbid the practice apparently did not affect its popularity. Evidence from the 1970s attests it was still practiced in various areas of the Middle East as part of folk medicine.[106]

Customarily, circumcision is performed on every Muslim boy. It is not a religious obligation, but is highly recommended nonetheless, after the model of the Prophet Muhammad (*sunna*). It is a ritual act that designates the person as a Muslim who believes in Allah, and is part of the Abrahamic monotheistic tradition. But circumcision was also practiced for medical purposes, and it is in this context that it is considered here. The nature of the operation was to remove an excess of skin from the male genitals. Thevenot said that in the case of many Turks, the extra skin was indeed considerable, and unless it was removed it could cause discomfort or even become infected.[107] Whether circumcision was for ritual or medical purposes, it was carried out by surgeons. Religious scholars were not involved with the actual operation (in contrast to Judaism, in which only religious officials have the authority to conduct the ritual ceremony and carry out the surgical cutting). Paul Rycaut, an Englishman, claimed that the Ottomans considered circumcision an improper and unclean task for the ulema, and it was relegated to surgeons. In the Ottoman palace it was the court surgeons who were entrusted with the royal circumcision of the imperial princes (an affair that was celebrated with much pomp) and of the freshly recruited Christian boys who became the sultan's slaves.[108]

Inoculation against smallpox was a "surgical" procedure common in the central regions of the Ottoman Empire. It was administered by older women specializing in folk medicine. They opened four or five veins in the arms, chest, and forehead of boys and teenagers (the sources do not specify whether the vaccination was given to girls as well). Into the open veins they inserted mucus taken from open wounds of smallpox patients. The children were ill after the treatment, and for few days ran high fevers, but recovered totally. The inoculation was especially popular during the fall months and was part of the rites of passage to adulthood among Turkish Muslim families, being celebrated with much festivity.

This inoculation received some attention in England before Edward Jenner (1749–1823) offered a different and less dangerous vaccine. It became known through Lady Mary Wortley Montagu (1689–1762), who accompanied her husband on his short tour as the ambassador of the Court of St. James to the Ottoman sultan, Ahmet III, at the beginning of the eighteenth century. Jenner suggested vaccinating human beings by infecting them first with cowpox, a related disease that attacks humans with much less intensity and fewer possible complexities than smallpox. The Ottoman method infected the children with smallpox itself, a highly dangerous and infectious disease. Lady Mary witnessed this popular vaccination given to several boys in Edirne and other towns in the Ottoman Empire. Lady Mary was highly impressed with the success of the Ottoman "vaccination." Her own brother had succumbed to the disease, and she too suffered from it, and although she recuperated, the pox disfigured her once beautiful face and smooth skin. This problem apparently bothered her very much, as this was one of the details she emphasized in her letters to her friends about the miraculous treatment: the fact that the Ottoman boys who went through the inoculation were not scarred. She chose to inoculate her son and daughter against smallpox, and the result was a great success.Upon her return to London she started a campaign in the popular press, in scientific circles, including the Royal College of Physicians, and at the royal court to adopt the Ottoman vaccination as a public policy. Although slowly the practice was adopted by royal circles in England and the continent, and generally among the people, it was still done sporadically.[109] It is interesting to note here how a popular medical practice in one society becomes part of learned medicine in another. In the transfer between societies and medical systems, inoculation became vaccination and received new legitmation from a different source. Jenner based himself on experiment and observation, the methods of investigation in medicine and science that had become the norm by his time, instead of the local tradition and custom to which Lady Mary was witness.

As a summation to the complex surgical realities in the early modern Ottoman world, let me point out again that surgery was common and accepted. Even in malpractice suits against physicians and surgeons the complaints were about the outcome, the failure of the operation to heal. The capabilities of a certain physician were blamed, or the choice of a specific procedure as the right choice for that ailment was questioned. Nowhere is it said (by the complainers as well as by the religious-judicial authorities) that the essence of the process—cutting into a human being's body—was forbidden. In fact, they seem quite blasé about it. The legal discussion revolved around damages, if guilt was established, not about the nature or essence of medicine and surgery. Two factors determined guilt: whether the defendant could prove he or she received permission from the patient beforehand to perform an agreed procedure and whether it was the medical norm among his or her peers. Unless these criteria were proved, the physician was not guilty (Moses Hamon was made suspect because of the second stipulation, as discussed above).[110]

There is evidence that even autopsies, a problematic surgical procedure because of its ethical-religious aspects, took place from time to time in various places in the Ottoman Empire. Rabbi Raphael Mordekhai Malki, a late seventeenth-century Jewish physician from Jerusalem, explained the context of autopsies. If someone passed away without an apparent cause, and had been under constant medical attention and received treatment, physicians could operate on the body in order to establish a concrete cause of death. But not every physician was entitled to decide about an autopsy on his own and carry it out alone. There had to be a consensus of three physicians about the need for autopsy in each specific case, and the deceased's relatives had to give their consent. Malki adds that autopsy was not to be performed on certain groups. Not surprisingly, all belonged to the elite: important personalities, the rich, and famous scholars—the right to medical treatment and autonomy over one's body changed according to social class.[111]

Malki was a member of a religious minority group in an Ottoman province, and he had been educated in a European university (he assumed a Christian identity and studied in Italy before immigrating to Palestine), but his Jewish medical situation was not totally removed from the situation in Ottoman Muslim circles. The sixteenth-century historian Mustafa Ali mentions autopsy as a means of demonstrating the inferiority of the local physicians to their European colleagues. While he was a clerk in the provincial divan in Aleppo in 1582–83, he came to recognize the greatness of a certain Christian physician who investigated the reasons of death in town of an acquaintance of the Venetian *bailo*. The physician insisted on opening the corpse's stomach and threatened to leave his post as the *bailo's* personal physician if not allowed to carry out this operation (the heads of the Venetian community opposed him). He received the permission and performed the operation, and the cause for the fellow's sudden death became clear: silkwormlike maggots had attached to his heart and had brought about his death. Ali was impressed and described the physician as a paragon of a learned and skilled doctor.[112] An educated Muslim Ottoman did not regard autopsy as forbidden or disgraceful.

Even if autopsies were carried out from time to time, they were not that common. This was apparently the reality encountered by a Scots physician by the name of C. Bryce who visited Istanbul sometime in 1830. As this was only the beginning of reform measures in the medical arena (the new European-influenced medical school had opened in Istanbul only three years earlier, in March 1827), his description is relevant to an earlier period as well. In his report to the *Edinburgh Medical and Surgical Journal*, Dr. Bryce says there was no legal impediment for autopsies for instructing students in the medical school. According to his local informants, a formal decree by the imperial head physician could allow it, although he would need the mufti's approval.[113]

Surgery as a whole was much more of a routine than autopsies, but likewise its clinical applications were more limited than the medical or legal authorities would have allowed. The surgery was usually light surgery. Rarely do we encounter evidence of intrusive procedures where the surgeon cut deep into the tissues, like the heroic scene encountered by Evliya. So the surgery usually practiced was not necessarily what we think of as surgery today. The common procedures referred to in the sources included cutting the bladder to take out stones, fixing hernias (*fıtık*), draining abscesses, curing various problems in the male genitals, and curing some eye ailments. Gynecology and obstetrics too included surgery-like procedures. These were mostly small operations, but they were done on a regular, daily basis. In the 1620s in the Asian district of Istanbul alone dozens of cases of hernia treatment were registered by three healers in the court protocols; two were male practitioners who bore the title of "surgeon," *cerrah*; the third was a female whose patients were males. One can only assume many more did not reach the pages of the court archives.[114]

CHAPTER 2

"In health and in sickness": The Integrative Body

Ottoman medicines shared several patterns. One of them was an integrative view of humans: a "whole" person is situated in a "total" environment.[1] Man was understood as standing in the center of a complex world with many diverse forces working on him and within him. The cosmic hierarchy was very clear, crediting human beings with having special privileges. Muslim theology regards man as God's supreme creation, for whose sake the entire bounty of nature had been created. Yet human beings are required to share the world with other of God's creations. The image is of man being the custodian of the natural world rather than of having the right to subdue and dominate it. The world of nature is occupied by both humans and nonhumans. This environment is made of both physical and symbolic realities, physical and material, on the one hand, and spiritual and divine, on the other. Although man is deeply affected by his mighty surroundings and the forces shaping him from the inside, he is not passive: he is able to leave his mark on his world. In fact, it is man's purpose on earth to cultivate the world, use it, and nurture it at the same time and thus sustain the balance God created. Ideally all forces should interact in a balanced manner and be integrated into harmony. Such an ideal balance (Arabic *mīzān*) is hard to find and create, as it changes from man to man; it is even harder to maintain. Yet man is supposed to dedicate himself to this multifaceted quest.[2]

Here we are concerned with the medical aspect of balance within the human body that corresponds with physical and mental health. The human body as a complex whole is composed of matter and soul. As a result, a physical problem could produce mental symptoms and vice versa. Other aspects of this balance are social and ecological, which are dealt with in the following chapters.

The term "holism" (from the Greek *holos*, meaning "whole") seems to explain the importance of balance in Ottoman medicine and the integrative outlook and man, his body, and his world. This term was coined by General Jan Christiaan Smuts (1870–1950) in his influential philosophical work *Holism and Evolution* (1926), although the intellectual heritage he based himself upon is much older. He used "holism" to designate a tendency in nature to produce wholes, like bodies and organisms, by grouping together units or structures. The synthesis makes the elements or parts act as one. The properties of a system come together and make a whole that is greater and more complex than the sum of its parts.[3]

Later philosophers of science developed from Smuts's term the concept of holism in science. It meant for them a paradigm or a philosophical outlook that facilitates the study of complex and integrated systems. It draws our attention to the wider or interdisciplinary contexts of our inquiry. This is a different mode of inquiry from the traditional one that analyzes systems by dividing them into their smallest elements and explains the whole system from its elemental properties (the mode was hence termed "atomistic" or "reductionist"). Smuts explained that the view of the world as consisting of separate interacting things is necessary for practical scientific reasons. The ability to think in such specific terms is a great invention, according to him. However, it is a limited way of considering the world, and separatism should disappear, to be replaced by an integrative approach.[4]

The term "holism" has also been adopted into certain scientific fields, like biology, cognitive studies, artificial intelligence, or dynamics. In applying a holistic approach, scientists try to harness large quantities of data to explain entire complex systems involving many variables.

Although holism has entered mainstream "orthodox" philosophy of science, responses to Smuts's term and theory are nonetheless varied. It is still regarded as controversial by many who criticize the concept as pseudoscience. The critics claim that employing this method results in a description rather than an analysis of a phenomenon. They further assert that it uses scientific-like language but not a scientific method. They contend that it gives leeway to religion and mysticism to infiltrate science. Indeed, Kenneth Earl Wilber, Jr., one of the best-known authors on holism and integral theories, currently claims that science should also accept knowledge derived from meditation and spiritual practice as valid evidence. Reliance solely on the five senses is too narrow a basis. He further claims that integrating science and religion is the most important challenge of our period. For him, science brings forth mere facts; it deals with value-free truths. These are meaningless without religion, which adds wisdom and values.[5]

"Holistic medicine" is the modern term to indicate a form of medical treatment that attempts to deal with the whole person and not merely with his or her physical condition. It integrates knowledge of the body, the mind, and the environment. Whereas conventional Western medicine identifies and attacks symptoms, holistic medicine seeks to identify the underlying conditions in the client's life that have caused the illness or allowed it to happen and then to alleviate them. A holistic approach to healing recognizes that the emotional, mental, spiritual, and physical elements of each person comprise a system. In addition to treating the whole person, it concentrates on the causes of the illness rather than its symptoms.

It is tempting therefore to use "holistic medicine" to refer to Ottoman medicine. What in our modern Western society is a provocative and "alternative" idea seems to be a fair description of the prevailing reality for the early-modern Middle East as part of its integralistic approach to health and medicine. However, "holistic medicine" is a problematic concept, not least of all because its application to the subject matter of early modern Muslim medicines would be anachronistic. Ottomans did not have a specific term equivalent to our concept of "holism." The word 'holism' was coined in order to oppose conservative scientific-technological medicine and critique modern Western society as a whole. Thus, the term evolved as a relative one, while for the Ottomans integralistic points of view were very much the accepted norm rather than an alternative outlook on their body and world. As this chapter will show, early modern Ottomans accepted integralism as a basic concept of the world and man's place within it, or as a natural way to understand them. For Ottomans, integralism did not require explanations or defense. The situation today is markedly different, as "holistic medicine" is positioned in contrast to modern science and medicine, which are characterized by their focus on one tissue (not even an organ), on one particular. As a result, today there is a need for a label in order to refer to and legitimize a different outlook on what health and medicine are.

Another problem is that "holism" is too broad a term to be a useful analytic tool. "Holism" means different things to different people. There are at least four different concepts of holism, as discussed in current biomedical literature: the metahistorical (health and disease are seen as developing from a distant biological past), the organismic (the body is understood a functioning unit), the ecological (the body is the outcome of a particular social and physical setting), and the worldview holistic (a metaphor for thinking about the well-being of society in general).[6]

In the framework of an integralistic worldview, the Ottomans, like other premodern cultures, positioned the human body in two parallel circles or cosmoses. The wider one dealt with the interaction between the surrounding world and the body—in other words, the environment. The inner circle was focused on the body as the exterior form of a complex cosmos within it. The discussions dealt with each cosmos and at the same time emphasized the intrinsic interactions between cosmoses and their reciprocal influences. These discussions were carried out within different discourses, or intellectual trends, raising different aspects ranging from the nature of the material world to theological and ethical considerations. For the sake of clarity, this chapter focuses on the individual body with its complexities and needs for a balance. The discussion of the wider circle, how the balance between man and his world was conceptualized and practiced in actual clinical settings, is picked up in the fourth chapter.

Ottoman integralism portrayed body and mind as meshed into one entity and positioned this entity in relation to its surrounding environment. This concept was discussed and debated among religious scholars, mystics, philosophers, and physicians. Their understanding of the individual human body allows much space to the soul. The exact nature of each component and the precise details of the complicated relationship between them were not agreed upon, but certain points were accepted. It was commonly believed that the relationship was not always harmonious. From the medical point of view, it resulted in the belief that one cannot be sick in the body and totally healthy in the mind, or to suffer mental problems yet be void of any physical discomfort.[7] The observation of Charles E. Rosenberg with regard to medicine in the United States is true here also: the explanations of the relationship of the emotional and physiological changed, but the clinical reality (that emanated from such integralism) was not doubted.[8]

Galenic humoralism was mechanistic medicine in that health and illness were explained as deriving from the balance (or lack thereof) between the physiological building blocks of the body, the four humors. These humors affected the human being as a whole—that is, balance was the basis for physical as well as mental well-being. The mixture of the humors is the temperament that dictates the operation of the body organs and shapes one's characteristic personality. Moreover, the sought-after balance was not affected solely by elements within the body. Rather, external elements outside man, the "six nonnaturals"—food and drink, sleep and waking, air, evacuation and repletion, motion and rest, and passions/emotions—were just as crucial to one's body and mental state.

Humoralism was based on the understanding that humans were composed of body and soul as two components affecting each other. Mukbilzade Mu'min's treatise dedicated to Murad II (reigned 1420–44, 1446–51) best exemplifies this union. This book, written in the 1430s, is considered an influential work in Ottoman medicine on mental problems. Mukbilzade catalogued the mental problems known to him, most of which are grouped under "Head Diseases," due to the organ in which they originate. He explains that physical trauma, like a head injury due to a fall from a high place, can cause a mental disorder, but some mental disorders are due to mental trauma. He mentions also other mental disorders, like hysteria, bulimia, or gluttony. Other types of mental problems discussed by Mukbilzade are sexual disorders and addiction to alcohol or opium.[9]

The view that humoralism presented of the duality of body and soul was part of a large philosophical-cum-psychological and theological discourse that tried to define what body (or physical circumstances) and soul (intellect or self) are, what each is made of, and to understand their connection. Like humoral medicine itself, this discourse originated in Greek discussions of these subjects and was transferred to Arabic and Islam. The translations from Greek to Arabic were in fact modifications to the point of producing new and original philosophical positions.[10]

The Greek philosophical heritage—modified or not—was exactly the problem that religious medicine had with humoralism. So although Prophetic medicine too offered an integralistic outlook of man and health, it differed from Galenic humoralism in order to present a Muslim whole, rather than one influenced by Aristotelian or Neoplatonic ideas. According to one Muslim thinker, "[L]ack of knowledge and the inability to internalize the holistic consequences of individual actions are symptoms of humankind's dissociation from Allah."[11] One issue that Muslim scholars commented on with regard to the body-soul relationships, the dichotomy between the material and terrestrial powers and spiritual/celestial elements, was the need to emphasize divine omnipotence.[12]

Instead of viewing man as a mental and material entity, a combination of body and soul, religious medicine highlighted another nonphysical component: spirituality. It accepted the efficacy of physical cures but pointed also to the power of the human person. It discussed excessive emotions like love, passion, grief, envy, and shame as a form of illness and how the health of the soul or heart and the health of the body were interdependent. This is why authors on religious medicine did not reject Galenic humoralism. As explained in the previous chapter, for them Galenism was not regarded as bad medicine; rather, it was perceived as lacking in giving room to the divine, and as a result inferior. These authors integrated the physical, the psychological, the spiritual, and the moral.[13]

The philosophical and medical concepts that married body and soul resulted in a therapeutic method that addressed the mental in order to treat both the mental and physical (and vice versa: physical treatments for mental problems existed as well). It was done by employing the senses, a treatment we would today call "psychotherapy." This term is taken from modern psychology, which started to evolve with Sigmund Freud in late nineteenth-century central Europe, and as such is an anachronism when applied to early modern Ottoman realities. Modern psychotherapy includes several schools of thought and methods, and the actual list of therapies includes a wide range of types of communication between the therapist and the client. The Ottoman therapeutic methods were different. The so common technique of discussion as a means of therapy, for instance, was absent in Ottoman medicine. But the modern term does help to draw our attention to the existence of a set of techniques within Ottoman medicine intended specifically to improve emotional or behavioral problems, to use modern terms. Peregrine Horden used a borrowed phrase, "a temple is as useful as a dam," to discuss urban health policies in medieval Christian context,[14] but it allows us to give due weight to the nonbiological or materialistic aspects of health and medical recovery in the Ottoman society as well.

In this chapter we shall focus on four examples that illustrate ecological concepts in Ottoman medicine. We will concentrate on the use of the human senses in medical treatment, the roles of hygiene in general and water in particular, the importance of belief and religion in therapeutics, and the conceptualization of health and sickness in general. These examples take us to the Ottoman conceptualization of what health and sickness meant as well as to actual clinical realities. So far, the scholarship on the Muslim concept of the human body has based itself on sources that tried to formulate norms. By their very nature these sources were idealistic and ahistorical. This chapter, however, presents concrete attitudes and practices pertaining to the human body in sickness and in health, set in the specific historical context of the early modern Ottoman Empire.

The Senses and the Sound of Music

Medicine embraces ample portions of the human senses. The senses are employed in diagnosis, where the doctors are supposed to act like detectives and interpret the clues about the medical condition of their patients through their senses. The doctor-patient encounter is about seeing, touching, and hearing. The senses are an important part of the process of studying, investigating, and exploring medicine. And sight, touch, taste, smell, and hearing are inevitable players in the healing process, both for the observing physician orchestrating the process and for the patient going through it.[15]

Middle Eastern therapeutics clearly tried to employ the sense of smell and sight. The previous chapter discussed the particular Ottoman use of the taste buds in food and medication. Indeed, the Ottomans used all the five senses. It was another aspect of Ottoman medicine being integralistic. Within this framework, music or sound generally is believed to play a fundamental role in shaping and rebalancing the forces at work in nature and the humors in the human body. Sound is energy, which is crucial to maintain health and cure sickness. The Ottomans believed certain types of sound had enormous power in healing and in maintaining bodily and mental health. In this sense music acts as both a generative and regulatory force in the body. It attunes individual and environment. The Ottomans recognized that creative activity has a therapeutic effect, and thus could support or be adjunct to other forms of treatment.

In the Ottoman context "music therapy" was a form of healing (that is, making strong and whole again), as well as a therapy (that is, a technique of intervention with distinct goals). Music therapy was very common among Turkish peoples throughout history. It was a cure for sickness and also a method for guarding one's health as part of a preventive lifestyle.[16] But Ottoman music therapy was grounded in combining three cultural-medical heritages. Ottoman scholars interested in music had the idea of comparing their own musical practices and ideas with the musical theories to which they had access. The fact many of these scholars came from far and wide and brought their cultural traditions with them facilitated such a cultural fertilization.[17] In addition to the Turkish one, there were also Arab-Muslim and Byzantine therapies. The Ottomans assimilated elements from these legacies as a basis for their own activity and creativity. The fact the Ottomans relied not on one tradition, but on three distinct ones in using music in a medical context made it all the more culturally possible for them to accept the theoretical concept and praxis of music as a therapy.

Like Galenic medicine, Arab-Muslim musical knowledge derived from translations and adaptations of Greek writings. Within the plurality of musical theories existing in this tradition, one prevailing concept was the belief in the overwhelming power of music over men and animals. Music was accepted as a model for human balance, physically and temperamentally. Musical theory was a means to put the world into order, harmony, and rhythm. It turns the shapeless and irrational universe into a manageable, intelligible, and less frightening reality. Without such a theory, the world seems to be in disorder, full of great dramas (both catastrophes and major successes) and frantic events brought about by God (or gods, as in antiquity), all of which seem to be beyond human grasp. It determines man's ethical and physical equilibrium and connects him to astrological forces (here music was connected with the zodiac).

Since antiquity, musical instruments have served as a model for understanding the behavior of man. Such models were needed especially for the mental and other internal aspects of human functioning, as the latter cannot be observed directly and need to be inferred from other signs. Aeorophones (in which sound resonates through cylindrical pipes) and chordophones (in which the performer plays on elastic strings) were prominent in this model.

Arab-Muslim music came to be understood to affect man's well-being. It was also developed into a concrete therapeutic means, for things like mental illnesses. A four-stringed instrument was played upon to symbolize harmony, as each string symbolized one of the four elements affecting the body, one of the humors composing the physical body, or one of the four temperaments. Like the ideal balance between the humors, so the music produced by the instrument, it was thought, needed to be harmonious and melodious. Music was part of the philosophical discourse on the world and humanity's role in it. It also suited the understanding of the human body as an automaton. Thus, music and musical instruments were related also to medicine as a theory and as a practical therapeutics.[18]

The sixteenth-century Ottoman doctor Dā'ūd al-Anṭākī included a chapter on music in his general medical compendium, written in Arabic. It is evident he was well read in music, which he used for medical purposes. Components of music—melody, harmony and rhythm—were diagnostic tools, exactly like pulse, indicating health and sickness. But music was also a cure. Al-Anṭākī introduced into medicine the notion of specific physical situations and mental modes with particular medical properties. From about the fifteenth century onward detailed tables of musical modes appropriate for each physical condition had existed; now with al-Anṭākī we can see that the concept of music therapy was also held by a physician. However, according to him, the professional who should administer this type of cure is the musician. Apparently al-Anṭākī did not envision a model of the *medicus perfectus* who was a master in music. Maybe this was so because for him music was (only?) a craft. The musician's task was to take the right melody from a known repertoire and apply it to specific circumstances, whether it was entertaining an audience, calming nerves, curing an illness, or stopping a quarrel. If the musician's aim was not achieved, it was because the musician apparently failed to choose the correct melody for the case. The musician was not required to be creative or artistic, or to analyze medically the music he was about to play. The musician was a technician, and all the information he needed to work with was given to him. This is why al-Anṭākī interpreted each of the eight musical scales according to its medical and astrological attributes and specified its main influences on humans. The scale *rast*, for example, is beneficial for hemiplegics, while *araq* can cure acute humoral imbalances, like brain diseases, vertigo, pleurisy, suffocation, and the like.[19]

The Byzantines, a third source of intellectual influence on the Ottomans, were familiar with practical music therapy. Music making of expressly therapeutic intent was present in Byzantine hospitals. Evidence from the eleventh century onward conveys the impression that the prescription of medicine and the prescription of music to patients were somehow connected, including within hospital space. Music formed part of the total healing environment of these hospitals.[20]

At least one Muslim observer, the famous Persian mystic al-Hujwīrī (died sometime between 1072 and 1077), relates that in his days the use of music in religious context as part of the arsenal of therapeutics in Byzantine hospitals was a regular procedure. According to him, it was well known that hospital patients were brought to a "concert" twice a week and listened to a string instrument playing for a length of time appropriate to their specific malady. This remark appears in his discussion of music and listening to music in a religious mystical context (*samā'*; chapter 25 in his treatise). Hujwīrī traveled around the Middle East. He also visited Syria, which lay closest to the Byzantine lands. In Syria, or maybe elsewhere, he could have seen a Christian hospital himself, or received reports from his informants on such procedures.[21]

These were not theoretical traditions alone; all were also implemented both in hospitals and by doctors treating their private patients. The Umayyad caliphs listened to music for therapeutic reasons on their weekly "wine days." The thirteenth-century hospital in Divriği, Anatolia, contained a fountain whose falling waters made melodious sound for the mentally ill. In the contemporary Manṣūrī hospital in Cairo, one of the designated expenditures was for musicians to entertain the patients daily. A fourteenth-century hospital in Aleppo employed musicians who played music in the courtyards for the inmates. One physician from the same period reported that some doctors used to take their patients' pulse while singing to them in corresponding rhythms.[22]

The Ottomans could rely on these theoretical and therapeutic traditions and used music in the course of their treatment, for example in some hospitals. (One could also claim that music in court served a medical purpose, in addition to its stated aim of pleasure and enjoyment.) There was no recognized body of professional music therapists, as in the modern context. The musicians employed in Ottoman hospitals were not qualified practitioners working with patients/clients who could not deal with specific psychological or physical conditions without professional assistance (the modern understanding of what "music therapy" is). Yet the people involved in music therapy in Ottoman hospitals were no amateurs. They were professional musicians whose employment was not incidental. It was an intentional policy on the part of the caregivers in the institution. No less than the famous imperial military band, the *mehterhane-i haqani*, performed in various hospitals, in addition to the "house musicians" employed by specific institutions. This may be a development of their twice-a-day concert in Istanbul that the traveler Evliya Çelebi tells about. Since the time of Mehmet II, two military groups played for the public every morning and evening from their quarters. One was stationed near the Iron Gate (Demirkapı) by the Palace Gardens, the other at the westernmost point in the city, the Citadel of Seven Towers (Yediküle).[23]

References to the intentional use of music as a medical procedure were made with regards to the hospitals of Beyazid II in Edirne, Mehmet II in Istanbul, and the one in the Topkapı Palace. Evliya Çelebi insists that the hospitals of Mehmet II and Beyazid II invited artists on a regular basis to perform for the lunatics. Evliya was also a trained musician in vocal and instrumental music. He won his position as companion (*musahib*) of Murad IV at court due to his ability to sing well. Later on he attached himself to the retinue of various officials in order to be able to travel around the empire; usually his position was chief of prayer callers (*muezzin-başı*). But Evliya was also versed in the theory of music. Hence his comments on music have particular value. Evliya devoted several sections to musicians and instrument makers in Istanbul, exalting their skills,[24] but his comments on musicians in hospitals are very revealing with regard to the intentional use of music as therapeutics.

Evliya's comment on musicians at the hospital of Mehmet II is quite short, but he elaborates with regard to a band of ten singers and musicians associated with the Edirne hospital. They played a concert thrice a week in the hospital, each time performing a *fasıl*, a complete musical composition containing a prelude and the development of a mode. The ten musicians comprised three singers and seven players of famous Ottoman instruments of the period, all of which were associated with court culture. There was one player for each instrument, which resulted in a very rich band. The instruments included the *neyzen*, a special version of the *ney*, a reed-flute with a bone mouthpiece, which had risen to great importance by the seventeenth century and was especially associated with Sufi and religious music; the *keman*, a sort of fiddle known also as *kemançe* played with a bow; the *musikar*, known also as *miskal*, an instrument created by attaching several reeds of different length together (the Europeans thought of panpipes upon seeing it); the *santur*, a dulcimer, or trapezoidal board with metal strings played by hammering on them instead of plucking; the *çeng*, a wooden harp influenced by the Celtic harp whose music was associated with delight, paradise, and the sensuality of the harem (it was a popular chordophone but disappeared between the seventeenth and eighteenth century); the *çeng santuru*, a hybrid of *çeng* and *santur*; and the *'ud*, a short-necked, unfretted lute that came in a variety of dimensions and was played by plucking the strings. The *'ud* enjoyed a central place for many centuries, but its role had diminished by the middle of the seventeenth century.[25]

The instruments, the changing rhythms, and the melodies were meant to rouse emotional responses from the patients: happiness, sadness, calmness, and so on. Evliya reports of the Edirne group that its music helped the patients. The band specialized in six scales and tonal models: *navâ, rast, dügâh, segâh, çargâh,* and *suzinâk*. He goes on to say that a combination of *zengüle* and *bûsalîk* scales gives life and energy, whereas all scales nourish the soul. Indeed, the various bands and artists performed different types of music and used particular instruments; they thus had different effects on the mental and physical condition of the patients. The military band used rhythms and instruments like drums or trumpets, which created stimulating music in marchlike tempos and high volume, as is needed for military purposes. As a result, it aroused the passions of the listeners and stimulated associations with war. Other bands might have performed a more relaxing type of music that soothed the patients. Moses Hamon, the private physician of Süleyman I, regarded soothing music as helping the princes to sleep. The different effect on the patients was due to the composition of the band (flutes or violins in contrast to trumpets and drums), and the modes and the exact time during the day when music was performed.[26]

Professional musicians judge the quality of music in aesthetic terms. Yet when it comes to music therapy, the quality is irrelevant to the process through which a person is healed, and this is the only desired outcome.[27] Here we can think of music produced by the patients themselves, in contrast to music performed for them by professional musicians. The sixteenth-century Ottoman bureaucrat Mustafa Ali described in distaste the mad patients in Cairo, who resided in filthy, run-down halls and lacked any understanding of their surroundings. He seems quite surprised that the lunatics could produce such music, which transformed the place into a house where a merry wedding takes place. Yet he wondered (and his irony is not hidden) who was actually listening.[28]

One particular instrument designed to make music is the human voice. Singing, either solo or choral, was a most important part of music. Instruments were played for their own sake, but many times they were used to accompany singing, as in the Edirne hospital. Singing could take many forms and contexts, including being part of religious services. Although all imperial hospitals incorporated prayer facilities, including a professional caller, it is from Jerusalem that we get a unique piece of evidence of the Muslim call to prayers used as a soothing tool. In Jerusalem, a sixteenth-century European observer reported, the first call at dawn was deemed especially beneficial for the sick patients suffering from insomnia. He did not claim that the early morning call to prayer was timed especially for the needs of the sick or that it was changed in any way to suit their needs. However, it is instructive to see that he was led to believe that the call to prayer was connected with treatment.[29]

Another means of putting the sense of hearing and human voice into action was storytelling. Certainly, treating the mentally ill with stories was a familiar theme in Arab-Muslim literature, as exemplified, for example, in *One Thousand and One Nights*.[30] Three of the Edirne artists were not musicians but orators who recited poetry and stories. This method was used also in the Manṣūrī hospital in Cairo, where dancers and other entertainers were brought in to amuse the sick.[31]

Discussion of other forms of music in a Muslim religious context are omitted here. Singing or reciting the Qur'an was a different task, separate from playing music. Incantations and magic spells in Prophetic medicine, for example, were intoned or muttered rather than sung. Their efficacy depended on their wording, not on any musical qualities.[32]

This abundant evidence of music therapy is impressive. As Evliya's discussion indicates, the knowledge of music as a medical tool extended well outside medical circles and infiltrated those of the Ottoman elite literati. His background in music may have given him easier access to it, but he was certainly not alone. The late sixteenth-century writer Mustafa Ali surveyed varieties of musical instruments and musicians. His focus was clearly music played in elite social gatherings, but some of his puns can be interpreted as hinting also to medical uses of music. His use of "rational" and "mad" to describe the audience of *kanun* music invoked the contrast between the listeners to music in general (*musiki*) and those who used it for devotion and ecstasy (*sema*). Alternatively, Mustafa Ali could mean here music played to calm the nerves of mental patients. In other cases he discusses several scales and modes and interprets them with relation to temperaments. He explains, for example, that the *uşşak makam* (literally "the lover's *makam*") is dry and thus suits the mood of hashish smokers.[33]

Despite the important role of sound in medical theory, and the knowledge thereof, music therapy was peripheral to other forms of treatment in Ottoman society. Let us recall Hujwīrī's description of music in Byzantine hospitals from the second half of the eleventh century. Even for someone who traveled extensively in the Muslim lands and was reported to have witnessed incredible things, it was a marvelous invention.[34] It seems the use of music in a medical setting, whether inside or outside hospitals, was not a common practice in the Muslim lands at the time. In contrast to what later local and European observers would like us to believe, the use of music in Muslim hospitals was the exception rather than the rule.

Even in Ottoman hospitals, where music was supposed to have been used quite regularly, musicians were employed by only *some* of the institutions. Description of these instances reveals that music therapy was indeed practiced; at the same time it attests it was a rarity worth noting. Yes, the comments talk about the high status of such a medical practice, yet we cannot ignore the possibility that it was its rarity that gave it an aura of an especially effective medical practice. Even in the hospitals where musicians could be found, they were not among the original staff decreed by the founder. We should be careful not to splice scattered references in partisan accounts too tightly together and make them a regular and accepted tradition in hospitals and outside. By and large, music was not in the regular arsenal of the educated physician. It is philosophy and mystical religion that make conceptual room for music therapy, but it seems marginal to learned medical authorities. It was available, but probably outside the best medical circles as these were defined by medical writers. In Europe, music was put on the same medicinal level as pleasant wine and conversation. Ottoman medicine continued the Arab-Muslim medical tradition that seems to have given music therapy a relative prominence in both theory and practice, yet here too the efflorescence should not be exaggerated. Music therapy still was fringe medicine (a term borrowed from Martin West, who discussed music in the Hellenistic context), even if one or two physicians or hospitals are recorded as having made some use of it. Theory seems more abundant than evidence of practice.[35] Mainstream medicine relied on other therapies: diet, exercise, drugs, baths, and, if necessary, surgery.

Music therapy was not widely practiced, because the attitude toward it outside of medico-philosophical circles was ambivalent. Music was the subject of a long controversy that has never been fully settled. Certainly music met with suspicion in religious circles. The ulema accepted the philosophical concept that music can affect the emotions, the character, and the ethical qualities of the listener. This was exactly the problem: some listeners react in a rather wild and free way, being thrown into ecstasy, and others remain quite and contemplative, but in either case one cannot be indifferent to music, which induces response, physically and mentally. Music could manipulate emotions and as a result be a dangerous tool. Music was believed to be so powerful that it could grow to magical or demonic proportions. Whether the scholar in question mostly permitted listening to music or mostly prohibited it, or took a middle ground, the consensus was that it should be controlled and supervised.[36]

The seventeenth-century clerk Katip Çelebi outlined in his *Mizan al-hakk fi ikhtiyar al-ahakk* (The Balance of Truth), the treatise he completed shortly before his death in 1657, various questions that at the time were causing violent controversy. One of them was music in various forms. The recurrent theme in this treatise is his rejection of what he saw as rigid religious sanctimony. He claimed it was pointless to force people to forgo their customs. Even if they are not in line with the spirit of Islam, it is best to let people keep their traditions, as long as they are not in clear contradiction of religion. His experience was that most often such an attempt is unsuccessful anyway.

Katip Çelebi explains that music and singing (chapters 2 and 3 in his book) have obvious effects on both body and soul. There should therefore be guidelines about what context music should be performed in and listened to and by whom. He added that the Muslim prohibitions in this regard are based on sound logic and wisdom. Here Katip Çelebi positioned himself opposite some Sufi religious scholars who claimed music had no harmful effects. Katip Çelebi asserted that one should pay attention to what is played and sung in order to not create undesirable or even destructive influences on the listener. He believed that the influence was greater (and thus more dangerous) if the listener was one of the simple folk, with no distinguished intellectual, mental, scholarly, or moral standing (Katip Çelebi was certainly an elitist). Therefore, the contents of the singing should not be of wine, debauchery, or lewdness—all against Muslim morality—and the music should be melodious. But music for the benefit of the community, such as playing the tambourine at weddings or the drums during a battle, is lawful. Within these guidelines the performance of music and listening to it are permitted.[37]

Indeed music therapy, at least in its more hypnotic and ecstatic cases, involves music, healing, and belief in magic and the supernatural. In certain Muslim mystic orders, like the Mevlevis or the Helvatis, the music (and dance) accompanying the sacred text were studied and performed with great care. This very belief that music has the power to affect individuals (man as well as animals), societies, and even the universe was exactly what made music in the forms of dancing, singing, or playing instruments such an important method for Sufis in their quest to reach ecstasy and unity with God.

Hujwīrī, a mystic himself, claimed that whoever denies the power and pleasure of music is either a liar or hypocrite. This is exactly why Ebu Su'ud Efendi, the influential head mufti under Süleyman I and his successor Selim II, issued several legal rulings (*fetvas*) concerning music and dancing. He was critical of both activities, especially in the mystical-Sufi context. His fear was that the mystics crossed the line when some orders claimed that dancing or listening to music were forms of worship. Ebu Su'ud rejected this belief, as it hinted that God had ordered those acts; for him this was apostasy.[38] Despite the criticism and Ebu Su'ud Efendi's disassociation from Sufi customs, the two groups found mutual agreement. Mystics too shared the ulema's anxiety over the influence of music; or rather, they feared the destructive influence of music in the wrong hands.

Hygiene and Hydrotherapy: The Power of Water

European travelers were impressed by the level of cleanliness the Ottomans regularly observed, both with regard to their own bodies and to the environment where they lived. Pierre Belon, a sixteenth-century French botanist and naturalist, crowned the Ottomans as "the cleanest people in the world." He was especially admiring of the way babies and infants were kept clean, and were not as smelly as European children were. Another sixteenth-century traveler to the Ottoman Empire, Guillaume Postel, a member of the Collège de France who arrived at Istanbul in 1535 to acquire oriental manuscripts for François I, wished that all the great cities of Europe had similar habits.[39] People removed their shoes before entering a house (or a mosque). Animals, such as dogs and birds, were considered to be unclean, and therefore were not allowed to enter private houses (although stray animals were taken care of).[40] The impression of European observers was that many Ottomans were punctilious about cleaning themselves after any unclean action, such as sexual intercourse or bowel movements, and did not merely purify themselves directly before prayer (all Muslims must be in a state of ritual purity—not the same thing as physically clean—before prayer).[41]

Water was used not only for general hygiene but also as a direct therapeutic tool. Medical qualities were attributed to both natural and artificial reservoirs of water, whether on the surface or subterranean. Bathing in different types of water sources was the subject of many illustrations in Ottoman illuminated manuscripts, such as the miniatures from a sixteenth-century work shown in figures 2 and 3.

These miniatures raise questions pertaining to privacy, such as where the boundaries between the private and the public domains in early modern Ottoman society were drawn, and how an Ottoman was supposed to behave in the public domain while doing something that is ostensibly intimate and private (here: bathing, being partially/fully naked). Privacy is man's right and need to be undisturbed, to have an emotional and physical sphere immune from public intrusion (or at least with restricted access to it). People who live in proximity have to adopt a set of guidelines to sustain the consent for this arrangement. The way a human group defines "privacy" is part of their specific lifestyle.[42] Privacy is a socially and culturally embedded phenomenon. The concept has evolved and changed from place to place, from time to time, and from certain social and economic circumstances to others. The *Oxford English Dictionary* includes references to uses of the term that go back to the middle of the fifteenth century, but not earlier, and the bulk of citations is from later periods.[43] What did the notion of "privacy" mean for Ottomans in the early modern period and what was its relative importance in the face of competing and contradictory legal, social, and cultural norms?

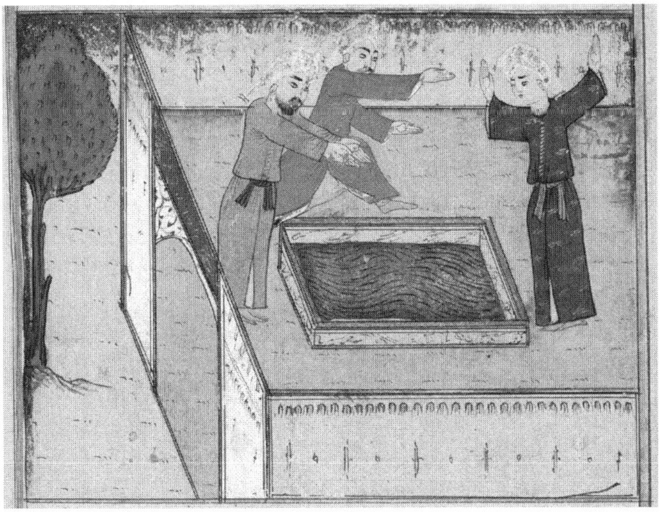

Figure 2. Three men standing on a roof planning to jump into water; the water is clean and medically beneficial. "Wonders of Art and Nature," manuscript held at the British Library, Harl. 5500, 124v. Reproduced by permission of the British Library.

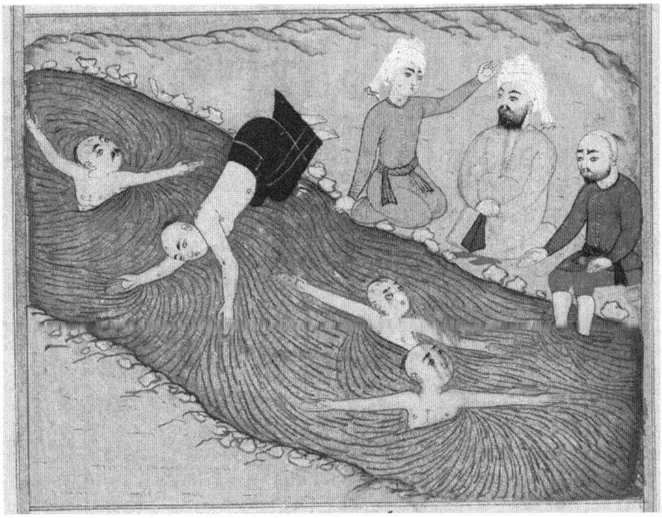

Figure 3. Four men are bathing in the river while three more sit on the bank. The river runs from the mountains, and its clean water is washing away dirt and sickness. "Wonders of Art and Nature," manuscript held at the British Library, Harl. 5500, 160r. Reproduced by permission of the British Library.

The Middle Eastern contexts of privacy have been studied so far by only a few scholars, starting in the late 1980s, who considered mainly the domicile and the neighborhood contexts of privacy. The first was Abraham Marcus, who studied eighteenth-century Aleppo, a crowded city by contemporary standards. Marcus discussed privacy within the context of social order and analyzed it as comprising two aspects: the physical privacy of the individual body; and personal privacy, or privacy of information, meaning the prohibition against interfering in the intimate affairs of another person. He concluded that it was mostly physical privacy that mattered, while neighborhood familiarity was taken for granted. Marcus argued that, although the urban poor maintained their own form of privacy due to financial constraints, the ideals of privacy and morality were those upheld and dominated by the elite.[44]

Shortly afterward Janet Abu-Lughod pointed out the intimate relationships taking place in a city alley. She continued the theme of privacy defined and maintained in different manners according to social class. Abu-Lughod deviated from Marcus in regarding the lower strata as creative and active cultural agents, promoting a culture of their own, rather than regarding them as merely responding to upper-class ideals. She demonstrated that the lower social strata regarded the public alley as a semiprivate sphere, as they could not maintain seclusion in their own domiciles like the upper class. This was one component in her refutation of the frozen model of "the Islamic City" as a chaotic entity.[45]

Dror Ze'evi, who studied seventeenth-century Jerusalem, followed Marcus's observation of the existence of two forms of privacy: a physical privacy alongside privacy of information. He argued that physical privacy was highly esteemed by Jerusalemites, who were willing to infringe on privacy of information in order to protect the physical privacy. Here Ze'evi ratifies Marcus on another point—namely, the gap between cultural ideals and social realities. People were willing to expose themselves intimately before the authorities as a means to minimize potential social and financial damage, if the authorities would not divulge that sensitive information. This explains why the people of Jerusalem used to tell the authorities about their neighbors when their behavior in private did not coincide with what they believed to be normal and moral, and why Jerusalemites endured their neighbors prying into their private affairs. Ze'evi sums up by saying that upholding physical privacy (including favoring it over other aspects of privacy) served as a basic principle in the consensual public order.[46]

Eli Alshech has added legal theory to the discourse about privacy. Marcus, Abu-Lughod, and Ze'evi studied court cases, whereas Alshech analyzed *fiqh* treatises that tried to conceptualize what privacy should mean rather than apply it to concrete situations. In his 2004 article, Alshech studied early Muslim legal thought and concluded that privacy, despite lacking a specific term, was a legal category. Furthermore, the notion evolved from the limited concept of privacy as tied to property rights to a separate legal category. His argument is that legal scholars adopted an instrumental approach to "privacy." It was not the final objective but a means to an end, that end being social control. Here Alshech echoes previous scholarly discourse that positioned "privacy" as a basic principle in maintaining a viable Muslim society.[47]

Paulina B. Lewicka discussed private acts in the public domains in her study of medieval Egyptian eating habits. She was interested in understanding why, contrary to common wisdom, no public consumption facilities like restaurants, taverns, or inns existed in pre-Ottoman Cairo. Although buying ready-made food was totally acceptable, negative attitude toward eating in the street as being undignified persisted. As Muslim legal sources did not restrict the eating premises to the private domain (and in fact inhabitants of Abbasid Baghdad often ate their meals in restaurants), Lewicka looks for the answer in the Arab customs and social practices pertaining to hospitality and territoriality. She concludes that eating was an intimate act. As such, food was supposed to be consumed, shared, and enjoyed in a private and friendly territory. Such sites were not only the private home but also a familiar public place like a neighborhood mosque.[48]

Most recently Iris Agmon revisited the definition of the term "privacy" and pointed out its weakness. While discussing family experiences in the Palestinian port cities of Haifa and Jaffa in the late Ottoman period, she argues that previous scholarship presupposed that the upper class defined cultural ideals about privacy and family. In this line of reasoning, the lower classes are portrayed deterministically as a materialistic construction whose own cultural preferences are the outcome of the lack of means to maintain the ideal. For the purpose of this discussion, I focus on her explanation that the very choice of the term "privacy" is misleading, as the cultural ideal was neither personal privacy nor the boundaries between the individual and the public. Rather, it was groups defined in terms of gender and family that were supposed to be separated. The issue at hand was female chastity and seclusion from nonfamily men, and not individual privacy per se. Marcus and Ze'evi had already brought this up, but Agmon is the one who highlights it.[49]

Now we add the medical context to the discussion of what privacy could mean to various Middle Easterners. Medical scenes like those we have seen above reinforce Lewicka's claim of the possibility of privacy in the public sphere—for instance, through a gendered definition of privacy, as Agmon has pointed out. In other words, private and public domains were not opposite poles but positions on a continuum.

Bathing is perceived (by us moderns?) as a private and intimate action, yet we see that it was done in the normal course of events in groups and in public. Even if the illuminated miniatures were artistic interpretation rather than documentaries of concrete realities, they attest to social norms. And these norms allowed Ottomans to bathe in places open to all, like public baths (or hammams), pools, and rivers. In such places other people were present as well. The boundaries between the individual and the public are blurred here. But in fact the danger of exposure to possible foreigners was limited due to various mechanisms. Bathing in these sites was arranged in a way that created an intermediate reality between total exposure and total seclusion.

A neighborhood hammam, for example, filled more than the functional role of providing bathing services. It was a friendly place where part of the neighborhood social life was conducted. The public bath was not private territory; it belonged to all. One could count on meeting people one knew for many years. Moreover, gender boundaries were meticulously respected. As we can see in the miniatures above and others like them, only men were present: men and women bathed in separate groups. Hence the hammam was willingly visited, well known, and safe.

Even in hospitals, where one did not know the other patients, privacy within the public domain existed. The physical structure of the hospital will be analyzed in detail in the fourth chapter, but here I can mention already that the intrusion of the outside world was checked with walls, gardens, and doorkeepers. Although privacy and physical isolation of the individual played a minor role in shaping the hospital's inner space, gender segregation (as discussed in the next chapter) was implemented and helped to create a sense of privacy.

These scenes are different from those in the literary and visual descriptions of Europeans, who were excited by the mystique of the hammam. Their imagination added erotic motifs to the descriptions. Such motifs are missing from Ottoman miniatures, which deal with the human body in the context of physical and moral cleanliness and hygiene, rather than eroticism.

The hammam was of great significance to the Muslim community—both healthy and ill. The hammam was a social and ritualistic center. People went to the hammam regularly, thrice or four times a week, according to European travelers. Ottomans believed that bathing there was healthy for them. Women, for example, bathed to keep their health and maintain their youth and beauty (as will be discussed below, physical appearance was an important characteristic of Ottoman society; it was one of the criteria for securing a position in the Ottoman administration). The cost of entering the hammam was reasonable, which made it easier for anyone to go there.[50]

The association of the hammam with health was prevalent in Ottoman popular lore. In Istanbul bath attendants bled their customers as part of the service, which included pummeling, rubbing, washing, body-hair removal, and massaging—or so claimed Salomon Schweigger, a chaplain to the Habsburg embassy in the capital during 1577–81.[51] In North Africa the institution was called "the silent doctor": its warm air and the increased perspiration it generated were claimed to cure various ailments, such as rheumatism. Pregnant women went to the bath to secure quick and uncomplicated delivery.[52] This theme of the benefit of hot water was echoed in religious literature and Prophetic medicine treatises alike. One tradition of the Prophet claimed that fever was caused by steam from hell, and should be extinguished with water.[53]

The advantages of the hammam were elaborated also by learned medical treatises of the time. Authors discussed baths as a means to return people suffering from "dry" symptoms to their "wet" balance. For example, bathing was a usual treatment for madness. Since madness was considered to originate in extreme cases of dryness in the patients' body, baths were supposed to return the needed moisture to the body. Thus, a madman needed to regain the balance of his humors, and, as a result, his sanity.

This is the context that explains why baths made their way into hospital practice. Hospitals employed bathhouse attendants (*dellak* or *külkhani*). Their task was also to maintain the personal hygiene of the patients in general, in addition to providing washing directly directed to the therapeutic process. The attendants shaved the patients and clipped their nails while washing them.[54]

Maintaining sanitary conditions was important in the hospital. This institution employed a team of people whose task was maintaining the bodily hygiene of the patients. In addition to the bathhouse attendants, there were launderers (sing. *cameşuy* or *ghessal*) who washed the patients' clothes and replaced their blankets and mattresses. The expenses of the hospital in Edirne at the end of the fifteenth century included grass for the mats (it also included soap, most probably for the bathhouse).[55] In the hospital in Manisa the washers' duty was double: to maintain the physical cleanliness of the patients in this world and to ritually cleanse their bodies after death.[56]

Other employees were responsible for cleaning the facilities and dealing with the regular and continuous physical maintenance of the hospital buildings. Sweepers (singular *ferraş*) picked up garbage from the floor and carried it outside to the nearest garbage dump. In one Istanbul hospital the two sweepers divided the work between them: one cleaned the hospital from within; the other cleared waste from the building.[57] A gardener (sing. *bakhçuwan*) nurtured the garden. A well-kept garden was an important part of the hospital physically and therapeutically (this theme is picked up in the fourth chapter). Renovators-cum-odd-job-men (sing. *mirimeti* or *mani'-i nuquş*) took care of the building itself to prevent the walls from falling down or getting dirty.[58] The cleanliness of the hospital and its immediate surroundings and the aesthetic of the building and environments were of great importance, and therefore money was invested in their upkeep.

Hammams operated inside many Ottoman hospitals. In some hospitals, the hammam was part of the original plan of the institution. This was the case in the sixteenth-century hospitals of Süleyman I, Hurrem Sultan, and Nurbanu Sultan, all in Istanbul. In others it was added as an afterthought. A hammam was added to the older hospital of Mehmet II in Istanbul, following the appeal of the chief physician, Haji Musa. His petition to the sultan, which he presented in person to the imperial council in October 1577, touched upon the welfare of his patients as the reason for his request. Haji Musa explained that a hammam was needed for the patients, and while all the other imperial hospitals had one, the hospital of Sultan Mehmet II lacked a bath. The doctor was clever enough to point out that as the financial management of the hospital was meticulous, there were enough surpluses for that project and no additional funds were needed. The sultan, Murad III (reigned 1574–95), granted his wish, but added a caveat: if the building of a bathhouse were to result in a shortage of medications for the patients, the person causing that would bear the whole responsibility of his misdeed.[59]

Medical qualities were also attributed to natural water reservoirs. Evliya Çelebi surveyed the hot springs associated with medical qualities all around the empire (hence the varied terminology designating such a place) and the popularity of immersion in them. He mentioned those in Istanbul, in the neighborhoods of Eyüp and Hasköy, along the Golden Horn.[60] It was Bursa, however, which was famous for its many springs and their virtues. Evliya mentioned the great popularity of visiting these springs from all around the empire. He wrote that sometimes the water coming from the depths of the earth was so hot that whoever bathed in it was "cooked." But even if the water was not that hot, bathing in those springs was healthy, and the longer one stayed immersed in these waters, the better for body and mind. Evliya graded the quality of the springs in Bursa. "The Old Spring" (on top of which Murad I Hudavendigar, who reigned 1360–89, built an impressive dome) was the most beneficial. The second in quality was the spring of Çekirge Sultan, whose water was especially beneficial for those afflicted with skin problems. Evliya also claimed that the wretched who drank from its water for forty days would be cured from leprosy (by God's will) for forty years.[61]

Legends were associated with the springs in Bursa and explained their qualities. One legend was mentioned by Thevenot, who visited there in August 1656. According to him, a princess was afflicted with leprosy and became ugly, and therefore no one would agree to marry her; she bathed in one of the Bursa springs and was cured.[62] This is a known literary topos. Because of its legendary character, it is connected to no specific place and time, and can be attributed to almost any place. Indeed, a similar legend was told about Urfa (today in eastern Turkey), where there were many lepers in Thevenot's time, the middle of the seventeenth century. The local lepers bathed in a special pool outside the city, next to the southern gate of the wall. They believed they would be cured by the water there, just like the legendary leper king of the city, a contemporary of Jesus. According to a popular myth, he bathed there and was healed. The king attributed his miraculous cure to a factor other than the water itself. Here Thevenot associated the power of the Urfa water with the Christian legend of the Veil of Veronica. Veronica was said to have wiped the sweat off the face of Jesus on his way to the Crucifixion. Thevenot claimed the king received messengers from Jesus. They presented him with a kerchief that Jesus had put on his face, and his image was imprinted on the cloth. For the king it was the blessed kerchief that delivered him from his disease, and he converted to Christianity.[63]

The last example illustrates that therapeutic water was legitimized by different traditions. This section started with a discussion of bathing in water and positioned hydrotherapy within humoralism. Here water was seen an external agent helping to achieve inner-body balance. But as the last example illustrates, regarding water as therapeutic was also grounded in religious belief and traditional customs.

Hygiene was presented as a Muslim way of life and was emphasized in Prophetic medicine writings. An oft-repeated saying attributed to the Prophet declared: "Clean yourself, and God will purify you all."[64] Another said, "Religion is founded on cleanliness." It was explained that the physical cleaning of external organs from filth leads to the inner purification of one's inner self from sins. On the one hand, hygiene was a personal matter connected to religion. On the other, and although religion was the primary motivation in the discussion of premodern Muslim scholars on this matter, they were not unmindful of the medical and aesthetic aspects pertaining to hygiene.[65]

Religion and Medicine, Religion as Medicine: A Placebo Effect?

This marriage of belief and medicine brings us to consider placebos. We would call the medical use of most of the practices described in the previous chapter and above as "mere" (?) placebos. A placebo is any treatment that is used for its ameliorative effect on a symptom or disease but that actually is ineffective or is not specifically effective for the condition being treated. The placebo effect is therefore the nonspecific psychological or psychophysiological therapeutic effect produced by a placebo, but may also be the spontaneous improvement attributed to the placebo. It may be used with or without the knowledge that a treatment is a placebo—for example, when a treatment is given in the belief that it is effective, but in reality it is a placebo by objective evaluation. A placebo may be inert (like a sugar pill) or active (such as an ineffective drug or a drug used at an ineffective dosage), although this division is perhaps merely academic, as even such substances as distilled water or lactose can cause bodily changes.[66]

In any case, the Ottomans believed them to be active medicinal substances. This explains why many dishes prepared in the Ottoman imperial kitchens included drugs disguised as condiments. Sweeteners like honey and sugar are a good case in point. These are two of the most important premodern foodstuffs. They were often used with sour ingredients (mostly vinegar) in order to create a balanced flavor. Honey was more widespread, also because of its being cheaper. But it became a popular substance because in addition to its nourishing value it could be used for preparing and administering various remedies. Honey was used as a kind of glue that transformed specific ingredients into one consistent and permanent compound drug. Sugar, in contrast, was believed to facilitate the acceptance of ingested drugs by the body and thus aid their performance.[67]

Another placebo believed to be an active medicinal substance was coffee, an everyday beverage (from the sixteenth century onward) to which therapeutic qualities were ascribed.[68] Drinking coffee became a social activity enjoyed together among a group of friends and was also popular as a remedy. The use of coffee as a medicine and a stimulating drug was quite common among Ottomans.

Coffee was believed to ease headaches and stomachaches and to assist digestion. It was drunk very strong, its black color standing out, and extremely hot.[69] However, the exact temperature was decided according to medical necessities. According to Thevenot, hot coffee cleaned one's head from poisonous vapors and thus prevented headaches, whereas cold coffee affected the body as a laxative. He summarized the situation by saying that the Turks held that coffee was effective for all kinds of medical problems, and its advantages were not less than those attributed to tea. It became clear even in the seventeenth century that drinking coffee suppressed tiredness. It is no surprise, then, that it became popular among students who wished to study well into the small hours of the night, or with merchants who used their nights to catch up with commercial correspondence.[70] Coffee acted as a placebo when serving as a basic liquid for concentrated medicinal solutions, helping to take them in. Toward the end of the eighteenth century the head mufti in office at the time was given something to calm him, and was instructed to swallow it with a drink of either water or coffee.[71] But despite the fact that coffee was common in popular therapeutics, and although it was discussed in learned treatises, it did not make its way into hospital clinical reality based on Galenism. Coffee beans were not purchased for hospitals.

A placebo uses the effect of imagination and belief, whether it is belief in the supernatural, in divine revelation, or in science, as the case may be. One should also remember that no treatment is sometimes the best treatment (Maimonides is credited with observing for the first time that the perfect physician is one who judges it better to abstain from treatment than to prescribe a treatment that might exacerbate the malady).[72]

Medicine, as we see, involves belief that takes various forms. One form is the patient's belief in himself or herself being able to endure the sickness and overcome a particular pain and malady. Another one is the patient's belief in the healing prowess of his or her physician. The phenomenon of the physician as a "walking placebo" has long been recognized. Galen already observed that the healer that cures most is the one in whom the patients have the most confidence. The healer is a strong therapeutic agent in his personality and his physical and mental interaction with the patient.[73] Founders of Ottoman hospitals thought also about this aspect, judging from the foundation deeds, which emphasize the personality of the physician and other hospital staff members. In addition to the clinical-medical expertise expected from them, healers had to present a certain moral and mental strength. This demand could be attributed to the integralism inherent in humoralism, and certainly added to the respect the physicians commanded from their patients and strengthened the belief in their therapeutic abilities.

A third form of belief manifested in a healing process is the patient and doctor's belief in God. Hospitals practiced humoral medicine, and on the surface ignored religious medicine. Religion, however, was nonetheless present in and around the institution. First, many of the Ottoman hospitals were located near central mosques and together formed grand imperial complexes (the location of hospitals in the urban landscape is analyzed in detail in the fourth chapter). Furthermore, hospital staffs included religious officials who offered religious services to the patients' community, like prayer and burial. Although the various foundation deeds do not include any mention of such activities in the institution in a formal manner, these employees appear regularly on the salary lists of several institutions. The fact that a special space within the institution was dedicated to the mosque attests that religious activity was indeed taking place there and that the appearance of religious officials on the lists was not just false pretences or a means to channel allowances to various people as salaries. The contrast with medieval Muslim hospitals is illuminating. This would seem to be a uniquely Ottoman approach in which hospital care was placed within a religious setting, whereas earlier hospitals in Muslim societies were secular institutions curiously devoid of religious functions.

The marriage of medicine and religion took also the specific form of regarding Allah to be the ultimate healer of all maladies. The Healer (*al-shāfī*) is one of his sacred ninety-nine attributes, or Most Beautiful Names. This is based on the Qur'an, where the following passage occurs: "[W]henever I am sick, [he] heals me, who makes me to die, then gives me life" (Qur'an, the Poets, 26:79). A famous saying of the Prophet claims that God did not create a sickness in this world unless he produced the cure as well. Indeed, many medical prescriptions carried God's name (*huwwa*—he) and started with the formula "In the name of God, the merciful, the compassionate." The authors added that only the all-knowing God knows precisely what the ailment is, and only with his help would the patient overcome his or her sickness.[74]

Amulets were used to call on the help and defense of God and ward off the evil eye. Belief in the evil eye was quite common, as many people believed spirits—capable of both evil and good—were real creatures present in this world.[75] Amulets came in every shape and size. The contents of the amulets were just as diverse as their outer appearance. They included written verses of the Qur'an (the Qur'an was an antidemonic power, in other words: the scripture was a form of exorcism),[76] or merely words, letters, digits, geometrical drawings, or special shapes. The *khamsa* (literally "five") is an example of a number and sign that is believed by many Muslims to possess magical value. It connects the use of the five fingers of the hand as a defense against the evil eye. It consists the stretching of the right hand with the fingers spread out. The *khamsa* has inspired various representations in the forms of jewelry ("the hand of Fatima"), amulets, and drawings.

Despite their variety, the amulets have two characteristics in common. First, they are very specific: they are made to help a specific person and a specific complaint. Second, amulets are secret. Their contents are known only to the maker, who does not share with the receiver what he wrote. They are usually worn in a small bag under the clothes or sewn to them discreetly or hidden somewhere at home. An exception is the talismanic shirt, which is visible and its contents (verses from the Qur'an, sometimes the Qur'an as a whole, with or without letters, numbers and shapes) known to all. It was a tight-fitting garment, worn as a sort of armor. It was supposed to hold back disease and the evil eye and protect from enemies on the battlefield.[77]

The strength of an amulet rests in the belief in God and respect for his word, whether written or spoken. Contemporary observers commented on the awe with which Ottomans treated scraps of paper that had God's names written on them. If such a note were found on the ground on the street, it was picked up, cleaned, and tucked into the cracks of buildings and walls. Even pieces of written text that could have included God's names were treated thus.[78] God's words were strong enough to be drunk, literally. Some amulets were meant to be drunk. The paper was soaked in water (sometimes with condiments like saffron), and the owner drank the water. Special bowls were made for this purpose. Such magical bowls were made of iron, and Qur'anic verses, prophetic sayings, and secret figures and texts were engraved into them to provide the amulet with extra strength.[79]

We have already seen how religion affects concepts of health, illness, and medicine, but faith also shapes the concrete course of treatment. Faith in a demanding established religion might require, for example, that one forgo the use of a certain substance that otherwise is perceived as medicinal and beneficial.

Alcohol could be such a substance. The prohibition of intoxicating beverages was seemingly clear-cut and well established. Yet transgressions happened all the time. The multireligious Ottoman Empire brought communities for whom the production and consumption of alcohol was permitted together with those for whom it was illicit. Moreover, large parts of the empire were agricultural land devoted to vineyards. In addition, the Ottomans built on previous traditions of literary wine-culture that had developed in various Muslim courts. All these were fertile grounds for alcohol consumption by Muslims, too.

Time and again the Ottoman sultans tried to enforce the prohibition in the public domain, to no avail. In the middle of the sixteenth century, Süleyman I ordered the burning of all the ships arriving to Istanbul with alcohol. Half a century later, Ahmet I (reigned 1603–17) ordered taverns destroyed. Murad IV was especially notorious for his harsh policy against wine, tobacco, opium, and coffee. He even sentenced to death those who ignored his wishes. The second half of the seventeenth century saw the rise of the influence of the Kadizadeli. This movement of popular mosque preachers, who called for a purified Muslim way of life, gained power at the Ottoman court and on the streets. They were one factor that motivated the authorities to demonstrate a hard line against Muslims who consumed alcohol. Toward the end of the eighteenth century, Selim III (reigned 1789–1807) closed the taverns yet again and banned the drinking of wine and *rakı* (an anise-flavored alcoholic beverage). These sultans tried to implement Muslim orthodoxy in the public sphere (they were less concerned with the private one). They were also concerned about public order. Like the use of drugs and narcotics discussed in the first chapter, consumption of alcohol as a social activity in public was perceived as a threat to the social and political status quo. Assemblies for what seemed like hedonistic behavior raised suspicions of promiscuity and the crossing of social, gender, and religious barriers. Lashes, fines, imprisonment, destroyed reputations (the annals of the Ottoman history are filled with references to the persecutions brought upon those who transgressed)—all proved to be ineffectual measures to stop drinkers from drinking.[80]

These complex social realities were mirrored in learned discussions in legal circles. The Qur'an condemns alcohol as an abomination invented by Satan (5:92). The prohibition is also connected with intoxication, seen as contradicting sincere belief and religious ritual. However, although condemned on earth, alcohol was promised to the believers as a prize in heaven. Legal scholars engaged in discussions about the classification of various beverages in order to determine what exactly was intoxicating, and hence forbidden. They considered the origin of the liquid (fruit, cereals, etc.) and the process of preparation (fermented or not, whether receptacles were added). Thus they could reach a conclusion (not necessarily unanimous) as to whether a specific beverage should be considered intoxicating and therefore prohibited. One point was clear in these discussions: intoxication and consuming alcohol for mere pleasure were forbidden for Muslims (although there were conflicting ideas about what was alcoholic); that was after all the whole point of reaching a legal definition of whether or not a certain liquid was nonintoxicating. When people prepared and consumed alcohol, it was understood by all as the transgression of a direct Qur'anic order.[81]

These two contexts—social realities and legal theoretical discussions—explain the multiple attitudes toward alcohol in medical settings, an issue addressed by both legal scholars and physicians. Under the title of treatment with forbidden things Muslim legal scholars discussed intoxicating drinks (*al-tadāwī bi-al-mukhammarāt*), as a special case. One school of thought maintained that alcohol was an ailment and could never be a cure. Adherents of this school insisted on the harmful effects of intoxication even as a treatment to a disease. These scholars claimed that God could not have made a cure out of things he prohibited, let alone one that is known to have ill effects on the human body, in addition to its moral perils. If alcohol is rendered desirable as a medication, it undermines the prohibition; consequently the substance should be avoided. Moreover, legal scholars who also engaged in Prophetic medicine (like the fourteenth-century scholar Ibn Qayyīm al-Jawzīyya) claimed that medicine—unlike food—was not a compelling necessity; therefore deviation from the legal norm was not justified. Other scholars claimed the opposite. They opined that medicine—like food—is necessary for preserving life. Moreover, they maintained that the use of intoxicating beverages for medical purposes was lawful. They based their claim on the reasoning that intoxication, the outcome of excessive use, was the thing prohibited; the substance itself was not defined as impure and illegal. Hence, one can consume unlawful drinks and foods under special and pressing circumstances; preserving one's life was seen as such.[82]

The medical discourse surrounding alcohol in a therapeutic setting mirrored these complex discursive and practical realities.

Standard medical compendia, authored by Muslims, discussed the benefits of intoxicating drinks while revealing opposing complex views of the matters. The sixteenth-century Arabic-Ottoman physician Dā'ūd al-Anṭākī presents the dual medical approach. Like so many other physicians, he discussed the medical benefits of various liquids on the border of alcohol. He used the category of *nabīdh* to refer to all intoxicating liquids save those made of wine (*kull muskir siwā al-khamr*). He acknowledges that Muslims are divided among themselves whether these beverages are permitted; they are forbidden for "us" (he refers here to the Shāfi'ī legal school, to which he belonged), whereas the Ḥanafī school (common among Muslim Turks) permitted it. He concluded this short entry by saying that such a debate is not of "their" concern, meaning not it is relevant to medical writers.[83]

It should be noted here that the medical discussion of intoxicating liquids did not differ much from the nonmedical discussion on the same issue, save in two respects. The first: the medical discussion of intoxicating liquids was conducted under the heading of benefits, thus emphasizing its usefulness rather than the ban surrounding it. The second: the medical discourse was not just a theoretical discussion but had concrete implications. Certainly the patients in the imperial palace hospital enjoyed alcohol as part of their medical therapeutics, as discussed above. What may seem puzzling to us today is that people who were sick and could not fulfill Muslim religious rituals that demanded some physical agility could avail themselves of nonreligious (antireligious?) means (such as the consumption of alcohol) in order to regain their health and resume full Muslim life.

Hospital therapeutics reveals that religion itself could be perceived as medicinal. Although religion as such was not an official part of Ottoman hospital practices, it was ever present in the daily routine and in the hospital atmosphere. In a nonformal way religious practices were part of the hospital therapeutics.[84] Hospitals were constructed around flourishing gardens (a theme picked up in detail in the fourth chapter). These gardens were interpreted also as hinting at paradise or heaven. The gardens were thus a constant reminder for the sick of the hereafter and invited them to ponder over their good (and not so good) deeds. Sick people, more than others, are conscious of their limited time on earth and tend to think of their destiny and God. The fact that the hospital personnel included the prayer leader, or imam, and the caller to prayer, or muezzin, can be attributed too to this concept.

What Is Health Then? What Is Illness?

Societies define health and illness in different fashions, and symptoms that are accepted as evidence of illness in one society may be ignored in the next. Definitions within the same society may also change over time.[85] We finish this chapter therefore with the question: how did Ottomans understand "health" and "illness" in the early modern period? We shall see that the integralistic outlook that was one factor shaping medical therapeutics also played a central role in defining these terms—that is, "holism" affected how Ottomans thought about and understood them.

Today we are accustomed to think of "disease" rather than "illness." "Disease" is a biomedical definition using terms like "germs" and "viruses." It assumes "disease" is a biological concrete condition that can be verified and classified in a definite manner through laboratory tests or other forms of clinical examination. In this context "health" is understood as a polarity, meaning simply the lack of disease. "Illness," however, is quite a different thing. It is a social and cultural concept, recognizing a situation that goes beyond medicine and the state of the body when a person cannot fulfill his or her normal roles adequately. This understanding of "illness" is reflected in the official definition used by the World Health Organization (WHO) of what "health" is. According to it, health is complete physical, mental, and social well-being, and not merely the absence of disease and infirmity.[86] In other words, "disease" tends to refer to doctor's definition within a Western medical framework, based on structural or functional abnormalities; "illness" refers more to the patient's experience of a social and cultural event.[87]

Putting the emphasis on illness rather than focusing on disease, or on being ill instead of underlying symptoms determining abnormality, allows us to conceptualize health at three different levels. The functional explanation refers to what can be done physically and mentally (or is allowed to be done) when one is healthy or ill. The representational level focuses on the physical outer image of the body. At this level we consider, for example, how health and sickness are expressed in art, or how people dress and choose to look when healthy and sick, or what they do in order to be perceived as healthy or sick. At the semiotic level our concentration is on the meaning and perception of health and illness. The focus is on the social significance of health, as health is associated with social activity, good behavior, and self-worth. Illness threatens one's position in society. Illness can remove one's ability to function as usual, and as a result one might fall into financial hardship. Sickness and physical disability have the power to prevent us from earning a living, pushing us toward poverty; poverty, for its part, is a fertile breeding ground for illness due to low standards of hygiene and nutrition.[88] Moreover, due to illness it is possible to lose our social, cultural, and political standing. Illness here is understood as damaging not only to our physical condition, but also to our ability to lead an effective and full social life. It follows, therefore, that health allows us to go on living at our expected physical, financial, and mental level, and to raise that level.

The Ottomans appreciated the whole gamut of social and cultural aspects of sickness. We can see it, for instance, in the emphasis by members of the Ottoman elite on their physical constitution. This emphasis is understandable when we consider the religious, moral, and theological consequences of illness. Health and sickness had religious and moral repercussions. Keeping one's body healthy was highly desirable, as it was the vehicle through which one worshipped Allah.[89] Ill health could hinder one's ability to fulfill religious duties that call for physical exertion, like prostration during the five daily prayers or fasting from sunrise to sunset every day during the month of Ramadan. The pilgrimage to Mecca and Medina, even in this age of airplanes and buses, can tax one's health. Health is a gift from God, and by keeping in shape one glorifies his creation.[90] In the words of the sixteenth-century Ottoman historian and bureaucrat Mustafa Ali: "[A]s long as man is not secure of illness through the healthiness of his constitution he is not able to lead a life of piety and worship and [cannot] acquire knowledge and learning."[91]

The Ottoman preoccupation with body (bordering sometimes on obsession) can be seen in their attention to physiognomy (*'ilm-i qiyafet* or *'ilm-i feraset*), the art of judging character from the general features of the face and the physical shape of the body. Arab-Muslim civilization inherited the study of physiognomy from antiquity. Physiognomy of various kinds (based on bodily features, expressions, and movements, on gender and race, on environment, on biology, on similarity to animals, and on divine inspiration) was mentioned in numerous anecdotes in legal, literal, mystical, and medical texts, as well as in distinct treatises.[92] According to Islamic medical and philosophical thought, the human body is conceived as clothing that envelopes and protects the soul. It follows that by studying visible physical traits and organs, such as the eyes, ears, hair, and hands, it should be possible to deduce character and temperament—or in other words, to determine the moral and inner qualities of a person, which are concealed by nature (whether intentionally or subconsciously)—by studying a person's outward appearance. Katip Çelebi, the seventeenth-century bureaucrat and scholar, explained in his vast bibliographical encyclopedia in Arabic that physiognomy (*firāsa*) is "a science by which one learns of the character of people from their external qualities, like colors, forms, and limbs. It is a deduction from the external makeup to the inner nature."[93] It was widely accepted that there was a correlation between physical and aesthetic perfection and noble and moral character; and, correspondingly, physical ugliness, deformity, illness, and handicaps are all indicators of a mean character and villainous personality.[94]

Physiognomy continued to be studied in the early modern period in Europe,[95] but it was an especially important branch of knowledge for the Ottomans. Although physiognomy was slow to enter into the canons of Islamic science, and not before the late twelfth century do we see the first texts in Arabic devoted exclusively to physiognomy,[96] the Ottomans embraced this branch of knowledge. If we take as a yardstick the number of treatises composed on this subject in Ottoman-Turkish in the Ottoman Empire during the fifteenth to seventeenth centuries, it is noteworthy that at least thirteen were composed; between 1530–85 nine manuscripts were copied, most of which were prepared for the reigning sultans.[97] In the middle of the sixteenth century, Yahya, a Jewish physician from the imperial medical corps in Istanbul, decided to practice in Jerusalem. He presented himself at the Muslim law court there with a letter of appointment signed by the sultan specifying his daily wages to be drawn from the treasury in Damascus. The letter counts his virtues: excellence in medical science and physiognomy (*feraset*).[98] *Feraset-name*, a sixteenth-century Ottoman manuscript on physiognomy, which includes a section on chiromancy (*kitab-ı feraset-ül-yad*, the art of reading the palms of hands). starts with the explanation that this branch of knowledge was intended originally for sultans and viziers. Yet this science should not be restricted only to those in high places and could benefit others as well.[99]

In the sultan's court physiognomy came to be an *applied* science, a practical technique, not merely an abstract theory dealing with systemization and classification of visual human signifiers. Physiognomy thus became a means to include or exclude individuals and groups. A sixteenth-century physiognomy treatise prepared from Arabic and Persian sources explained that the sultan should "acquire the skill and expertise to discern their inner character from outward behaviour, and from their external appearance the true nature of his *kul* [servant slaves] . . . and those in the hierarchy of government, and even his subjects [*re'āya*] . . . thereby appointing each to according to his worth, whether he is fit for the [offices of] *vezāret, sanjak, aghālık*, or for trust."[100]

Indeed, decisions on the buying of slaves, on appointments of officials in the Ottoman palace, and in military and administrative institutions were based on, among other things, physical attributes. Physiognomy became a practical aid in the art of government. Mustafa Ali, the Ottoman historian and bureaucrat of the sixteenth century, explained that an expert on physiognomy was included in the selection of the young Christian recruits to the army and Ottoman bureaucracy (*devşirme*).[101] European diplomats from the sixteenth and seventeenth centuries were familiar with the palace policy of practicing physiognomy and convey the impression it was regular policy in their times. They corroborate that there was an official in the palace who was in charge of this selection. He bore the title *qiyafet-şenas* (from Persian: someone who is master of the science of *qiyafet*).[102] It seems, then, that the Ottoman palace employed professional practitioners of physiognomy. In previous centuries, such experts were referred to in the sources in vague collective terms. It is likely there were astute men who were consulted from time to time about matters concerning character assessment, rather than individuals who made their living by practicing it.[103]

Some of the causes that may have driven the palace bureaucracy to use physiognomy on a regular basis are explained by Ali. He claimed that lazy and lying servants are also unclean and wear soiled garments; the faulty in appearance is faulty also in truth. Meanwhile, good servants who fulfill their duties quickly and faithfully are always tidy and well behaved. European diplomats add that the selection procedure, which was not based on a long examination, tried to deduce intellectual ability and moral standards from bodily perfection and muscular strength. Some of the sultans supervised this process personally. One of the commentators was Ghiselain de Busbecq, the Habsburg ambassador to the court of Süleyman I. He emphasized the meritocratic nature of Süleyman's court. He told how Süleyman considered at each appointment whether the designated appointee was suitable for his position according to his abilities, character, and disposition.[104] Another one was Paul Rycaut, an English diplomat of the seventeenth century, who explained: "[T]hese Youths must be of admirable features, and pleasing looks, well shaped in their bodies, and without any defects of nature; For it is conceived that a corrupt and sordid soul can scarce inhabit in a serene and ingenious Aspect."[105]

Here we see the equation of beauty and health: something or someone is beautiful because he or she looks healthy, and is healthy because his or her physical image is aesthetically pleasing. This motif existed in Ottoman culture for centuries. Dr. Bryce, a medical doctor from Scotland, claimed that even during his visit to Istanbul in 1830 the Ottomans paid much attention to their physical appearance. They were ready to use medication while healthy in order to look after their bodies and maintain a healthy and shiny skin.[106] This was the social practice of Ottoman-Egyptian elite as well, as observed by French physicians and pharmacists accompanying Napoleon Bonaparte's expedition to Egypt. They noticed that the wealthy Egyptians (with some variety among Muslims, Jews, and Coptic Christians) used certain medical preparations only in periods of good health in order to keep their physical good state and high spirits. Such medications could include opium and hashish preparations, theriacs, and various fattening agents.[107]

Illness could cost an Ottoman official his social, economic, and political position and the livelihood of all the members of his household. Such was the background to the petition of one Mevlana Abd al-Latif to the sultan in May 1565. He introduced himself as a teacher (*müderris*) in the *medrese* adjacent to the Üç Şerefeli Cami (i.e., the Mosque of the Three Galleries/Balconies) in Edirne, built by Sultan Murad II. He complained that because of his illness he had left his position in Edirne and traveled to Istanbul to seek treatment there. Now that he was well again he asked to reoccupy his position. The sultan ordered the governor (*mütevelli*) of the charitable endowment supporting the institution (Arabic *waqf*, Turkish *vakıf*) to employ Mevlana Abd al-Latif and supply him and all his students (!) with a reasonable salary.[108]

The Ottoman archives contain several petitions from Ottoman officials to the sultan asking for their commission (and salary) back. Take Mustafa, an officer in the Ottoman army in eastern Anatolia who was assigned to the expedition to Cyprus in 1570, but made it only to Iskenderun, a port town on the Mediterranean shore. Thereafter Mustafa was stripped of his considerable fiefdom (worth of twelve thousand silver coins [*akçe*] per annum) in the province of Arapkir in eastern Anatolia, which was transferred to another officer. Now, during the spring of 1571, Mustafa petitioned the sultan asking for his fiefdom back. He claimed that the sole reason he had been left ashore was his sickness. Although he could not accompany his soldiers, he did send them to Cyprus, where they had served the sultan well. The sultan ruled in his favor. Mustafa was reinstated as a *timar*-holder retroactively from the day it had been taken from him.[109] A similar lot awaited also the rank and file of the Ottoman army and bureaucracy. Hasan, a soldier in the Arabian Peninsula, petitioned the sultan in June 1571 and described himself as a simple guard in a fortress in the Hijaz province whose daily salary was no more than seven silver coins. On his visit to his family he fell sick and failed to return to his post, which was then given to another.[110] The nature of Hasan's request from the sultan is not specified in the document, yet we can assume that, like Mustafa, Hasan wished to be reinstated.

The background to these two petitions, and others like them, seems to have been quite similar. The soldiers had failed to carry out satisfactorily a command issued to them, and had therefore lost their commissions. An Ottoman without a position in the army or bureaucracy (as in Mevlana Abd al-Latif's case) could not sustain his household, and without the members of his household he could not hope to perform well enough in the field to win a new commission. The Ottoman experience was that illness caused harm not only to the sick person himself, but also to his or her dependants. These petitions originated in the fear of this vicious circle.[111]

The petitioners claimed that only illness and not insubordination to the sultan was the cause of their negligence. It was not an act of justice, therefore, to remove them from office on these grounds. They tried to emphasize their medical problem in order to convince the sultan they had valid reasons for their ill performance, and at the same time they tried to belittle the same physical incapacity. The petitioners made it clear that whatever malady they had suffered from, they were now fully recovered and could resume all their responsibilities—and enjoy their material gains. It is instructive to note that the sultan ruled in their favor.[112] Illness was an acceptable reason for failing to carry out a sultanic command. Knowing that, illness could have been brought up by the petitioners as an excuse for their ill performance. Faking an illness was by far a better strategy when approaching the sultan than admitting to lack of willingness or ability to perform well.

Officers and soldiers fabricating medical problems to explain their inadequate performance were one type of medical pretenders. Another type was the pages in the imperial palace in Istanbul. They claimed to be sick in order to be admitted into the palace hospital in the first court of Topkapı at the right side of the Bab-ı Hümayun (the Imperial Gate). While the physical distance was rather short, there was a major difference in lifestyles between the private (third) court and the public (first) one. The severe rules of conduct of the third court, befitting those close to the sultan, were not enforced as heavily in the first court. This was one of the reasons why the hospital was attractive to patients. Seventeenth-century observers maintained that in their period, the hospital had been transformed into a sought-after recreational center where many a tired servant wished to stay even while healthy.[113] The French traveler Jean Baptiste Tavernier explained that due to their high status as the sultan's personal servants, the pages from the third court enjoyed extremely comfortable conditions at the hospital. The usual period of hospitalization was ten or twelve days, during which time the patients could amuse themselves with vocal and instrumental music performances for hours, sometimes even at night. Moreover, for medical reasons the hospital allowed the drinking of wine, which is of course forbidden for Muslims under other circumstances. According to Tavernier, it was the wine, more than the music, that encouraged the pages to look forward to their convalescence period in the hospital.

The "hospital turned convalescent home" became a literary topos in Muslim societies. An anecdote told by an Egyptian traveler to Damascus in 1427–28 echoes a similar phenomenon. Khalīl b. Shāhīn al-Ẓāhirī wrote in his *Zubdat kashf al-mamālīk*, a treatise on the Mamluk sultanate, about the visit of a high-ranking Persian to the Zangid hospital in Damascus at the beginning of the fifteenth century. The visitor was so impressed with the excellent diet at the hospital that he decided to try it himself. He pretended to be sick and asked to be admitted into treatment. The head physician checked his pulse but detected no malady. Yet he possessed enough of a sense of humor to play along and admitted the visitor into the hospital. The doctor put the Persian on a diet that included tasty and sweet-smelling syrups, tender meat, and fresh fruit. When the doctor wrote down on the recipe that "hospitality is for three days only" (another topos), the pseudopatient took the hint and discreetly left the place.[114] We cannot establish what the European description of the palace hospital owes to this literary motif (if at all), yet several European observers in the early modern period claimed that the Topkapı hospital had such an attraction. For the pages, the hospital offered refuge from the very regimented and hectic life they led at the inner court of the imperial palace. By voicing medical problems they were secured a well-deserved vacation that otherwise would not have been granted. It is not surprising, therefore, to see that the hospital had a waiting list; the minute one patient was discharged, another was waiting to be admitted in his stead.

There is another context in which we can understand the petitions to the sultan on medical grounds or the cases of pretenders: that of employer-employee relationship. The examples illustrated above portray how professional groups within the Ottoman state—bureaucrats, military, and palace pages—survived as employees and guarded their interests in the period before labor unions. There were no organizations to defend the rights of the workers and instruct them how to behave and claim their prerogatives. Despite the lack of collective action, employees were able to devise strategies as individuals to exploit the system for their benefit or at least to survive within it. This was part of the never-ending bargaining between the state as an employer and its employees. They acquired the knowledge of what to claim and how to present their claim in order to make it work. Here we see that invoking medically related excuses was such a mechanism. But of course we cannot assume that all these petitioners were making false claims. Some of them were presumably indeed sick. One way of minimizing the damages resulting from illness was to petition the sultan invoking medical reasons—faked or real—after the harm had already been done (that is, they were removed from their post and lost their livelihood).

Exactly because illness posed a grave hazard for one's social standing in Ottoman society, preventing such harm from occurring in the first place by way staying healthy was an enticing option. Early modern people, Ottomans included, could not but have been aware of the abysmal success rate of the medicines available to them. Curative medicine was a very dangerous business indeed. A sick person could enjoy a variety of healers and therapeutic procedures, but they would not necessarily lead to full recovery. Failures were not attributed to medicine as such. Nonmedical people were not necessarily aware of the limits of the available medical knowledge and techniques; the blame rested with the shortcomings of the practitioners. It was better, therefore, to do one's utmost to keep in health in the first place, thus avoiding physicians all together. And indeed preventive medicine was commonly practiced.

CHAPTER 3

"Feed the hungry, visit the sick, and set those who suffer free": Medical Benevolence and Social Order

The title of this chapter is a famous saying attributed to the Prophet Muhammad. Several versions of this saying exist, each of which emphasizes different acts of benevolence. The inclusion of aid to the sick in a Prophetic saying signals it as a highly regarded and important pious act. Visiting the sick, the specific act mentioned here, is but one means of medical assistance. What else was done to help the sick in the early modern period in the Middle East within the context of charity? By whom was medical charity offered? How was it organized? And what was its importance, and what role did it play among other existing avenues of charities?

Medical charity was far from being the only form of benevolence practiced in early modern Middle Eastern society. Individuals, communities, and states were busy with charity: it seems that almost everyone was occupied with either giving or receiving charity. Recently Amy Singer summarized the wide spectrum of motives for giving charity in the Ottoman context.[1] There is a human tendency to give, out of kindness and sympathy/empathy. But charity was also a functional means to a particular end.

Charity was inspired by spiritual, social, economic, and political motives. By giving to people the donor wishes to communicate with God and strives for atonement, expiation, and absolution. Scholars have commented on the financial benefits reaped from the endowment of property to charities. These scholars have claimed that the main reason that donors endowed property was their hope to use this mechanism as a loophole in the Ottoman policy of confiscating personal property upon death or dismissal from office. The donors were seeking financial advantages through tax reductions and protection of property. Philanthropy included self-interest and ambition. Social historians have highlighted philanthropy as a means of classification and stratification. The practice of endowment and building patronage was a visible act of confirmation of one's power, social status, and image. It was a venue for the representation of oneself in a manner that demanded the acknowledgment of rank and status. It was the visual expression of one's achieved status and status hoped for. The motives were competition, rivalry, show, and a desire for greatness and wealth. Attaining paradise in the hereafter and social status in the present world, consolidating the support of constituencies—all were possible motives for benefices.

In addition to various motives attracting private individuals, Muslim states also used charity as a key tool in their policies. Welfare was used by the ruling elites to direct settlement trends, affect urban life, tie rural and urban interests together, spread specific brands of religious ideas and mysticism, and generally further the interest of the ruling classes. The Seljuks used this method in the eleventh century to strengthen orthodox Sunni Islam after a period of Shi'i revival. The Ottomans in their turn contributed to various mystical orders and institutions in their process of absorbing newly conquered territories during the fourteenth and fifteenth centuries. In this way they also allocated financial and human resources to important urban centers.

Ottoman philanthropy encompassed many types of charities, either humble or grand, ranging from mosques and schools, to food distribution, to supporting poor pilgrims or orphans. It included formal, public, and institutionalized forms of charity and hidden and spontaneous ones, like giving aid (food, clothes, money) from the back door of one's house or almsgiving to a passing beggar on the street. Students of the past tend to focus on formal giving, as our information on spontaneous forms tends to be anecdotal. Public exhibitions of giving and getting, in contrast, are visible, and they were better recorded.

Philanthropy created and sustained social patronage, hierarchy, and obligation. The framework of gift relationships, or the "gift exchange" as described by Marcel Mauss (1872–1950), can explain the web of relationships and their binding forces as created by Ottoman imperial benevolence. Mauss built on the work of Bronislaw Malinowski (1884–1942), who argued in the 1920s that gifts are given because of the expectation they will be returned someday; gifts are returned because of the fear they might otherwise stop coming. This is Malinowski's "principle of give-and-take." Mauss went further and demonstrated that gifts are never simply given and returned. Rather, the exchange of gifts is a social activity; at the same time it also has economic, juridical, moral, aesthetic, religious, and mythological meaning. What may appear to be voluntary, disinterested, and spontaneous is in fact obligatory. The behavior of both giver and receiver is formal, self-interested, and dictated by social necessity. Both of them are empowered by the exchange, and both giver and taker are now in debt in honor and prestige to the other who allowed them to fulfill their role. Giver and receiver are equally important, and by giving to each other they publicly proclaim that they are worthy of each other and bound in partnership to each other. One gives because one is forced to do so, because the recipient has a sort of propriety right over everything that belongs to the donor. The recipient has the obligation to accept presents and has no right to refuse them. He repays by giving equivalent value—for example, by praising and appreciating the giver. This creates personal relationships, and also connects man to the deity. Gifts to men were intertwined with gifts to God, pleasing him by showing generosity, moral justice (excessive wealth is deplored), and sacrifice.[2]

The notion of reciprocity was expanded and refined in later anthropological literature. Among other things, Mauss was criticized for overemphasizing the spiritual aspect of give-and-take. It was also demonstrated that the social ramifications of gift exchange are even more complex than portrayed before, that sometimes there is no "equivalent return," to the point that there can be no expectation of any return. Since the 1980s, the concept of "giving while keeping" is the new approach. Gifts are individually owned and never fully leave the donor. The objects given cannot be alienated from the giver. Although the donor loses actual possession of the gift for a limited period of time, it will come back to him or her eventually. New studies thus argue that people in fact give in order to protect special possessions that are central to their identity and social status. Recent literature also emphasizes that at the simplest level, gift exchange is a personal relationship between giver and recipient, but at the same time the act of giving is aimed at a wider audience and wishes to deliver a public message.[3]

Following the "gift exchange" theory with its numerous refinements, the chapter will show how Ottoman charity nurtured a two-sided obligation. The beneficiary had to acknowledge graciously the position of the giver, to be obligated to him or her till the debt was repaid, and to accept his or her respective positions on the social ladder. At the same time, the giver was now tied to the beneficiary. The giver was indebted to the beneficiary for allowing him or her to act as the benevolent one. The giver was obliged to support the beneficiary and had to endure this dependency.

I will argue that medical charity creates especially strong bonds because of the nature of the relationships included. True, medical charity was only one avenue for welfare activity, and its dispensing resembled other philanthropic acts. It was given publicly and directly—for example, in hospitals that were endowed institutions. Medical charity could also be a secondary objective of a public ceremonial act. Such was the case when the sultan celebrated his son's circumcision and arranged for poor boys to be circumcised on the same occasion by palace doctors. Medical charity could also be granted behind the scenes—for example, when a physician treated his patient pro bono. But whatever specific form of medical charity was involved, it had to do with health and sickness, and as such was inherent to major life events. On top of that, many times medical aid required intimacy and physical contact between giver and receiver.

Ottoman medical charity could thus take many forms, some of which may not be considered today as "medical." As we have seen in previous chapters, taking *care* of people (who may have been still healthy) was just as important as offering a *cure* to a sick patient. Nursing and nurturing were yet another aspect of medical treatment, its continuation rather than its opposite. For example, food, clothing, and shelter can be considered "medicine" for those who lack them. Being sufficiently warm, protected from the elements, and nourished are all part of making people healthy when they regularly lack such possibilities. Here we are concerned with a narrow kind of medical charity, one that may originate with lay benefactors but is aimed specifically at helping the sick by way of medication administered by medical professionals.

Medical charity that involved professional healers was relatively rare in the early modern Middle East in comparison to other forms of philanthropy. Those few who did engage in medical philanthropy, or rather were documented in our sources as doing so, are a select elite. The state of the research so far does not allow us to expand further the picture of those involved in medical charity in the Ottoman world. For instance, the sources so far have provided us with only hints of evidence of certain guilds managing sickness and disability funds.[4] The reality that only few are involved in medical charity is what makes this kind of charity distinct from other types of philanthropy open to all in which the size of the purse and one's ambition were the sole criteria. In medicine, however, we do not seem to find the small-scale donation of the sort one finds in mosques, for example: adding a lamp, a sweeper, supporting a Qur'an reciter. In medicine big money was involved, which narrowed the pool of people who could act in that arena. But the identity of the people who were involved with medical charity reveals that the pool of actors was even narrower. It was restricted to the imperial family; moreover, not even all members of the family were allowed to take part. Social and cultural obligations and assumptions shape the decisions to give, and mold the actual act of giving (what, where, when, how, how much, and to whom). Medical charity thus tells us more than other types of charities do about why people engage in philanthropy and how they choose their specific charity.

This chapter first portrays the ethos of medical giving and then analyzes the more formal ways of giving in the medical scene in the early modern Middle East. It thus tries to answer why so few engaged in this activity, why those who did were the ones involved, and what they tried to achieve (taking care not to fall into the intentional fallacy—that is, endowing the private thoughts and wishes of the donors with undocumented intentions).

The discussion of the motivation to donate funds for medical charity also bears on the sense of community and its borders in the early modern Middle East. Relief is extended only to a narrow category of "deserving." The restriction of philanthropy is not unique to Ottoman society, but the exact definitions of "deservedness" in general and in the medical context in particular are products of the Ottoman understanding of a community and mutual obligation. Mosques, a prominent target for philanthropy, served the whole community. Other communal charitable institutions were targeted at specific social and economic groups deemed worthy of public support. The "other" in the case of medical charity—the sick and disabled person—is regarded as needy and deserves help and support, meaning he or she was regarded as part of the community. A special case of the sick—the lunatics—pushes this further. Madness was marginalized, yet although it existed on the fringes, the mad were always within the borders of the community.

How medical charity brings together the helpers and the helped and thus makes the community cohesive is one theme of this chapter. Although the figures for size and total number are small, Ottoman hospitals were thus very relevant to early modern Ottoman society and left their mark upon it. Another theme connected with the previous one explores yet another aspect of medical charity and social order:

the close links between medical charity and control mechanisms. Medical institutions were visualized as not only expressing charitable instincts or relieving the needy, but in doing so also bringing about regulation. Humanitarian motivations do not exclude the inclusion also of more cynical and hypocritical motives. The connection between medical help and control brought Marco van Leeuwen, building on Michel Foucault and moderating and refining him at the same time, to view welfare institutions, medical ones included, as arrangements for risk. Poor relief is a control strategy of the elites and a survival strategy of the poor.[5] Medicine and control/order are discussed in the last part of this chapter.

The Imperative of Health and Medical Care in a Muslim Context: A Religious Duty and a Philanthropic Act

Of the various things that shaped Ottoman medical charity, one was religious impulses. "In an age which was profoundly dominated and shaped by faith, I find it difficult to accept that religion should not have shaped the public and private approach to the way the poor and the sick should be treated," claimed Ole Peter Grell with regard to early modern Protestantism.[6] This was true also for the early modern Ottomans, for whom the spirit of medical charity combined a religious duty with a benevolent and moral act.

The sayings of the Prophet Muhammad, hadiths, were an important source for Ottomans who wanted a reference for what was considered normative or desirable Muslim behavior. The authoritative collections date from the Middle Ages, but the canonical collections of *aḥādīth* of al-Bukhārī (d. 870) and Muslim (d. 875),[7] continued to be consulted by Ottomans and were known by religious scholars as well as by lay Muslims. Special institutions (*dar-ül-hadith*) were dedicated to the studies of such collections, and al-Bukhārī's collection received special attention by professional Ottoman scholars and students.[8]

Al-Bukhārī organized his hadith compilation by subjects. Prophetic sayings concerning medicine were collected in the chapters called "The Book of the Sick" (Kitāb al-marḍā) and "The Book of Medicine" (Kitāb al-ṭibb). The sayings contained in these two chapters and other similar collections form the basis for the Islamic medicine known as Prophetic medicine (*al-ṭibb al-nabawī*) discussed in previous chapters.

An important theme in "The Book of the Sick" is the religious duty to assist the sick. In section 4 of this book al-Bukhārī quotes two sayings. In the first, Muhammad encouraged the believers to feed the hungry, visit the sick, and set those who suffer free. In the second, Muhammad prohibited seven acts (among them wearing gold rings, wearing silk clothes, and betting) and recommended seven others. Among Muhammad's recommendations are attending funerals, visiting the sick, and spreading peace (i.e., Islam). The following sections list more sayings dealing with specific aspects of visiting the sick.

Ibn Ḥajar al-'Asqalānī (d. 1449), the jurist, historian, and famous commentator on al-Bukhārī through whom many Muslims became familiar with al-Bukhārī's collection, discusses the limits of this duty. Al-'Asqalānī opens his remarks with hadiths that claim that visiting the sick is a communal duty (*farḍ kifāya*), not an individual one (*farḍ 'ayn*), but also questions to what extent this duty is indeed obligatory for all. The hadith al-'Asqalānī quotes do not agree, as some narrators believed that visiting the sick was a duty, while others claimed that it was less than a must.[9]

One important aspect of al-Bukhārī's collection (one in which he is followed by al-'Asqalānī) deals with the question of whom medical charity should be extended to. It seems that many regarded visiting the sick as a kindness that should be offered only to other members of the *umma*, the Islamic community. This can be deduced from section 11 in "The Book of the Sick," which deals with the matter of a Muslim who visits a non-Muslim (*mushrik*). One of Muhammad's servants, a young Jew, was sick and the Prophet visited him. After wishing him a full recovery, Muhammad invited the young boy to embrace Islam, and the servant agreed. One can understand from this anecdote that a Muslim is to visit a non-Muslim only if that person is in the process of converting to Islam, has expressed his willingness to do so, or at least seems open to it. Al-'Asqalānī, however, makes it clear that opinions on this issue are far from unanimous. Indeed, according to one school of thought, visiting a non-Muslim invalid was not considered a duty and a kindness, whatever the circumstances. Others claimed that visiting a non-Muslim is an important duty, as in addition to helping a sick person it may turn out to be beneficial to Islam by leading to what the Qur'an terms "reconciliation of hearts."[10] The Shāfi'ī jurist al-Māwardī (d. 1058), for example, insisted on the view that the reward for visiting a *dhimmi* equals the reward one gets for striving to get closer to God by charity and kindness (*qurba*) and from living near holy sites (*jiwār*).[11]

The obligations to visit any sick person regardless of sex and the type of the illness were discussed by al-Bukhārī. Al-Bukhārī includes in his collection hadiths maintaining that women are allowed—even obliged—to visit sick men.[12]

As for types of disease, apparently the duty to visit the sick includes those invalids who are unconscious as well. Some hadith scholars claimed that the phrasing of this duty was intentionally vague, as the Prophet meant to include all types of illnesses. According to others, the friends of those who suffer from toothaches or eye pains are exempt from visiting them.

It is noteworthy that the hadiths recognize the needs of the family in addition to those of the patient. For example, al-'Asqalānī explains that visiting the sick is intended not only for the benefit of the sick but also to alleviate the distress felt by the family of the sick person. Al-'Asqalānī also makes it clear that one should not stay long beside a friend's sickbed or visit at inconvenient hours (and he cites multiple and sometimes contradictory opinions to explain what constitutes inconvenient times): after all, the aim of the visit is to check on someone's condition and help in the process of recovery—not to tire the sick or exhaust the family.[13]

The delicate question of how to balance the needs and interests of an individual patient with those of his family has surfaced only in recent years in our modern society after years of silence. One situation that now attracts attention from legal advisors, health practitioners, and deontologists is the delicate one that arises when the best interests of a patient clash with those of his family, who are obliged to take care of him, or the one that arises when the family has the right to intervene, but friends who have no legal standing are closer to the patient and are better familiar with his true wishes.[14]

Another example of the spirit of medical giving was the expectation that physicians would cultivate a moral and ethical code according to which the interest of their patients would come before the personal gains of the physician or the wishes of family and friends. Although Ottoman healers were very diverse in the world they belonged to and in their clinical expertise, they were united in their common attempt to improve the lot of the sick. Most of them were genuinely devoted to healing people, and the social expectation was that healers would place the interests of their patients before their own. The discussion around what the balance between the needs of the patient and the healer should be was part of the larger discourse on medical ethics and the debate on the merits and defects of medicine as a science, art, and craft.

One aspect of the relationship between healer and patient was the discussion surrounding the amount of the physician's fee, and whether a doctor should demand a fee in the first place. Some authors maintained that if healing is a noble vocation, it is appropriate that physicians derive no material gain from it. Doctors were not supposed to earn worldly benefits from this lofty duty/call/destiny. The ideal of medical doctors working pro bono appears in many premodern sources. Their livelihood was to be gained only from their well-to-do patients or even from nonmedical activities.

The exemplary physician who waived his fee was contrasted with the greedy doctor. Belles lettres and ethical literature from the Middle Ages onward included both satirical and philosophical remarks (some of which were themselves satirical) about money-loving healers. Stories were told about charlatans who ill-advised their patients and harmed them out of ignorance, stupidity, or laziness, or even harmed them intentionally.[15] Even artists addressed this theme, as in the story and illustration disussed in chapter 1 of a sadistic bloodcupper.[16]

Other authors claimed that the doctors' demand for appropriate remuneration does not diminish the moral standing of their work. A popular saying has it that practicing medicine assures one's path to the hereafter, and this aim does not preclude considerable luck and financial gain in this world as well.[17] Not surprisingly, many practicing physicians adopted this position, since it enabled them to make a living through medicine.

Physicians, of course, played an active part in the discourse about the virtues of their vocation. They wished to defend the honor of their profession as a noble art and the social status associated with it. Their problem was twofold. They had to deal with critics from outside the profession, and they also needed to construct the boundaries and standards of their profession more rigidly in order to safeguard it from competition from within. This is the context in which physicians, too, condemned quack medicine and tried to disassociate themselves from it. They claimed that the charlatans were others—ignorant physicians, foreign physicians, and in any case not trustworthy persons like themselves. This complex situation put physicians in a delicate position: waiving their fee could certainly enhance their claims with regard to their noble intentions in practicing medicine for the benefit of humankind. And, indeed, deontological treatises authored by physicians also promoted the notion that it was great charity to treat poor patients. However, medical doctors did not want to lose the financial returns they had come to expect. So they also included in their ethical manuals practical maxims about setting fees—claiming, for example, that the higher the fee the higher the patient's respect for the physician. Biographical dictionaries celebrated the examples of eminent healers who showed generosity and refused payment. These examples are few, and they could be legendary, anyway. Moreover, even these rare stories reveal that such behavior occurred only when the physician in question earned his living from a different profession or business.

Formal Medical Aid and the Donors

The alms tax in Muslim societies (*zakāt*) is obligatory because of a Qur'anic injunction. It explicitly demands that all Muslims who possess a minimum level of wealth should allocate part of their income annually to charity. However, voluntary welfare endeavors (*sadaḳa*) were the social and legal vehicle for organized charity in Muslim societies.

One especially popular form of voluntary charity was the endowment (*waqf* in Arabic and *vakıf* in Ottoman-Turkish). The expressed goal was to draw closer to God (*qurba*) and attain a place in paradise. This was achieved in the endowment because the founders transferred the title of their properties to God. The donors gave up the properties permanently for the benefit of a specific purpose. The deed was an irreversible act. It was made public and binding by preparing a legal written document (Arabic *waqfıyya*; Ottoman Turkish *vakfiye*) supervised and signed by the local Muslim judge. The document included the following details: the endowed property, the beneficiary from the revenues, and the identity of the person who would run the endowment. It was also an eternal charity, and the ultimate beneficiaries were stated to be "the poor" as an alternative in case the original ones died or disappeared.[18]

In Islamic societies medical aid was a recognized and accepted form of action in the arena of benevolence; and institutionalized medical treatment via hospitals was only one of a number of forms of medical care in the Ottoman Empire that included lay and professional, outdoor or indoor assistance.

Some scholars have followed the sources in accepting this view of the philanthropist hospital. Norman Stillman, in his "Charity and Social Service in Medieval Islam,"[19] discussed what he saw as the primary Muslim attitudes toward philanthropy and what he regarded as the principal institutions of social welfare supported by Muslim philanthropy in the Middle Ages. According to him, the hospital was "perhaps the most impressive institution of social welfare or charity in the medieval Muslim world."[20] Stillman was impressed by the pivotal role in Muslim society played by hospitals in the medieval period. We may regard Stillman's statement as poetic exaggeration, but it does draw our attention to this important institution.

But what factors made this particular medical charity so important for a Muslim society? Stillman seems to hint that medieval Muslims were astounded by the philanthropy embodied in hospitals, which seems too simplistic. It is true that hospitals were more visible than other forms of medical charity as a symbol of how the benevolent founders deployed their wealth for the welfare of the community, and as a result drew more attention by contemporaries. Yet, hospitals were founded in the early modern Ottoman empire for many different reasons, varying with the specific times and places of their foundation and according to the different personalities involved in the initiative.

The founders of hospitals and their future managers were likely to create an image that they believed to be attractive to the community and to persuade the community that what they did was good and worthy of support. Ottoman hospitals depended on the support of the local community and therefore struggled to capture for themselves the loyalty of the community.[21] The ways donors organized their hospitals were far from random. They wanted to make a success of their institutions and planned them in accordance with what they believed would be appealing to the community. Hospitals were not the only expression of this. Whatever the *vakıf* institution—a hospital, a mosque, a *medrese,* or anything else—the donors wanted it to be used. An empty building does not perpetuate the donor's memory and enhance his or her patronage, whereas a living institution, where people come and go, keeps the memory of the founder in the users' minds all the time. As a result, hospitals were molded according to an image the donors had of what would make "their" hospital popular. The philanthropists may wish to "seduce" the public by offering a range of services that they estimate the community needs or wants in order to draw the community in. This is not to say that personal preferences, whims and considerations of fashion, as well as true interest in the well-being of needy individuals, did not play an important role in molding these images. Ottoman medical charities thus tell us something about the beneficiaries. Philanthropy hints at the existence of need, whether material, emotional, or spiritual. Such needs may be also those of the donors. Or, in some cases the donors are primarily responsible for creating a perception that such needs exist.

One reason for regarding Ottoman hospitals as charitable was the hospitals' foundation as institutions of *vakıf,* whose legal format created an administrative and financial mechanism for charitable institutions in premodern Islamic societies. Moreover, Ottoman hospitals offered medical treatment free of charge, in contrast to the practice of European hospitals. Evliya Çelebi praised Viennese hospitals for their medicine and their abundant food and drink (although not their taste). He claims these institutions were extremely rich, which allowed them to offer such splendid services. Pots, plates, trays, candelabras, and skewers made of various metals, from copper to silver and gold, were visible signs of the hospital riches. However, the wealth of the hospital was the result of patients paying for services rendered by donating to the hospital.[22] In this respect, hospitals in the Ottoman Empire were not different from similar institutions in other Muslim societies.

The first hospital to be established in the Ottoman Empire by a member of the Ottoman dynasty was built in Bursa by Beyazid I (reigned 1389–1402).[23] The second one was established in Istanbul, then a new capital, by Mehmet II.[24] His son Beyazid II had one erected in Edirne.[25] In the sixteenth century three hospitals were erected in Istanbul. Both Süleyman I,[26] his favorite concubine (*haseki*) and later wife Hurrem Sultan,[27] and Nurbanu Sultan, mother of Murad III,[28] included hospitals in their complexes in the capital. As already mentioned, Ahmet I had an imperial complex erected in the center of Istanbul at the beginning of the seventeenth century. One of the dependencies of the mosque, in addition to the *dar-ül-hadith*, was a hospital.[29]

Hospitals built in the provinces were *vakıf*s too. One example is the hospital in Manisa initiated by Hafsa Sultan, mother of Süleyman I, while she accompanied her son, then a governor of the province.[30] Other examples are the imperial hospitals built in Mecca by the famous vizier Sokullu Mehmet Paşa at the end of the sixteenth century;[31] and a hundred years after him, Gülnüş Sultan, the favorite concubine of Sultan Mehmet IV and later the mother of two sultans—Mustafa II (reigned 1698–1703) and Ahmet III (reigned 1703–30)—had another one erected.[32] The hospital established in seventeenth-century Tunis by the local Ottoman governor was a *vakıf* as well.[33]

However, there were also exceptions to the rule that hospitals in a premodern Muslim society (here, early modern Ottoman) were established as *vakıf* institutions: hospitals in the imperial palaces. In Topkapı, for instance, there existed a hospital for the pages in the outer court founded in the fifteenth century (it burnt down in 1856); in the harem compound there was a hospital for the female slaves founded in the sixteenth century after the imperial women entered into Topkapı, and a harem was added to the compound; and along the Marmara shore of the palace there existed a third hospital for guards (*bostancılar*—namely, gardeners, thus called for growing vegetables for palace consumption in addition to their guard duties). There were also other hospitals or infirmaries in the old palace in Istanbul (*saray-i atiq*) and in the palaces of Galatasaray (Pera/Istanbul), Bursa, and Edirne.[34]

The funds for these hospitals came from the palace budget. For this reason, there was no need to come up with a different mechanism of finance, like the *vakıf* system. The staff in these hospital—medical personnel and others alike—were all on the palace payroll. The hospital for pages in Topkapı, for example, was run by a large staff headed by a eunuch from the palace service. The sources give contradictory information on the identity of this eunuch. In a sixteenth-century miniature of the first court included in Loqman's *Hünername*,[35] the administrator of the hospital is depicted as a black eunuch. Contemporary European travelers, however, claimed that as a department of the Palace School, the hospital came under the jurisdiction of the chief white eunuch, who added "medical director" (*timarhaneci*) to his numerous titles.[36] But whatever the exact identity of the eunuch, it is clear his post was an integral part of the palace staff, and did not belong to an "extraterritorial" independent *vakıf* institution that happened to be within the palace.

Hospitals in the imperial palaces were not part of the *vakıf* system but were considered nevertheless an expression of philanthropy. *Vakıf* was only one means of action in the arena of medical benevolence. Palace hospitals, much like *vakıf* hospitals and other acts of beneficence, expressed the commitment on the part of the sultan to the members of his household, and were therefore considered charity. The sultan's commitment to his sick servants is attested to in the description of the sultan's visits to the hospital in the outer court in Topkapı. In this palace thousands of people, in addition to the imperial family, worked, studied, and served; the hospital took care of the pages among them. The French merchant and traveler Tavernier visited Istanbul in 1688. In his treatise on Topkapı he described the hospital within the palace compound as a well-organized and efficiently administered institution, thanks—among other things—to frequent visits by the sultan to check on the patients' state. The sultan would interview the patients and inquire whether they were being treated well by the physicians and staff.[37]

The act of founding a hospital as a *vakıf* and laying down its future functions was expressed in terms taken from the language of religion and morality. Basically, *vakıf* is a legal format to finance various large projects for the benefit of the community as a whole.

The intent of benevolence was added later on, but by the Ottoman period the two were well tied together. Philanthropy was expressed in elaborate terms integrated into the legal text of the endowment deed. If the survival of the donor's good name after his or her own death was the chief worldly motive for philanthropy, the desire to approach God was the otherworldly motivation.[38] Endowment deeds explain that this act is a *qurba,* as for example, in the endowment deed of a hospital in Tunis in the mid-seventeenth century the donor is exalted in the following phrases: "May his name be praised, with concern for his great policies and sound leadership, he who seeks to draw near [to God] by means of sacrifice, by providing charity for the needy and for those in want, with ample, continuous alms, and everlasting, virtuous *hubus* [*waqf*]. His lofty zeal is devoted to it. His noble view was directed toward it."[39] Hafsa Sultan was described as "[t]he queen of queens, royalty among royals, distinguished among mankind, the pure among the purest women, the beloved lady, the mistress who is a guarantor of tradition, the cream of the august women, the prop of the respected ladies, the protector of male and female Muslims, the possessor of sublime characteristics and good fortune, the 'Aisha of her time, the Fatima of her period, the rising jewel of the radiant sultanate, the pearl of the bright caliphate."[40] The praises associated with Hafsa recalled her status as a respectable married woman and recalled one of Muhammad's titles as "Chosen of Allah" (*Ṣafī Allah*).

The above two motivations—perpetuating the donor's name and desire to approach God—are personal. There could be also collective motivation. Here the founder thinks not of himself or herself as an individual but of the interests of his or her social group (usually elite) or society as a whole.[41] An example is the presentation of hospital foundations as a response to a communal need (the term *haca,* "need" or "necessity," appears quite frequently in the documents). Demands are presented as the driving forces shaping welfare policies. According to this structure of supply and demand, if hospitals are founded (or not), it shows the population was (or was not) in need of their services.

Could it be that only a few hospitals were founded throughout the Ottoman Empire in the early modern period because the population did not suffer any grave medical problems? Istanbul of the sixteenth century—one of the largest cities in the world at the time, with an estimated population of several hundred thousand people[42]—had only five hospitals, with a total of few hundred beds altogether. In Cairo and Aleppo, the two next-largest cities in the Ottoman Empire, the situation was the same.

The history of natural catastrophes in the Ottoman Empire is yet to be written, but the few plague and earthquake studies published on the early modern period (epidemics and earthquakes being two of the most devastating catastrophes, the third being famine), suggest natural disasters and their intensity did not decline in the Middle East during this period. Likewise, the sources do not claim that the population was healthier and the number of sick people was not lower than the average norm in previous or later periods in the area.[43] The hospital at the Süleymaniye complex in Istanbul was founded in the middle of the sixteenth century, shortly after another hospital was opened in the nearby complex of Hurrem, Süleyman's wife. The sources do not claim that in that particular period there was a greater than usual need for medical services in the capital.

Even if there was no "real" need for founding hospitals, presenting a new hospital as a response to need provided a plausible explanation or socially respectable reason behind the project. When a hospital was founded in Manisa, a later addition to an existing sultanic complex there, the *vakfiye* (the foundation deed) stated that local people were in dire need of such an institution: it would organize the therapeutic facilities and methods in the town and treat the injured and those in pain. The document states that the benevolent patrons and the administrators of this complex were acting in compliance with petitions sent by local people to the "exalted and mighty threshold" asking that a hospital be erected.[44] The authors of the document wished to describe this act of philanthropy as an answer to a request from below.

The claim that the presentation of a hospital was "an answer to a need" ought to be taken with grain of salt. This rhetoric may cover other motivations for hospital foundation that were not readily acceptable. In the case of Manisa, perhaps Süleyman wished to strengthen the imperial presence in this important urban center. He may have been nostalgically attached to a provincial town where he had previously served as governor, a post to which his mother accompanied him. This may explain why Süleyman had a hospital added to the complex already existing, which his mother, Hafsa Sultan, had erected several years prior.[45]

Personal wishes and needs may not necessarily be documented and known to us. Individual circumstances could bring a donor to be involved in medical and health activities, but these were rarely documented. How many figures were there to match al-Malik al-Manṣūr Qala'ūns (reigned 1279–90)? This Mamluk sultan supposedly founded his grand hospital in Cairo to repay a moral debt to the physicians who had previously cured him of a grave illness. This is the story as told by Taqī al-Dīn al-Maqrīzī (1364–1442), the Mamluk historian. According to him, Qala'ūn, still an emir, was sent in 1276 by the reigning Baybars to raid Anatolia. Some sickness delayed him in Damascus. Local physicians treated him with medication brought from the twelfth-century hospital in town. When he recovered he asked to see the institution and was amazed at its marvels. Qala'ūn took an oath that when God made him the sultan he would build a hospital. When Qala'ūn took over the sultanate he endowed much property to establish a hospital in a spacious building (maybe imitating the Zangids and Ayyubids and trying to outdo them).[46]

Al-Maqrīzī's story is apocryphal, but not implausible. There might have been those who, like Qala'ūn, came to be interested in medicine after personal experiences. Such was the case of Katip Çelebi, the Ottoman financial bureaucrat, as he explained in his work *The Balance of Truth*. The treatise contains quite a number of autobiographical details. In the concluding chapter Katip Çelebi tells us about his career as a clerk (*katip*) in the army audit bureau, his studies, his teachings, and his writings. He mentions that he quarreled with the chief clerk in his department: Katip Çelebi asked for promotion but his boss refused, claiming there was no vacancy. He then took a leave of absence. For three years he was without employment, devoting his time to his studies. During this period he suffered a bad bout of sickness, as a result of which he became preoccupied with medicine (mainly spiritual) in order to restore his health.[47]

Many might have been interested in medicine and health, but only for a few was it a springboard for active involvement with medical charity. Despite the many merits in this world and the next accruing from medical benevolence, those engaged in it in a formal and public way in the early modern period included only five sultans, two mothers of the sultan, two concubines, one vizier, and one local governor. The small size of this group is remarkable. It is apparent that it is made of selected and exclusive members in and around the Ottoman court. It was so exclusive that not even all members of the imperial family were included. Could it be that despite the rhetoric, medical charity was not considered such a pious deed in comparison to other possible philanthropic projects? Maybe it was not fashionable enough? Maybe the cost effectiveness was not great enough, so potential benefactors chose to direct their endeavors elsewhere, where smaller investments could reap more in worldly and religious benefit? Or perhaps, medical charity was not in fact open to all.

Subtle cultural and social rules determined who founded what, where, for whom, and on what scale. Maybe there was something that forbade many to deal with medicine. We need to pay attention to who appears on the list of contributors and who does not. The absence of male members of the imperial family save the reigning sultan is very conspicuous. Not even sons of the sultans, the heirs apparent, appear on them. Leslie Peirce pointed to a process of exclusion of male members of the royal family in the imperial philanthropic projects—for example, in the foundation of mosques. Princes threatened the sultan, competing with him over legitimacy, creating their image as a possible ruler, and therefore their charitable activities were restricted.[48] I suggest the restriction encompassed medical charity, like the foundation of hospitals.

Charity and philanthropy in a Muslim society are theoretically decided by the donor's wish as to what to give, how, where, how much, and when. The rationale behind the right to freedom of action was that it was the benefactor's capital at the root of the benevolent action. However, the decision in practice was not entirely his or her own. For example, there might be sudden crises due to natural disasters, like hunger and famine, floods, plagues, or earthquakes that needed to be addressed. Even in regular, less dramatic, times the donor had to cope with constraints. The founders were influenced by precedence, fashion, social expectations, and cultural norms.

The Medically Disabled as Needy and Entitled

Students of Europe in the early modern period claimed that the major context of health care provision in the early modern period was poor relief. Studies of Europe claim that the richer classes donated funds to medical relief, yet never drew on it themselves. The rich made their own medical arrangements in their homes and rarely attended hospitals as patients.[49]

The Ottoman sources mention the "poor," the "miserable," the "needy," and the "weak" as the entitled beneficiaries of endowed institutions. The separation of patients according to social class is an old tradition in many medical systems. As today in our Western society, so in the early modern Middle East, those with means had more medical options. In many studies, hospitals have been portrayed as reinforcing/emphasizing this separation. It is almost a commonplace to assert that (only) those who could not afford private medical treatment at home went to hospitals. Hospitals were thus associated with poverty, poor medical attention, and death, seen as a final option or last resort. When people of means (the richer) did eventually enter hospitals in the twentieth century, a second form of separation occurred: now patients were separated within the buildings according to social class (which included also race). A patient's ability to pay for service and his or her insurance coverage became factors that determined the nature of care: the particular hospital, and even the wing, ward, and room in which a patient was placed.[50]

On the surface it seems Ottoman reality is yet another example of separation of patients according to social class. Patients of means were treated at home by physicians who came to them; they did not visit physicians at their clinics, let alone undergo hospitalization. The story of a sick person who is cared for at home by his loving family and close friends is a literary topos popular also in the genre of biographical dictionaries. Hospitals as a place of care are but rarely mentioned in biographies of Ottoman dignitaries even as an option.

Evliya Çelebi included in his book on his extensive travels in the Ottoman Empire in the middle of the seventeenth century the biography of his relative and patron, Melek Ahmet Paşa, a senior Ottoman official. In the winter of 1656, while serving as the governor of the province of Özü to the northwest of the Black Sea, Melek Ahmed's neck swelled up and he fell sick. A pustule developed, and after five to ten days his neck became red and as thick as a loaf of bread. Many physicians, surgeons, and phlebotomists were brought to the paşa's bed, and although each of them prescribed a different treatment, the paşa's condition deteriorated: he lost his voice and could only hum like a bee. Many in his household believed his end was near. Some officers in his entourage left to look for a new patron. Melek Ahmet Paşa himself was sure his time had come: he dictated his last will and his funeral arrangements using sign language (Evliya does not elaborate about the signs). However, Evliya Çelebi, the faithful companion, dreamed a dream whose interpretation gave the paşa new hope. Once again a surgeon was summoned. The surgeon opened the paşa's collar, drained the pus, and removed the rotten flesh. New medications were sent to Melek Ahmet Paşa from the imperial palace, and within two months he had fully recovered.[51]

From these and other pieces of evidence one could deduce that poor people were admitted into hospitals where medical care was distributed free, whereas the well-to-do contracted private doctors and were treated in the privacy of their own homes. Many studies make this deduction, but I believe the reality was different. It is true that hospitals offered medical treatment free of charge, and thus probably were quite attractive to the materially poor, but in the Ottoman context the word "poor," which refers today primarily to those who have little money and as a result may not be able to obtain the necessities of life, may have several possible meanings. In cases where it is possible to determine the identity of Ottoman hospital patients, it is clear that a considerable percentage of them were actually well-off. They may not have been the richest people in town, but they were not in need of free medical service. The social status ascribed to them placed them higher up, toward the middle of the social ladder. But still they were accepted into hospitals free of charge. There were other, nonfinancial, circumstances that could bring someone to a state of neediness. Hospital patients, rather then being financially needy, were perceived as deserving help and sympathy due to their merits, social status, and specific circumstances.[52]

The identity of hospital patients is not unlike the identity of those granted permission to dine at the Ottoman soup kitchens. It is clear that a considerable percentage of them actually belonged to elite groups. The categories of those entitled to a free meal were many and varied, whether such entitlement was based on religion, social standing, or vocational activity. Religious scholars, employees of the institution, Sufis, poor people and those retired from military or palace service might all dine side by side in a soup kitchen, although the imaret meals were very hierarchical and they did not necessarily dine together at the same table, dine at the same time, or eat the same amounts and dishes.[53] However, it is interesting to note that being entitled to medical and food support was expressed in terms referring to economic, social, and physical hardships.

Sultan Süleyman expected that people carrying with them money and goods would be admitted into his Istanbul hospital, and instructed what should be done in such cases: he ordered the clerk (*katip*) in the hospital to record in detail the belongings that patients brought with them when admitted; special attention was to be given to recording money and other valuables. The clerk's duty was to return to the patients leaving the institution whatever they had brought with them according to his records.[54] A special area in the hospital was reserved for the treasury (*bayt-lü-mal* or *hazine*), which no one was allowed to enter except the head physician. The hospital funds and the patients' valuables were kept there.[55]

The attraction of affluent patients, therefore, was not only the expectation of the donors about who the future beneficiaries would be. The affluent actually came. We have already mentioned one Aḥmad

b. Muḥammad from Damascus, known by his nickname Ibn al-Munqār (d. 1623). According to his biographer, Muḥammad Amīn b. Faḍlallah al-Muḥibbī (d. 1700), a family member of a later generation, Ibn al-Munqār, became famous as a poet before he was twenty years old. He was renowned for his expertise in both science and the Arabic language. After his father's death in Istanbul, where he had held the position of a judge, Ahmad traveled to the Ottoman capital to claim his inheritance. His fame spread in the capital as well, and the head mufti of the empire made him his assistant. But soon Aḥmad succumbed to melancholy and lost his reason, and his speech became slurred. He was first put in the hospital but later was sent back to his hometown, accompanied by some other Damascene notables returning from Istanbul. In Damascus a house was rented for him where he was under constant care and supervision. He was allowed only to leave the house when accompanied by a guard and for limited periods of time. He never regained his reason and after thirty years died, still a madman.[56]

In sum, a simplistic explanation of who was entitled to free medical services based solely on the social and economic standing of poor hospital patients versus rich people treated at home does not reflect the realities of the early modern Middle East. Neediness was decided upon the establishment of poverty, which was described as the lack of something crucial. That could include the lack of *material* objects, but when it came to entitlement to free medical services it seems the second category was at least as important: the lack of *social* objects, like skills or family that allow one to rise from one's position. Need may result from circumstances imposed from outside or from a choice to live in an ascetic way (like the Sufis). Poverty can be structural—that is, it could be the result of a long social and economic process that affects groups; poverty can also be a temporary situation, a specific case that can be easily remedied and from which recovery is possible.

Who, then, were the majority of patients in hospitals? We should remember that the sources used here are the product of urban Ottoman elite groups, and therefore it should not come as a surprise that the "heroes" of these sources are members of these same groups. The wretched and the miserable, whether socially or financially, are anonymous and invisible in sources of this type. However, although the sources provide almost no direct evidence on the identity of hospital patients, they do speak to us and reveal who were deemed worthy of medical support in early modern Ottoman society. Unlike in our modern hospitals, in early modern Ottoman hospitals social status determined acceptance, rather than medical diagnosis. And in contrast to the popular image of premodern hospitals as almshouses, those who could expect care in Ottoman hospitals did so on social grounds, not economic ones.[57]

The Nonpoor Foreigner as Entitled to Medical Help

The specific mission of Ottoman hospitals was to help the sick, the injured, and those suffering from mutilations and pain. In this sense, hospitals were part of a group of institutions to which imarets, hospices (*tabhane*), and hostels and inns for the wayfarers in towns and along commercial routes (*han* and *karavan-seray*) also belonged. This group of institutions had two aspects in common. The first is that all distributed physical help. The second is that this group of institutions was intended to serve people who for a number of reasons could not take care of themselves. They might have lacked financial means, health, and strength (physical and mental), or supportive family (through accident or physical or emotional distance). But it was not necessarily because of a continuous poor situation, that a person availed himself or herself of charitable medical services. Under certain circumstances even a member of a famous and well-off family could use free medical services.

Medical treatment and care were usually distributed within the family. If the family was the prime agent in distributing health and medical care, hospitalization, then, signaled the absence or the dysfunction of a family. Here "family" is understood in a wide context. Family here is more than blood or marriage ties. It encompasses also those who are close, which allows also us to consider also "strangers" like friends, companions, and associates from work or a religious order, as providing care and affection to a patient and taking responsibility for him or her in times of medical need.[58] The function of the hospital institution together with, or in addition to, the family exemplifies the balance (and sometimes rivalry) between different supportive agents: family, the neighborhood, and the community at large.[59] People of means were patients in hospital if they had no family close by to support them. They may have had no family at all or they may have been strangers in a faraway place.

"If travelers and wayfarers are sick, they come to the hospital of Sultan Mehmet the Conqueror and they treat them."[60] This was the description by Evliya Çelebi—a traveler himself—of the patient population in the hospital established in Istanbul by Mehmet II. The English traveler George Sandys described the hospitals in the capital at the beginning of the seventeenth century as a place where foreigners were entertained.[61] In Istanbul, the Ottoman capital, there were many foreigners, who came there for many different reasons: they included merchants, immigrants from the provinces, scholars, adventurers, and others.

Strangers to Istanbul who owned property were among the patients in the hospitals in town. When patients died in hospitals, as in other cases of deaths of people of means, the *kadi* (judge) was asked to manage the estate. He would write down a detailed list of the estate of the deceased (*metrukat defteri*), record who the rightful heirs were and what their share in the inheritance would be after settling debts (including sums owed to the spouse, like the remainder of the bride price), and pay for burial costs. These lists were included in the Muslim court registers, and indicated where people died, whether peacefully at home or in special circumstances, such as during the pilgrimage of Mecca. The very fact that people who died in hospitals appear on such lists testifies that they left some property when they died, otherwise the *kadi* would not have been asked to intervene in his capacity as settler of inheritances. Yet the estates of such hospital patients were rather modest.

In the deceased lists from seventeenth-century Istanbul, four people are recorded as having passed away in hospitals in town. Their property was composed of movables only. One of them was Ahmed Efendi bin Hasan Beşe, who died in the hospital of Mehmed II. He owned three male slaves (*ghulam*). This hints at his being a man of wealth, but apparently their quality was mediocre at best: their value in January 1617 was estimated at 11,450 silver coins. It was a modest sum in comparison to the prices of other slaves recorded in these lists. He also left behind several unsettled debts, in the amount of 1,150 silver coins. Osman Efendi bin Mehmed Bey, a religious scholar (*'alim*), passed away in the Süleymaniye hospital. The head physician tried to gain control over his estate, but his riding animals and beasts of burden amounted in December 1649 to the humble sum of 3,400 silver coins. He owed 640 coins to a man who had loaned them to him previously. The estate of Façli Beşe, who also died in the Süleymaniye, was settled in the summer of 1656. It included cash in the amount of 1,100 silver coins and merchandise worth an additional 905 coins.[62]

Two of the four patients who died in Istanbul hospitals during the seventeenth century left no heirs. One of the two who did leave heirs was survived by five family relatives, including a wife, two daughters, and two brothers, but the head physician tried nonetheless to gain control over the inheritance.[63] Could it be that he thought he could get away with it because these relatives were not present? It is telling that the possessions of all four of the patients who died in the hospitals included no immoveable property; rather, their assets were all moveable items: cash, slaves, and merchandise. Perhaps this is evidence of their identity as visitors to the city.

In addition to the capital there were other urban centers that were magnets for foreigners. The Holy Cities, Mecca and Medina, attracted thousands of Muslims from all corners of the world. They flocked there both to fulfill the duty of the hajj and to study. The long road and its hardships proved too difficult for many, and they fell sick or died along the way, or else arrived sick and died there. Rapacious local governors and leaders of caravans certainly tried to seize the belongings of people who died along the way.

This was the context of a complaint sent by 'Umar, the caretaker of the holy sites in Medina, to the sultan about certain leaders of hajj caravans. According to him, they had taken charge of the property of dying pilgrims and embezzled it. Instead of taking only the outstanding share for expenses of the convoy and transferring the rest to the imperial treasury, the leaders had taken an extra share for themselves, robbing widows, orphans, and other heirs who should have benefited from these funds. The sultan sent a decree to the provincial governor and head judge in Damascus to investigate this alleged crime. The decree says that if 'Umar's complaint proves to be valid, the culprits should be removed from their posts in the hajj caravan; all excess charges levied by them be recovered and transferred to the treasury.[64]

Those lucky pilgrims who reached Mecca and Medina unharmed were obviously exhausted. Even the healthiest and strongest among the pilgrims and travelers were foreigners in town, and when they fell sick some of them had to seek help at the local hospitals. They did not know the physicians there and could not rely on supportive friends and relatives. Thus, the patients in the hospitals in these cities might be rich people who would have contracted a private physician in their hometown—they certainly could have afforded one—but on their travels to foreign lands used hospital services that were given free of charge. Several hospitals existed in Mecca and Medina, which were founded in the pre-Ottoman periods. The hospital founded by 'Imād al-Dīn Zangī (d. 1174)—who also erected medical institutions in Syria, his seat of power—functioned as a hospital in the sixteenth century as well, despite financial hardships as the endowment supporting it shrank.[65] To these were added Ottoman institutions, like the hospitals of Sokullu Mehmet Paşa and Gülnüş Sultan, mentioned above.

It is conceivable that there were also wealthy foreigners among those who died in the Meccan hospital, deaths that became the subject of two identical decrees. In March 1568 two decrees were sent to the Ottoman judge in Mecca at an interval of two weeks. The sultan ordered the judge to inform him in detail about who had taken charge of the personal effects of dead patients in the hospital there. The judge was to explain what had been done with them, how and to whom they were sold, how much was received for them, and how that amount was spent.[66]

The palace pages in Topkapı Palace who were treated in the hospital there, which served only members of the palace service, shared some characteristics of the travelers. The pages did not have immediate family close at hand, since they were the product of the periodic levy (*devşirme*) of Christian youngsters from the conquered lands. Despite being far away from their biological families, they were not alone in their illness. In contrast to foreigners admitted to hospitals who found themselves in a strange land in their time of illness, the palace hospital was situated in the first and outer court, to the right of the Imperial Gate, a mere few hundred meters from the pages' private rooms in the inner, third court. The palace pages could thus rely upon the friends and colleagues with whom they lived and worked. European travelers in the seventeenth century who visited the palace (but were not patients in this hospital) described how as soon as he fell sick, a patient was brought there from his room in a small cart covered with a red curtain dragged by two servants. On seeing it, palace members and visitors stopped and cleared the way, as did the sultan himself.[67]

When a patient in the hospital in Topkapı died, the imam of the nearby wood depot was summoned. He cleansed the body and prepared it for burial. In the presence of the friends and colleagues of the deceased, the body was taken out of the palace and carried to a special cemetery in Kasımpaşa or in Karacaahmet (neighborhoods on the European and Asian shores of the Bosphorus, respectively) dedicated to the palace servants. The late seventeenth-century Ottoman bureaucrat and historian Abdallah b. Ibrahim Üsküdari described in his *Tarih-i vakiat-i sultan-i süleyman-i sani*, which dealt with Süleyman II's period (reigned 1687–91), how in the absence of a biological family peers from the palace school and service created an alternative "family," at least at the funeral.[68]

Regarding foreignness as one of the things that can cause someone to lose a comfortable position and viewing the foreign traveler as someone who might especially need medical aid were not new in Ottoman society. Medieval Muslim-Arabic society was also well acquainted with this problem. In his article on the stranger in medieval Islam, Franz Rosenthal described the stranger as a literary, religious, and philosophical topos and examined the reality in which strangers lived. Based on an analysis of the literary conventions used by several authors to describe strangers and strangeness, Rosenthal pointed to wretchedness as a constant companion for strangers. Two possible sources of wretchedness are poverty and ill health. These conditions are always hard, but they are especially difficult to bear when one is in a foreign place.[69] The tenth-century *Book of Strangers*, a collection of verses of graffiti collected by an anonymous Iraqi traveler, has one dominant theme: lost happiness. Foreign and strange travelers vent feelings of homesickness, lovesickness, longing for a happy past or better future, anxiety, fear, and deep melancholia. They complain about being miserable and helpless without friends and kin.[70] The Geniza offers evidence that medieval Jewish-Muslim society also associated being a stranger with poverty. Foreigners, whether they were wayfarers, immigrants, captives, or refugees, were perceived as lonely, needy, and deserving of help. The Egyptian Jewish community was therefore encouraged to act in a charitable manner toward them.[71]

Ottoman hospital policy targeted foreigners as clients and showed willingness to accept the stranger. This attitude coexisted with an opposing one that cultivated wariness of the unknown and advocated preferential treatment of one's own kin and familiar faces. Ottoman society struck a balance between these two tendencies. Striking a balance between priorities was an inherent feature of the institution of endowed charities, which could be used to support public utilities, to support the poor, or to provide regular income for the founder's relatives and circumvent succession rules. Hospitals themselves turned to both locals and foreigners. Accepting foreigners did not exclude the locals. In fact, some of the hospital activities were intended for the local community, like hospital physicians making house calls or dispensing medication on the special days when the hospital acted as an outpatient clinic. There were also clear stipulations that medication should not be dispensed too widely.

Religious Affiliation and Entitlement

Hospitals were open to foreigners, but not all of them. Religious affiliations restricted the open arms of hospitality considerably. Ottoman hospitals were not a place where different religious communities mixed as patients and staff. Previous studies of premodern hospitals in Muslim societies have exalted hospitals as secular institutions, an anachronistic term. They depicted hospitals as born of—and functioning according to—medical-scientific considerations; a hospital, according to them, was the only space in Muslim societies where people of various faiths could meet as equals for the service of science and humankind.[72] Even if this observation of Muslim hospitals reflects a concrete historical reality at all, rather than romantic wishful thinking, it cannot be applied to the Ottoman case.

It is true that Ottoman hospitals were a charitable institution in which the benefactor could include also non-Muslims. Early versions of the endowment deed for the hospital of Mehmet II in Istanbul specified that medical doctors should be hired solely on professional grounds, irrespective of their religion. And salary lists from the fifteenth century prove that this stipulation was indeed implemented: Jewish and Christian physicians worked side by side with Muslim doctors. However, the inclusion of non-Muslims was not more than a possibility, and it never became a popular policy among founders and hospital administrators. Even the inclusion of non-Muslims as hospital physicians did not last. In most cases (and from the sixteenth century this became the norm), staff members in the hospital of Mehmet II and other hospitals were Muslims only. Moreover, patients, it seems, were always Muslims.

Staff members in Ottoman hospitals and patients were Muslims only, and they created a Muslim community. They did not live their lives in accordance with a monastic code, as was the case in Europe—such a code did not exist in Muslim societies, anyway. Their mission was to heal the patients medically. Although spirituality played a role in Ottoman medicine (as described in the previous chapter), this institution was not a fulfillment of a religious idea, as was the situation in contemporary Europe. However, as members of a Muslim community, hospital staff members did observe the religious-legal code incumbent on all Muslims.

Foundation deeds, which specify the aims of endowments, usually refer to the benefit provided to Muslims among the advantages of hospitals. The *vakfiye* of Mehmet II states that Muslims can avail themselves of hospitals,[73] and the *vakfiye* for the complex of Beyazid II in Edirne specifically says that the hospital is intended for the religious (i.e., religious Muslim) poor.[74]

This admissions policy goes hand in hand with the religious services of various sorts offered to Muslim patients in hospitals. On the hospital staff there were imams and muezzins at the special space within the hospital building reserved for a mosque, and *ghassal*s who prepared the dead for Muslim burial. Non-Muslims were cared for separately: Ottoman Jews had autonomous hospitals run by the community.[75] Near the hospital of Mehmet II in Istanbul there was an institution especially for *dhimmis*, according to Evliya (we have no reference to this hospital other than Evliya's).[76] In sixteenth-century Jerusalem there were hospitals that served the Jewish community (or subcommunities within it) exclusively.[77]

The separation between Muslims and non-Muslims in Ottoman hospitals should not come as a surprise. As we have seen in previous chapters, medical practice can contradict religious beliefs at various levels: medical theories, therapeutic procedures, and even seeking the help of medicine and doctors rather than that of religion and religious scholars could (and still can) contradict religious beliefs. One can assume, for example, that one reason for Jews to stay away from Muslim hospitals was fear of the food in the institution. For many, medical exigencies were not sufficient to transgress dietary regulations.[78]

*Dhimmi*s generally did not wish to use the "state" hospitals, although this "boycotting" was not necessarily practiced in all periods. Apparently a religious division among hospitals did not always exist. Material from Crusader Jerusalem reveals that at the end of the twelfth century Jews and Muslims, and not only Christians, were admitted to the Hospitallers' medical institution in the city. This is the testimony of an anonymous Christian patient who claimed to have stayed at the hospital for quite some time. Although the hospital was founded by a Christian order for pilgrims and Crusaders, it did open its doors to Muslims, regarded by the Franks as infidels from whom the Holy Land must be saved. Soon after the Crusaders' conquest of Jerusalem in 1099 Jews were forbidden to live in the city; the order was fully enforced, as we know from Jewish travelers like Benjamin of Tudela in the twelfth century.[79] Nevertheless, the articles of the Hospitaller order from 1182 stipulated that patients who cannot eat pork should be given chicken. This stipulation presumably referred to those whose religion forbade them to eat pork (i.e., Jews and Muslims).[80] It also strengthens the hypothesis that dietary regulations could on occasion prevent Jews from going to non-Jewish hospitals, Christian or Muslim. But it is difficult to know whether the intracommunity medical system was a substitute for quasi-state hospitals that were closed to Jews. Possibly, too, an ideology of communal autonomy was the reason for ethnic and religious separation in hospital admissions policies.

Staff members of various faiths also did not intermingle in Middle Eastern hospitals in the early modern period. This was a different situation from previous centuries. The Cairo Geniza includes numerous references to Jewish physicians practicing their craft in hospitals, even if there is not a single reference to Jews being patients there. In the fifteenth century non-Muslim physicians are mentioned on the salary lists. This was in accordance with the hospital foundation deeds, which detail the criteria set up for doctors' employment. The criteria included professional excellence and high moral personality. Religious faith was either ignored or explicitly mentioned as something that should be ignored. However, salary lists from the sixteenth and seventeenth centuries yield no non-Muslims. Ibrahim or Musa could really be Abraham and Moses, yet the lists did not include the religious titles that the Ottoman bureaucracy used regularly in other documents (like *dhimmi*) to indicate non-Muslims. It is reasonable to assume therefore that all the employees in hospitals—medical, administrative, and menial staff—were Muslims only.

Outside institutionalized medical treatment, division between the different religious and ethnic communities existed, but the Ottoman medical system outside hospitals was characterized by constant crossing of such borders, if one was so inclined. The possibility to do so always existed. While some sick people favored a doctor from their own religious, ethnical, and/or linguistic community, others did approach physicians from other communities as well. Court records from all over the empire reveal constant medical relationships across religions. These were accepted as routine. Thus, we see that in malpractice suits where the accused healer was not of the same faith, and even when the injured patient was Muslim and his/her physician was not, neither the formal complaint nor the judge refer to the religious affiliation other than as a means to identify the personalities involved in the case.[81]

Male and Female in Medical Neediness

Another factor that determined entitlement to free medical services was gender. Women were usually described in the sources as needing special attention and help from family and society at large. Women were perceived as having an especially weak position in society and economics. Yet when it comes to formal medical aid, it seems that in actuality males were those who received such help, not women.

Ottoman foundation deeds do not include any reference to the question of gender. Here these documents depart from earlier Mamluk *vakfiyes*, which stressed that there should not be any kind of discrimination against those who wish to be admitted into the hospital, including discrimination that is based on gender. The evidence, however, suggests patients in Ottoman hospitals were usually male. It is only in rare cases that female patients are mentioned specifically. In other cases they are not mentioned at all. Moreover, the sources do not mention any special consideration of the Muslim moral code and its insistence on gender separation.

The moral code in traditional Ottoman society—in Muslim and non-Muslim communities alike—laid down segregation of the sexes. This of course had direct bearing on the contents and management of medical treatment. The crux of the matter was that male and female patients could not have been treated together in the same space. The aspect of privacy was discussed in the previous chapter, where we saw that privacy as a cultural idea was understood to be about the boundaries between the genders.

Indeed, in the rare cases in which there is a direct reference in the sources to female patients in a hospital, it is said specifically that there was a special space dedicated for women within the all-male hospital or even a building solely for their use. Patients in the palace hospital in Topkapı were mainly male; the few female patients in the institution were taken care of in a room of their own.[82] The mid-seventeenth-century writer Evliya Çelebi claimed that in a corner near the hospital of Mehmet II in Istanbul there was another hospital—one dedicated to women.[83] It is not clear what Evliya was referring to here, as other sources do not mention a special institution—or a wing in the main all-male hospital—specializing in the treatment of female patients, except in Topkapı. Moreover, this is the same institution referred to earlier, for *dhimmis*. It is interesting that according to Evliya this second hospital served both women and non-Muslims, not necessarily female ones.

Evliya Çelebi reported that in Cairo, too, there existed a hospital dedicated only to female patients. This institution was situated near the Manṣūrī hospital for men (the Mamluk hospital from the late thirteenth century that continued to function well into the nineteenth century): "On one side of this *darüşşifa* [hospital—MS] is a *bimarhane* [hospital—MS] for women. It is also a magnificent, sumptuous building. Moreover, all the servants [in it] are also women, but the [male] physicians are allowed inside. [The physicians] enter [the building] fearlessly and without scruple and give medication according to the different illnesses."[84] Evliya Çelebi mentioned several terms for "hospital" that can be used interchangeably without hinting at the existence of specific terms for female or male hospitals.

Here we encounter another medical-ethical related problem caused by the moral and physical separation of the sexes: should women be treated by male staff? Was medical treatment by a member of the opposite sex permissible or desirable? There was not any division of labor based on gender among Ottoman healers. The Ottoman case seems to show what Monica Green demonstrated with regard to medieval Europe:[85] there was no simple gendered division of labor with men practicing only on men, or women only on women. This does not mean that there was no moral discussion on the desirability of such a situation. Maybe the practice only intensified the theoretical discussion on the issue. The clinical reality as well allowed such an interaction to take place in a variety of ways that seemed acceptable to the various healers and patients involved.

The physicians in the Manṣūrī hospital for women were described as *maḥram*, a legal term denoting people in close biological-family relations that forbid them to marry each other.[86] By this legal stratagem the problem of privacy between doctors who were male and patients who were female was avoided. The male physician treating a female patient was not considered to be transgressing, but was given the status of a close relative in order to sanction their proximity. In other cases it was mentioned specifically that the staff included female attendants as well.

The legal and moral solution accepted in the Manṣūrī hospital was not good enough for the women closest to the Ottoman sultan. In the Ottoman women's world there was stratification with respect to wealth, family, community support, and the effectiveness of the restrictions placed upon women. Female members of the elite enjoyed much greater scope for activity in comparison to women from lower strata. Some of the roles played by them in fact lay in a very gray area between male and female spaces. These were fortunate and sometimes powerful and wealthy women,[87] but hand in hand with the variety of possibilities came also restrictions: female members of the elite, especially the women in the imperial Ottoman harem, had to be more committed to gender separation and their isolation in the harem than other women.

This social-moral code had a direct bearing on the medical care given to palace women. The female servants in the harem were not taken to the first court of the palace. The sick among them were treated in a separate hospital situated under the harem living quarters, thus maintaining the segregation of the sexes in the palace.[88] If even those nonranking women in the palace received special medical treatment (special in its administration, not necessarily in its quality), certainly those of high status received medical care subject to strict surveillance. Here we encounter a paradox that although these women enjoyed much power and vast financial means, their access to medical aid was far from easy, maybe even more so than for supposedly less fortunate women. The moral-ethical code of behavior that had a lot to do with gender shaped the medical options feasible for the Ottoman sultanas. Thus, the female members of the Ottoman family living in Topkapı were not treated even in the female hospital within the harem compound, but only privately by the palace doctors.

Otaviano Bon, the Venetian *bailo* in Istanbul for two and a half years at the beginning of the seventeenth century, described the inherent complexities of medical attention for the female occupants of the palace. When one of the women in the harem fell sick, a physician was sent to treat her, but only after the sultan's approval had first been obtained. When the sultan gave permission for the physician to enter the harem, he was accompanied to the patient by one of the black eunuchs, while all the other female servants retired to their rooms so as not to be seen by him. The patient was covered from head to foot except for one arm, so that the doctor could check her pulse. After examining the patient the physician gave the eunuch accompanying him instructions about her medication and diet and immediately left the harem. However, if the patient was the queen mother (*valide-i sultan*) or one of the sultan's wives or concubines, the arm given to the doctor to check her pulse was covered with silk: it was forbidden for any men, physicians included, to touch the bare flesh of these women. Talking with her was prohibited as well. Therefore, immediately after checking his patient the physician was removed from the sickbed, and gave his instructions to a eunuch in another chamber. Moreover, if this patient was in need of a surgeon she had to suffer her pains patiently: modest covering of her body was not possible in the case of surgery, and as a result a surgeon was not allowed to treat her. In contrast to this, a normal female servant in the harem who needed surgery was simply transferred to the old palace and received there whatever treatment was necessary for her recovery. Medical attention that did not include surgical intervention was given at the harem in Topkapı, and therefore there was no need to transfer the female servant to another hospital.[89] Due to their close proximity to the sultan, his mother, wives, and concubines enjoyed as much power and status as society could confer on individuals of either sex, but this same advantage hindered their access to certain types of medical treatment.

Although these women were denied access to male doctors, they could benefit from the skills of a different group of healers: female attendants. Bon, being a man, was possibly not aware of a sophisticated female medical system operating in the harem itself. A budget report for the household of Süleyman in the year 1513, while he was still a prince, reveals the existence of a female doctor (*hekime khatun*) among the employees, alongside a Jewish physician and two trainee physicians.[90] Midwives, wet nurses and other women with therapeutic experience and knowledge and skills lived either in the harem itself or outside but enjoyed access to the compound. An example of the latter is the *kira*, a Jewish woman who routinely acted as an agent for the mother of the sultan outside the harem in the sixteenth century. These women served the queen mother in various capacities: they entertained them, executed all kinds of transactions on their behalf (especially in connection with luxury goods), and represented them in all dealings outside the harem. The *kira* also advised the queen mother on medical subjects.[91]

The extreme case of female patients in the Ottoman palace demonstrates the effects of deontology on distribution of medical aid. But reality was not just gendered. Social standing played a decisive role as well in limiting accessibility to medical treatment and restricting the medical options available to the patient. One aspect is that seclusion and its effects in the medical realm applied also to the male members of the royal family: the sultan was certainly not hospitalized but was treated in his private chambers.[92] Another aspect is that those on top of the social pyramid, who financially could afford any type of medical treatment existing, were in fact quite limited, medically. This is the opposite of what one would expect. The realities for the female palace dwellers were not that different from those of their servants. The first chapter revealed the extent to which one's diet was controlled by cultural norms. Cuisine cultures differentiated between social classes, but in addition to the social function, these gastronomical realities had health ramifications. Gender was another factor that society considered in order to decide who was entitled to medical care in general and what kind of treatment in particular. The basic social expectation at the time was that women would be treated in their family circles or within the household, as the case of the palace females demonstrates. Women were not supposed to be in a situation where they were strangers far away from home and in need of support from the locals, as males quite frequently were.

The Age of Entitlement

The situation of children mirrors that of gender. Ottoman foundation deeds of medical charities do not include a direct reference to the ages of patients or a possible connection between their ages and the admission policy. Mamluk documents did include specific instructions that age was not to be used to discriminate between patients admitted into hospitals. Thus, we find the following flowery statement in the *vakfiye* of the Manṣūrī hospital: "Into the hospital there will enter groups and individuals, old and young, adults and boys."[93] Several pieces of evidence, however, indicate that those admitted as patients into imperial Ottoman hospitals were not young boys, but mature men.

The endowment deeds do not refer to a situation in which the institution would have to adjust to the presence of young boys—for example, by supplying special food or clothes of smaller size, and the donors seem to have expected that their future beneficiaries would be adults. Let us consider the roles of the hammam attendants in the hospital. In Süleyman's hospital they had to shave the patients, a task that would not have been required if the patients were children.[94] Among the evidence there is a miniature included in an album prepared for Sultan Ahmet I in the beginning of the seventeenth century. This miniature depicts a scene in a hospital for the insane. The patients are all bearded men.[95] In addition, circumstantial evidence (weak as it is), for example, in Evliya's *Seyahatname*—corroborates this. Evliya writes that "old and young" populate the hospital in Edirne,[96] but he does not add anything concrete to explain his figure of speech. When talking of Cairo, Evliya takes the trouble to mention that in the hospital for women adjacent to the central Manṣūrī institution some female patients had given birth. He tells the story of a boy born in the hospital who was named "Health" (*şifa*)—a pun on the name of the institution: the literal meaning of the term "hospital" (*darüşşifa*) is "the house of health." From Evliya's description it is clear that giving birth in a hospital was a rare occurrence.[97] Apparently what Evliya had heard of was a boy born to a female patient, and not a child patient in his own right.

The material that we have, which suggests that children were not supposed to be among the patients in a hospital, echoes the social norm that children should remain in familial or household surroundings—the female private space in the family, to be exact—and therefore could be on their own only in extreme cases; in such cases they had to be treated in hospitals. We should remember that the transition from childhood to adulthood in modern Western societies today is considered to happen at an older age than is usual in traditional societies. According to the sharia rule, fifteen-year-old teenagers were considered legally mature (*bāligh*); external physical marks or the declaration of the teenager in question could bring the court to regard even younger boys as adults.[98] Today, teenagers are treated in special hospitals for children. It is thus possible that young males of such ages were indeed patients in Ottoman hospitals but were regarded as adults. This too confirms the image of hospitals as an adults-only institution.

This notion that underage children should be treated within the household is related to another phenomenon—namely, the absence of orphanages and foundling homes in early modern Ottoman society, as in other premodern Muslim societies. Raising small children was understood to be the responsibility of the family rather than an obligation of society at large. This task was carried out in various ways. Orphans (Arabic sing. *yatīm*, plural *aytām*—that is, underaged infants or children whose father and/or both parents had died) were generally absorbed into the extended circle of their nuclear family. They were to be absorbed by the wider household and offered a place within a related family that would take over their guardianship. Formal and legal adoption (*tabanni*) was not sanctioned by Muslim scholars, although in practice it seems the custom did exist. The finder of a foundling (sing. *laqīṭ*, pl. *luqaṭā'*—a minor child whose parentage and whose legal status, free or slave, is unknown) was obliged to assume personal responsibility over the child. The responsibility was conferred on him by the wider community, with financial help from the public treasury. We see here how several social authorities shared the responsibilities surrounding abandoned children. This was the spirit of the classical Hanafi legal discourse.[99] As with the case of gender, the expectation that youngsters would not be in need of formal, communal, nonfamily medical help reflects a family-oriented society.

Illness as a Precondition for Defining Entitlement

Those entitled to free medical care in hospital were sick. The foundation deed stated clearly that the institutions were for only for "the sick, the wounded and those who suffer injuries and aches."[100] The administrators were expected to make sure that no one entered the hospitals on false pretences and misused hospital funds. The eunuch administrating the pages' hospital at Topkapı stood vigilant at the door to keep out those wishing to enjoy the free services at the institution. Certainly a common theme in contemporary literature was of people treating hospitals like hotels (in European languages these words ultimately derive from the same root). In this context I am reminded of an anecdote told by the fifteenth-century writer Khalīl bin Shāhīn al-Ẓāhirī about a noble Persian who was witty and had a sense of humor. As mentioned in the previous chapter, the man pretended to be sick in order to be admitted into the Zangid hospital in Damascus and enjoy the full service. After three days the doctor who recognized the scheme hinted that hospitality was only for three days, and the "patient" left the institution discreetly.[101]

Ottoman hospitals were expected to admit all patients regardless of their medical problems. This policy may be deduced from the composition of the medical staff, which included various specialists like internists, oculists, and surgeons. Yet many Ottoman sources mention madmen among the patients and to a great degree totally disregard other sorts of patients. The foundation deeds refer to the possibility of lunatics among the patient population,[102] and travelers described the antics of the mad in the hospitals.[103] The fascination of the sources with this group of patients should not come as a total surprise: lunatics are, after all, more picturesque than people who suffer, for example, from dysentery.

Lunatics could be found in "regular" hospitals throughout the empire. In the Zangid hospital founded in Damascus there were many madmen.[104] In the Ayyubid hospital in Jerusalem founded by Saladin, Dā'ūd b. Muḥammad al-'Ajamiyya was appointed at the beginning of the seventeenth century to the position of caretaker in the hospital to treat the sick and the lunatics; Dā'ūd had inherited this position from his late father.[105] According to Evliya, some of the female patients in the Manṣūrī hospital in Cairo were mad.[106] For Thevenot, the French traveler, the patients in that hospital were first and foremost lunatics; almost as an afterthought he adds that there were also sick poor people in the institution.[107]

The hospitalization of lunatics in "regular" hospitals is not unique to the Ottoman institutions. Treating the madmen alongside the physically ill suited the medical theory of the time, according to which both physiological ailments and mental illnesses were caused by problems in the body and the soul. Michael Dols claimed that the devotion of special space to the mentally ill in the "regular" hospital was the most notable characteristic of hospitals in Muslim societies. Dols's research into marginal groups in the social and medical senses (like lepers and madmen) reveals how much these groups lived at the margins of the mainstream of society but at the same time were incorporated into it, especially the madmen.[108]

What did the patients in hospitals receive? First and foremost, patients received treatment, inclusive of warm and clean beds, food, and physical and mental therapy. And as already been mentioned, in cases where the treatment proved ineffective and the patients passed away, the dead were looked after as well: the institution had the bodies cleansed and buried in shrouds.

Patients in Ottoman hospitals were indeed sick. Here hospitals differed from similar institutions in early modern Ottoman society like the *han*, the *kervan-seray*, and the *tabhane* discussed on page 121. All offered physical aid including temporary lodgings. But hospitals were unique in that the lodgers were sick, not healthy, people. It is possible that in the various hostels for merchants and other wayfarers there were exhausted people to be found also, people who needed bed and board in order to recover their strength or their health. Yet such people did not make use of professional healers there, or at any event this kind of service was not officially offered by institutions other than hospitals.

Hospitals differed from hospices and inns in their policy on the length of stay permitted. Patients were allowed to stay in the hospital without limits on the length of time. Hospices and inns, in contrast, enforced the maximum three-day-stay rule, after which the visitors could no longer enjoy the free services of the institution.[109] We should not underestimate the possibility of an unlimited stay in a hospital. Foreigners who fell sick far away from home had no permanent abode in the place where they became ill. For them the hospital was also a hotel, and thus they were spared the need of looking for a suitable lodging.

The "patients only" policy distinguished Ottoman hospitals from their European counterparts. During the Middle Ages and the early modern period in Europe, the institution called "hospital" was not necessarily associated with sickness and medical care. The clear identification of hospitals with ill people who are treated medically in the institution is a relatively recent phenomenon in the Western world. It should be remembered that the medical knowledge of the time and its application often prescribed no more than rest in a clean and warm place with a nourishing and balanced diet without medication; in consequence, even for "real" patients hospitals could often not offer much more than hospice services. The nonobligation of an institution named "hospital" to treat sick people allowed some hospitals whose mission was to treat sick people to shirk their responsibilities because of budgetary considerations. In other cases, hospitals put into force selective admissions policies, for the same reasons. The managers of Florentine hospitals in the sixteenth century preferred to concentrate their limited resources on the acutely ill rather than the chronically sick, as it could be expected that they would either recover quickly or succumb to their illness; either way, the bed would soon become available for another patient. Illnesses like fevers (a common term for a number of acute infections), fractures, wounds and bites, hemorrhoids, exhaustion, cataracts, dysentery, smallpox, typhus, and constipation (all appear in patients' dossiers) have one thing in common: none are chronic conditions.[110]

An Instrument for Social Control: The Other Side of Charity

The decision about deservedness was based on a combination of criteria. One precondition was being sick, to which other criteria like age, gender, and religious affiliation were added. Here, however, I would like to stress the "pro-foreigner" tendency. Early modern Ottoman society was family-oriented, and as a result the stranger was an alien, not belonging to the community. Being foreign was an abnormal and undesirable situation, yet it was a common phenomenon due to various life constraints. Hence, formal medical charity targeted this specific group as entitled to aid. In their admissions policies hospitals favored the stranger rather than the local community. But medical charity balanced several considerations and communal needs. If the admissions policies favored the foreigner, other aspects of the same institutions discussed below favored the local community.

When considering the full range of services offered by hospitals, we can see that they were quite generous: hospitals served a large number of people.[111] Here we realize that admitting the entitled sick into the hospitals was only one aspect of formal medical charity. Ottoman hospitals (not unlike Italian and English hospitals)[112] offered different types of services to different individuals and groups within the community they served. This "package deal" allowed the donors to reach a vast range of social groups. Moreover, the intentional balance between social groups and needs was meant to bring about social equilibrium. Medical charity in the form of hospitals was transformed into a means of social control.

This is the other side of charity: by giving help, there is much control over those who can—or at least are perceived as able to—threaten the social order. It was Michel Foucault, of course, who argued there was an intentional drive to remove social misfits from European streets. "Dangerous" elements (madmen, beggars, unemployed, criminals, vagabonds, or poor) were confined in institutions like factories, prisons, or hospitals. More broadly, Foucault argued that medical institutions (hospitals, clinics, and lunatic asylums) had more to do with incarceration, exclusion, and authority and its assertion than with medicine and health per se. This reality intensified from the seventeenth century onward when medical perceptions and medical institutions (although masquerading superficially as "harmless" charitable institutions) became intertwined more and more with power and social order.[113]

Foucault has been widely criticized for being ahistorical and all-embracing. Studies more focused in time and place, and on non-French cases (Foucault based himself exclusively on French ones), have suggested another reality.[114] Yet the crux of his theory that knowledge (here: medical knowledge) was used to "mark" marginal groups and reaffirm power and social control has been widely accepted. In this manner hospitals in early modern Europe are explained as vehicles for the reintegration (rather than the isolation) of the sick and poor into the workforce, and thus into society, as productive and self-sufficient people instead of being a burden on welfare services.[115] But this is in fact just another mechanism to achieve control over certain social groups that were deemed by the elite, the hospital founders, as potential threats to the social order. American hospitals were likewise understood as serving a multiplicity of purposes, which included control as well as healing; medical care itself was sometimes incidental to the hospital's larger social purpose.[116]

In early modern Ottoman society, too, medical charitable institutions were used to assume social control. The Ottoman way, however, to reach this goal was quite different from the path outlined by Foucault. Instead of exclusion of specific groups within society, the patrons of Ottoman hospitals chose to be as inclusive as possible. They tried to reach as many people as possible in order to bring them into the fold—that is, into the social patronage of the elite-member donor of the hospital. This subtle (yet binding) method was complemented by other means that were more aggressive and obvious. Indeed, in certain cases the mechanism involved more than virtual obligation, with more direct control, whether physical or financial. At the same time, medical institutions were a fulfillment of duties by the head of the household towards his protégées. The donors revealed their interest in preserving the social status quo, and their use of medical charity was a springboard for achieving this. This dual obligation and mutual dependence, the gift relationship, resulted in a cohesive society.

Ottoman hospitals offered a variety of services in which medical treatment was only one component among many, not necessarily medicine-related. Ottoman hospitals were aimed at sick patients who needed medical treatment. However, these patients were only one of the groups that used the institutions' services. Hospitals reached beyond their walls in their services. There were several concentric circles of services around the hospitals.

The first circle contained those patients admitted to the hospitals who had to spend time there. The prosopography of this group was the subject of the previous section. That discussion dealt with the intertwined questions of who were deemed worthy of medical help by benevolent patrons and who were the patients in their hospitals in reality. One conclusion is that the patient population in hospitals was rather varied. It included patients from many social and economic strata and different age groups who suffered from a variety of medical problems. Most patients were male, but a few institutions catered—separately—to women as well. Yet the patients were certainly more homogeneous than is implied in the foundation deeds and travelers' descriptions. The *vakfiye*s describe an institution open almost to all. The phrasing used by Evliya Çelebi, for example, refers to old and young, poor and rich, but his more concrete description creates the image of a rather homogeneous group of adult "middle-class" men. It is possible that both the authors of the endowment deeds and Evliya Çelebi aimed to give the impression of an ideal situation—or perhaps wished to present a high standard to Ottoman philanthropists. In reality, however, only certain groups in society were represented among hospital patients.

The tendency toward homogeneity in the patient population was due to a double selectivity. On the one hand, the social and cultural codes accepted as norms in Ottoman society restricted the variety of people approaching hospitals and the circumstances in which they did so. On the other hand, some hospital administrators directed their limited resources toward the more deserving among their patients (at least in their eyes). I would like to suggest here that presenting the stranger as worthy and entitled could have stemmed from the wish to put an end to his status as a stranger. As a stranger he had no local affiliations. He was transparent and thus outside the control mechanism of the community. By allowing him into hospitals he was put in debt to the local community, which now knew of him, about him, and could oversee him.

Another example of using hospital admittance policy in order to control a specific, potentially dangerous, group was the case of madmen who were confined in various institutions. This was done not to madmen as such but to madmen who were considered by the state to be politically or socially dangerous to the social order. In various instances dealing with cases of madmen, both among ordinary people and among the sultans, physicians were not consulted; bureaucrats, religious-legal scholars, and judges were those involved. Practically, madness was defined and constructed by the state. This is Boaz Shoshan's main criticism of Michael Dols's seminal work, *Majnun*; Shoshan pointed out that Dols in fact does not define the phenomenon of madness in medieval Muslim societies.[117]

Evliya Çelebi reported that the madmen of Edirne were put in chains and were brought to the city hospital. These were "love fools," the victims of the spring malady, and had nothing to do directly with politics. Yet the authorities had them removed forcibly from the streets, maybe because they were deemed able to disrupt the social order. Nonetheless, many madmen in Istanbul roamed the streets freely and were part of this colorful city. They wandered naked and barefoot on snowy days, danced and played tricks for an audience, or frightened Jewish mourners at funerals when they spat on them and knocked over the gurney bearing the body. These examples of improper sexual, social, and religious behavior (they were supposed to be lunatics, after all) apparently were considered harmless by the authorities.[118] Another Istanbul case did end in confinement because it happened in Istanbul. The behavior of the madman was not that eccentric, but his thoughts and public speeches were. This was in 1653, when the authorities of Istanbul arrested Şeyh Mahmud, originally from Diyarbakr in eastern Anatolia, on the order of the imperial council (*divan*). He was hospitalized at the Süleymaniye hospital. The man was proclaiming that the solution to the empire's misery was the remarriage of Turhan Sultan, the mother of the sultan Mehmet IV, and her removal from the imperial harem. The great lady, although a widow, was still a young woman. The old *şeyh* gathered many admirers in Istanbul, who considered him to be a saint. The contents of his sermons, his growing audience, and the fact it was all taking place in the capital made his preaching politically dangerous in the eyes of the divan.

The example of the madmen illustrates that local people, rather than only foreigners were entitled to receive services from the hospital. Another avenue was to be an "outpatient"—that is, a sick man who was not formally admitted into the hospital but was entitled to make use of hospital services. This is the second circle of patients served by hospitals. Generally, the endowment deeds admonished the administrators of hospitals to refrain from financing the medical needs of people outside the hospital: medication and food should be given only to patients in the hospital. However, the same *vakfiye*s also clarified the circumstances in which administrators could depart from this rule. In an early *vakfiye*, Mehmet II stated that physicians must not distribute food, drinks, or medications to people other than those staying in the hospital. There was an exception, though: if some particular medication was not available outside, the doctor was indeed allowed to give it. Although the warning appears in both versions, the exception is found only in the fifteenth-century version.[119] This suggests that the exception may have caused too much expenditure and as a result was later revoked. In Hurrem Sultan's Istanbul hospital the two physicians were instructed to hold "open days" twice a week, on Mondays and Thursdays. Those in need could come and ask for their help. But the donor stressed that also in these cases medication was to be given only to the really needy (and deserving), not to just anybody.[120]

Those who received treatment and medication at home constituted a third circle of patients around the hospital, as is suggested by the provision included in the *vakfiye* of Mehmet II that a herbalist was to make special medications and take them to the "assigned places" (a detailed explanation is not provided). The foundation deed also stipulated that once a week the administrator, the head physicians, and the clerk should convene in the hospital to discuss medical cases of sick people at home who were not strong enough to call a doctor or who had no money to pay for a private physician and the medication that he or she prescribed. To these people a doctor was to be sent with medications from the hospital's supply depot.[121] This should not be understood to mean that treatment at home was considered better than that at the hospital. Rather, if a person was so sick at home that he could not leave his bed to purchase his medications, there was no need to transfer him to the hospital: for these severe cases doctors from the institution conducted house calls.

Hospitals catered also to the healthy members of the community. They fulfilled a public role. In the hospital in Manisa the head physician in the sixteenth century used to prepare a medicinal paste (*ma'cun*) based on a secret recipe. The paste was very famous in the area, and it was believed to have magical therapeutic properties. Its medical components were discussed in the first chapter, and here its public and ceremonial aspects are highlighted. The paste was distributed during public ceremonies on special occasions like the Nevruz celebration for the Persian New Year's Day.[122]

It seems that Ottoman hospitals offered some kind of education program for physicians and medical students, perhaps following previous traditions, as we have hints that Seljukid hospitals in the Anatolian towns of Konya and Tokat served as medical schools,[123] although the extent to which Ottoman hospitals played a role in educating future physicians is still a matter of debate. In premodern societies medical knowledge was gained by various means. One could study in a "formal" way with a family member, with a private tutor, in public classes in hospitals or in mosques, or in the very few designated medical schools (in the early modern Ottoman Empire there was only one school formally designated as a medical school, the school at the Süleymaniye complex in Isṭanbul). Autodidactic learning and apprenticeship with a practicing physician were popular too. Non-Muslims could also study in European universities (this option was open mainly to Christians, as Jews were usually excluded from this institution). One could also skip organized study altogether if one claimed professional legitimacy due to supernatural qualities and initiation. All were deemed of similar quality in educating future doctors, although physicians raised professional ethical claims against their competitors in order to gain the upper hand (and social and financial gains). The Geniza suggests that in medieval Egypt, Jewish medical students awarded extra prestige to hospital posts and vied for them during their specialization.[124] The Ottoman case is less clear-cut.

Several Turkish scholars took it almost for granted that hospitals played a pivotal role in rearing the next generation of physicians according to the highest standards. A tone of pride accompanied their claim. However, their evidence seems to relate mostly to one specific hospital, that of Mehmed II in Istanbul, and this evidence is too sporadic and anecdotal to generalize from. An example is a reference in the endowment deed to two medical students attached to the hospital who were allowed to dine at the nearby public kitchen like all hospital personnel; yet there is no mention of them in the section related to the hospital itself. Yet another piece of evidence is a tradition of appointing students to this hospital during the eighteenth century.[125]

Who was this medical student? Was he a student or someone further up in his career as a physician? His vague identity demonstrates the problematic evidence pertaining to the educational functions of hospitals. The Ottoman term used in the documents, *şakird*, is ambiguous. It can mean a pupil, but the term also carries the meaning of a novice or an apprentice (in a shop, workshop, or a bureaucratic office). In the context of the Ottoman medical institution I suggest it is more appropriate to identify the *şakird* with the medical intern rather than with a student. Medicine was not unlike career paths in other Ottoman institutions. When a student finished his studies in a *medrese* and aspired to a career in the religious institution (*ilmiyye*) as a *müderris* or a *kadi*, he had to serve first as a candidate (*mülazim*) before receiving his first appointment to a real position as a religious scholar. This in-between rank was a means to control the increasing numbers of students vying for a much smaller number of positions. Likewise, in the central administration (*kalemiyye*) there was a position of junior clerk in an office (*şakird*). The medical *şakirds* worked beside a senior practitioner in hospitals and palaces. Upon the opening of a new job in the Ottoman medical establishment, they were promoted to junior positions.[126]

The presence of several interns in some hospitals allows us to say that hospitals took an informal and sporadic role in the education of medical doctors. Even if they were not a prime site for medical education, hospitals nevertheless served the medical community at large. This explains why many medical treatises were to be found in the hospital of Mehmet II in Istanbul. The were probably for the doctors at the institution and perhaps also to be lent to other physicians.[127]

The most obvious way in which hospitals served the healthy members of the community was by being an employer. People of different types of education and manual capabilities—medical and otherwise—earned their living in hospitals. Whether doctors, attendants, builders, or gravediggers, hospitals increased their employment opportunities in a world characterized by chronic financial risks. Moreover, workers at the hospitals of the empire were organized in a clear professional hierarchy, expressed through wages. Here we can see the more obvious means of using medical charity to bring about the social order: this was achieved by controlling their wages and their moral and professional behavior.

Physicians were supposed to integrate the theoretical knowledge of medicine with the experience and professional skills needed to diagnose and heal according to their respective disciplines (there were three: "general" practitioners, surgeons, and ophthalmologists), while their personal character remained unblemished.[128] The high standards demanded of physicians can be understood in the context of medicine being perceived also as an art of knowledge (*ilm*) and wisdom (*hikmet*). The classical view of medicine as a liberal occupation included an image of the ideal physician as a philosopher. However, that does not explain why high standards of professional and moral rectitude according to their rank and function were expected of all personnel, from the lowest menial worker who emptied the chamber pots by the patients' beds (*ibrizi*) up to the head physician. The foundation deeds gave instructions as to how each duty was to be fulfilled. The *ibrizi*s, like the male servants (*hadem* or *qayyim*), the cooks (*tabbah*), and the bakers (*habbaz* or *neqib-i nan*), were directed to approach the patients with a pleasant smile and gentle talk to ward off melancholy. The hospital clerks in charge of provisions (*vekil-i harc*) and the budget (*katib* or *emin-i sarf*) were to be honest. Their account books were regularly scrutinized.[129]

As discussed in the previous chapter, the process of diagnosis, treatment, and recovery, and hygiene procedures in general, brought healers and patients into intimate physical contact. This demanded extra attention to the moral character of the people involved in order to preserve modesty in the physical and moral sense. This was done by presenting an ideal high standard in deontological discussions combined with actual attempts to implement it. And indeed, Evliya Çelebi remarked that most (but not all . . .) staff members in hospitals were good, pure, and pious.[130]

Physicians who had not fulfilled their duties for the patients of the hospital were admonished. If after being warned once and twice they still did not mend their ways, they were dismissed. This was the fate in 1606 of Ismail, a junior physician (*tabib-i sani*) in Hurrem's hospital in Istanbul. He was found guilty of not paying the appropriate attention to his duties. He did not even concern himself enough to arrange for a replacement (*naib*) during his (nonauthorized) leaves of absence. He was dismissed from his post and replaced by Mustafa.[131] Ali, another junior physician, this time from the Istanbul hospital of Sultan Ahmet I, was dismissed in November 1679 after being reprimanded. Abdül Rahman from the hospital of Süleyman I was promoted and received his post.[132]

Physicians were transferred from one post to another, sometimes without their consent. Hasan, a physician from Amasya, refused to move to the Konya hospital where he had been reassigned. His explanation was that being a native of Amasya he preferred staying in the local hospital in town. In summer of 1574 his demand was approved. The reasoning put forward by the central bureaucracy is telling: it was feared he would incite the staff in the hospital to which he was sent. The administration chose to capitulate to Hasan's demand instead of confronting him over his audacity in order to keep the personnel content in both institutions. Aladdin, who had been meant to replace Hasan in Amasya, was sent in his stead to Konya.[133]

The variety of services weaving together various social groups means that medical charity was used as a means to create and nurture ties of loyalty in Ottoman society. Likewise, the regular visits of the sultan and the chief black eunuch were an intimate expression of patron-client relationships. Like the *majalis*, the social and cultural meetings in a ruler's salon, the meetings in the hospitals were a scene where formal interactions based on personal and face-to-face meetings took place. These meetings reaffirmed patronage ties, acting as a subtle means of regulation and keeping order.[134]

CHAPTER 4

Spaces of Disease, Disease in Space

Concepts of illness and health form our understanding of space and our use of it. In particular, etiological theories (attempts to explain the causes of illness) affect our perceptions of movement through space. These theories shape the directions of human movement, because they define certain places as dangerous. History offers numerous examples of occasions when people, including healers, evacuated their place of residence at the first sign of deadly plague in the neighborhood. Etiological theories can determine even the possibility of movement—for example, when these theories lead to the isolation of people and goods in quarantine. While illness restricts only the freedom of the ill, etiological theories affect the healthy as well. Etiologies are human creations, but in turn these theories also constrain human beings.

This chapter discusses urban space in Ottoman towns in the early modern period and how this space was shaped by such concepts and ideas. Drawing on social science literature going back to Durkheim and Mauss, the discussion revolves around spatial organization and medical knowledge. It deals with the interrelationships between medical knowledge, social practice, and physical design. The working hypothesis is that space and architecture are socially produced rather than naturally given. They are not absolute passive concepts, but rather are active ingredients in society. As a result, spatial divisions and categorizations are understood as an arena for the interplay of symbols. The same applies to architectural styles: although they are the product of individual creativity, they are not solely the product of personal imagination. The design is an inherent part of its social world and reflects a discourse with regard to the building. Buildings are artifacts of culture as well as individual constructions. They reflect morals, ideas, needs, social understanding, and conduct.[1] Every building is a domain of knowledge and a domain of control as it orders categories and boundaries in space. In the words of Jonathan Hughes, "Architectural design is not a neutral, value-free resource from which architects draw as desired. The layout, design, and styling of buildings can manifest the geographically- and temporally-localized thinking, aspirations, and prejudices of their designers and clients . . . the conflict of clinical, social and architectural ideas, which justifies . . . the development of a particularly influential architectural solution."[2]

The materials analyzed are learned medical treatises, legal discussions, and lay references in various genres of literature touching on spatial organization and medical knowledge as well as one specific medical institution that physically embodied abstract discussions—namely, the hospital. Hospitals are a special case of buildings, and embody principles of medical knowledge. They disclose concepts of health and illness and can reveal changing objects of medical attention. Hospitals in their physical format and inner space reveal not only what people thought of or discussed in theory, but which—and how—medical concepts were shaped in actual instances of human use of medical institutions and spaces. Decisions about where hospitals should be located in space and about how their inner space should be constructed reflect what a given society recognizes as the main causes of illness.[3] In any society there may exist several competing theories about the causes of illness and the nature of health. Theories discussed in learned medical treatises may not be the ones that are actually accepted by the society at large.

The physical aspects of hospitals founded by the Ottomans in their capitals—Bursa, Edirne, and Istanbul—are the focus of our study, including their locations in the urban space and their individual structure. However, the aim is not to focus on the architectural aspects of these buildings as such, but rather to discuss how contemporary Ottomans perceived these buildings as revealed by chronicles, biographical dictionaries, and pictorial miniatures. I shall also compare the physical attributes of Ottoman hospitals with those of their European counterparts, following in the footsteps of European travelers in the Ottoman Empire. European visitors to the empire were both astonished and puzzled by the medical institutions that they saw there, and they have left us a number of valuable descriptions of the contrasts between what they saw in the Orient and what they had left behind at home.

The discussion raises two fundamental questions. The first is this: how did medical conceptions about health and illness common among Ottomans in the sixteenth and seventeenth centuries shape their decisions about where to locate hospitals in specific urban spaces and about how to construct the individual buildings? The Ottomans understood human beings as a composition of body and soul. An integralistic understanding shaped the Ottoman understanding of health, illness, and medical treatment. These conceptions affected decisions as where to situate a hospital and what its environment and physical characteristics should be.

The second question at the center of this chapter asks what can be discerned from hospital locations and building characteristics about the attitudes of Ottomans toward the ill "other." Those defined as mad are a special case: they drew much attention from contemporaries, local Ottomans as well as European visitors. The patients in hospitals became one of the marginal groups in the Ottoman society, yet the physical and emotional closeness contemporaries felt toward them was quite considerable. Moreover, madness and physical illness catalogued a person as "other" only temporarily: once people recuperated and left the hospital, the ex-patients were once again equal members of the majority group in the Ottoman society, the healthy.

Ottoman Medical Institutions as Urban Institutions

Understanding the siting of Ottoman medical institutions—hospitals, convalescent homes, and doctors' private clinics—poses a methodological problem for modern students. The benevolent founders, the architects, or contemporary observers of these hospitals did not leave us written explanations of their reasons for choosing particular sites. The discussion that follows is therefore a retrospective reconstruction of what those considerations might have been.

The Ottomans situated their medical institutions only in cities, and generally only in major urban centers at that. In the early modern period hospitals, for example, were founded in Bursa, Edirne, and Istanbul, the three imperial capitals. Some hospitals were founded in important provincial towns as well, like Manisa, Mecca, and Tunis. In other towns, like Damascus, Aleppo, or Cairo, hospitals had existed in the pre-Ottoman period, and they continued to function, despite financial hardship, well into the eighteenth century at the very least. The rural population in the Ottoman Empire had different organizations for medical aid despite the fact that land was cheaper in these areas in comparison to dense cities. And certainly the rural population was ill as well.

Why did the founders insist on founding medical institutions only in the cities? The answer lies in a combination of financial considerations and cultural and social motivations that create unique relationship between medicine and urban life. These shape the structure and functions of medical institutions and practice in an urban context. As in other European cities,[4] medical institutions played multifaceted roles in Ottoman cities.

Historically, urban life has the reputation of being unhealthy.[5] It was partially true. Towns displayed a greater need for formal medical aid than rural settlements (or the need was perceived as greater in cities). Students of nineteenth-century European and American cities observed that poverty and charity went hand in hand as integral parts of urban life. And although the supply of charity varied with political and intellectual fashions, economics and demography meant that the demand for charity was more constant and pressing. They point out that urban artisanal work experienced a remarkable inconsistency, not unlike agricultural labor with its built-in unreliability due to seasonality, crop failures, and limited marketing opportunities. However, urbanites had fewer support systems, and as a result could experience more financial catastrophes.[6]

Granted, the lack of safety valves in early modern Ottoman society did not lead to a situation as intense as in nineteenth-century European and American cities. Yet the comparison does point out the characteristics of urban communities that resulted in real, as well as imagined, pressing needs for new forms of medical aid. Although the population in the rural countryside was not necessarily healthier, its social composition was simpler. Big towns, maybe more so than villages, include many people who cannot take care of themselves medically: either they lack the necessary financial means or do not have a social network of family or friends to rely on in their time of need. Consider the case of the many visitors to the towns: students, merchants, workers, travelers, or adventurers. They all lacked local support. Foreigners were indeed one group of patients entitled to hospital care.

Another type of a social need in urban centers was felt not by the hospital's possible clientele but by their founders. Hospitals were aimed to further their interests as well. Here, in cities, especially the central ones, the elite was more pressured socially and politically to supply clear visual symbols of their dedication to the welfare of the community. They were expected to justify their status and privileges. For the founders, situating a hospital in towns publicized their actions more widely and maximized their gains from their investment. After all, an urban institution enjoys a wider visibility.[7]

Combined with the greater needs, urban communities also possessed greater abilities to supply those needs. As far as finances are concerned, medical institutions and especially hospitals, then as today, are costly. They demand a high investment in human and financial resources. The investment needed for day-to-day operation is considerable as well. Stable surplus for such projects can be found only in cities, not in villages or even in small provincial centers. Hence, in a global context, hospitals—as an idea and a durable reality—were possible usually in urban economies.[8]

Hospitals were established in several major urban centers in the Ottoman Empire but not in all of them, not even in all the towns that had special political, military, or economic importance, or in all the larger towns. Ottomans generally chose to build their hospitals in places where there were no previous hospitals. When they did build where hospitals previously existed, it was in areas where Christians had operated. A prime example is Constantinople. Prior to 1453 several Byzantine medical institutions functioned in the city, yet the Ottomans founded five more of their own.

Even if the Ottoman policy regarding the issue of hospital location was clear—it was certainly consistent—the reasons behind it are not. One could suspect that the Christian flavor connected with the Byzantine hospitals prevented the Ottomans from integrating these institutions into their own medical system. Certainly, the Ottomans were not the first Muslim dynasty to forgo the use of conquered Christian medical institutions, yet they were not averse to recruiting the Christian medical personnel to their personal household or the medical institutions they patronized. We can find an example in Saladin (d. 1193). He did not use the Crusader hospital in Jerusalem but initiated another one in a converted church. He did hire, however, Christian physicians from the Crusader institution.[9] However, we know the Ottoman policy was to Islamize churches and transform them into mosques. It was a symbolic act claiming superiority. The Ottomans had to invest quite a lot in order to make a church into a building capable of serving as a mosque (adding minarets on the outside and a prayer niche in the inside, and whitewashing the religious scenes illuminating the church, to name only the most obvious steps that were needed).

The problem of conversion of buildings did not arise when it came to incorporating hospitals surviving from previous Muslim dynasties. The Ottomans refrained from erecting new hospitals in several important cities in Anatolia, where pre-Ottoman institutions functioned. However, they did continue to use the Il-Khanid hospital in Amasya and the Seljuk ones in Kayseri and Sivas. A similar situation existed in Aleppo, Damascus, and Cairo, the three important centers in the

Arab provinces, where Zangid and Mamluk hospitals continued to function during the Ottoman period as well. The difference between the Christian hospitals and the pre-Ottoman Muslim ones lies in the fact that the latter resembled those which the Ottomans established themselves in their administration and medical practice. These hospitals were established under the auspices of a *vakıf* system—that is, they were endowed charities, and practiced humoral Galenic medicine as interpreted by Muslim doctors.

Mecca and Medina, the holy cities of Islam, are a special case. The Ottomans "inherited" a Meccan hospital from Nūr al-Dīn Maḥmūd Zangī (d. 1174), who also founded hospitals in Damascus and Aleppo.[10] But during the sixteenth and seventeenth centuries three more hospitals were added to the city. Hurrem Sultan, the concubine and later the wife of Süleyman I, erected the first one in the middle of the sixteenth century.[11] Toward the end of that century the Ottoman grand vizier Sokollu Mehmet Paşa established yet another medical institution. A century later the concubine of the Ottoman sultan Mehmet IV, Gülnuş Sultan, had a third hospital established in her name. Mecca and Medina were the destination of many pilgrims all year round, but especially so during the hajj season. A town with so many strangers might well have needed more medical facilities. Combined with this motivation was the fact that any form of philanthropy in a pilgrimage place attracts that much more publicity not only in the Ottoman lands but in many other parts of the Muslim world as a whole. Therefore there was strong motivation to choose Mecca as the site of charity, seemingly with no regard to the already existing institutions.

Hurrem's two hospitals in Mecca and in Istanbul, respectively, suggest adding hospitals to those already existing in Mecca was more complex than simple. Hurrem attracted much attention and controversy in her time, and the details surrounding her Istanbul project are abundant. The sources, however, are silent when it comes to the hospital in Mecca. Could it be that they were not aware of Hurrem's charitable act in the holy city? Did they not care about or appreciate the bountiful donation? Or maybe it was the result of the sources being authored by Istanbulis who were interested in the capital to the point of ignoring of anything outside the imperial center.

As mentioned, the most famous hospitals were built in the imperial capitals: Bursa, Edirne, and Istanbul. Most of these institutions were commissioned by the reigning sultan. However, sultans did not necessarily choose their capital as the host site for their hospital. Mehmet II, Süleyman I, and Ahmet I built in Istanbul. Yet Beyazid I erected his hospital in Bursa toward the end of the fourteenth century, although shortly before that the capital had moved to Edirne. Beyazid II built his impressive hospital in Edirne around 1500, when Istanbul had already been the imperial capital for fifty years. Although Beyazid II established a rich endowment in Istanbul as well, it did not include a medical institution. The building projects of Beyazid I and Beyazid II hint that Bursa and Edirne still enjoyed imperial status, at least to some extent, even after the official seat of government moved elsewhere.

One can point to a common denominator of the three sultanic complexes (Turkish, *külliye*) in Istanbul, which included hospitals: they established a new standard in the city and in the empire as a whole for imperial architectural grandeur. Each was constructed so as to be grander than preceding hospitals in its size, design, ornament, and the value of the building materials used. Their unique structure and visibility in the landscape complemented the policies of the founding sultans: the hospitals were a means to an end, enhancing the image that the sultans wished to project in public.

The sultanic complexes, and other projects financed by Ottoman elite members imitating the sultan, transformed the city into a center of Ottoman and Islamic knowledge and monumental structures. The complex of Mehmet II in Istanbul spearheaded a vast project of building a new capital and reviving the recently conquered city. The complexes in the new capital of Istanbul were thus one proof of the Ottoman claims to be worthy heirs to the Byzantine heritage. The Süleymaniye, named after its builder, Sultan Süleyman I, included several educational institutions, mostly teaching Islamic subjects, but included a hospital and a medical school as well. The complex symbolized Süleyman's policy of enhancing orthodox Sunni Islam throughout the empire and reaffirming his own legitimacy.[12] Ahmet I commissioned a hospital in his complex in Istanbul at the beginning of the seventeenth century. Ahmet I's extravagant complex created some public resentment when it became evident that its mosque boasted no fewer then six minarets: the maximum number for a sultanic imperial mosque until then and thereafter was four.

The sultans focused their building efforts, including hospitals, in the imperial cities. In the provincial cities the hospitals were built by other members of the Ottoman elite: female members of the imperial family, viziers, and local governors. The hospitals in Mecca built in the sixteenth and seventeenth centuries have already been mentioned above. We should supplement this list with the hospital in Manisa added to the complex of Hafsa Sultan, Süleyman's mother; the hospital in Ottoman Tunis commissioned by the local governor (the only one in town); and other hospitals built in Salonica, Belgrade, and Budapest.[13]

There are two more hospitals of interest, both of which were established by imperial women in the sixteenth century. These hospitals, built by Hurrem and Nurbanu, mother of Murad III, are unique in that they are the only medical institutions built by female members of the imperial family in Istanbul in the early modern period. In fact, only Hurrem's hospital was located in Istanbul proper. Nurbanu's was very visible on a high hill, but on the Asian shore of the Bosphorus, in Üskudar.

The establishment of a grand complex in Hurrem's name (to be more precise, under her title as Haseki, "the favorite concubine") in a central site in the capital did arouse controversy in the sixteenth century. Traces of this can be found in George Sandys's writings. Sandys, an English traveler who visited Istanbul a century after the events, claimed that the chief mufti of the empire refused to recognize Hurrem's project as a charitable act. The mufti was angered that a concubine—legally a slave—was allowed to endow a charitable institution, as one of the legal stipulations for endowments is that the founder be a free Muslim.[14]

Other critics did not concern themselves with the identity of the founder. Rather, they focused on Hurrem's decision to build a substantial complex in a prime location in the capital. They had an issue with her grandiose plan and the sultan's permission to act upon her decision to found what they saw as a megalomanic complex for a woman. Many imperial women before Hurrem were active in charitable activities, but their foundations were built separately; when they initiated complexes, those were located outside the capital. Hurrem's charity in Istanbul, however, rivaled in its size that of the major imperial charitable complexes in the city (though not that of Süleyman). It was the first of five big building projects during Süleyman's reign. The mosque within the complex was rather modest: attached to it was (only) one minaret, as distinct from other mosques erected by women of Süleyman's family, which were adorned by the two minarets allowed to members of the imperial family save the sultan who could boast four. However, the number of affiliated foundations and their size made a strong impression. On the one hand, the complex was built at a distance from the center of town and other imperial foundations for a reason. On the other hand, the site was deliberately chosen: it was associated with the nearby "Women's Market." To her critics, who bore a grudge because of her exceptional power in Süleyman's court, the unique complex symbolized the fact that Hurrem played by her own rules. Yet she was only the first of several strong and publicly active women in the Ottoman imperial family during the sixteenth century. It was a period of transition when the dynasty started to enhance the public role of imperial women, including their benevolent patronage, to compensate for the changing images of the sovereign and the withdrawal of the sultans behind the walls of Topkapı Palace in the period after Süleyman. Among these women, the *haseki*, the favorite concubine, was the first to gain strength. With her "the sultanate of the women" starts. Then toward the end of sixteenth century, power moved to the sultan's mother (the *valide-i sultan*), and the role of the favorite diminished as a result. Being the first visible female figure and a concubine whose position was elevated, Hurrem had to endure cruel public scrutiny.[15] The inclusion of a hospital in the complex, not a common feature of charitable endowments, was one factor that distinguished Hurrem's project from others.

Each social stratum and professional group in Ottoman society was identified by its unique clothes and architectural activity. The architecture of buildings revealed the social position of their founders. Size, site, dome dimensions, cost of building materials, richness of ornaments, and originality of planning—all reflected class.[16] Hospitals are a subtle stratifying element in comparison to minarets or domes, which are much more visible; in contrast to mosques, hospitals do not reveal their function unless one approaches the actual building and identifies it, with the help of inscriptions. Yet, the addition of a hospital to the more common institutions within a complex helped to single out the project as an imperial one, associated with a member of the Ottoman family.

Ottoman Medical Institutions within the Urban Landscape

The foundation of hospitals was thus the product of much thought and intention on the part of the initiators. As a result they were very revealing for Ottomans. Hospitals were signposts in the city and helped to make sense of the use and inner hierarchy of urban space.

Once the decision to erect a hospital was made, it was time to think about the actual site, and here several factors came into play. In addition to political considerations of hospital location, logistics had to be taken into account. An important issue was the accessibility of running water. Hospitals, like the hammams, were in constant need of considerable quantities of water. Water was vital for maintaining high levels of hygiene in the building and its surroundings; insuring its continued supply was an important task for the administrators. Water was used for cooking and for the gardens around the building. And if the treatment failed, water was needed to purify the dead to prepare them for burial. The managers of the hospital of Mehmet II hired several porters to carry water to the building (*saqa*).[17] Presumably, the amount of running water in the hospital was not sufficient, and there was a need to supplement it manually.

Hospital location and construction also had to take into account the need to drain sewage from patients' rooms, the latrines, the bath, and the kitchen. The sewage system in the Bursa hospital of Beyazid I was one of its unique features. An underground canal ran under the patients' rooms in the eastern wing, then joined the latrines to collect sewage in the building, exploiting the slope on which the building is situated. One hundred years later, a similar system was installed in the Edirne hospital of Beyazid II.[18]

The dependence of hospitals on running water and sewage systems may explain the inclusion of hospitals in charitable complexes. The Ottomans did not erect hospitals separately but incorporated them into complexes comprising several buildings, whether mosques, soup kitchens, or schools. Installing water supply and drainage systems was costly in terms of human and financial resources, and required an architect to plan them carefully. A comprehensive system had to locate water sources, collect water in reservoirs, perhaps far away from the site of actual use, and lay down networks of pipes, aqueducts, and distribution points. It was therefore more cost-effective and efficient to include hospitals in complexes in which several buildings shared an infrastructure. Dividing water at the site in order to distribute it to the different buildings required neither a basic change in plan nor a major financial investment, and the same applies to the sewage system.[19]

Urban Medical Institutions, Environment, and Gardens

There were many cultural considerations that affected hospital location. Hospitals thus can be very revealing to modern students of medicine and society. In situating hospitals in major urban centers of the empire, and in prime locations within the cities themselves, the Ottomans demonstrated a lack of fear of ill people. Ill people were an integral part of society.[20]

It is true that two imperial hospitals were built outside the cities. One is the hospital of Beyazid I in Bursa, located on a hill northeast of the walled city. Yet the hospital did not remain outside the city limits for long. The intention of the planners was not to isolate it totally; the complex was designed to serve as the locus of a new settlement, to be absorbed into the urban tissue as the city grew. Quite soon, more complexes were built outside the walls, drew the city limits eastward, and thus "closed" the open space.[21]

Beyazid II built his Edirne hospital outside the city, on the banks of the Tunca River. In fact, during high tides the water lapped at the foundations of the complex. Later on, a stretch of land between the complex and the river was filled in order to protect the buildings.[22] The architect who planned the complex anticipated that the clientele for this establishment would arrive from the land side to the west, and not across the river (from the city). Therefore the complex was situated with its back to the river, although the view of the banks at this point is especially engaging.[23] Yet Evliya Çelebi, the renowned Ottoman traveler, observed that the hospital was well known to the population in town who regarded strolling to the complex as an enjoyable excursion.

Hospitals originally within towns became located in central junctions in the city. The sites played on several layers of meaning in the urban fabric—for example, in cases where the chosen location carried importance from earlier periods. Mehmet II founded his hospital in such a place. The hospital was included in a complex erected on a hill by one of the main thoroughfares in the capital, which connected Edirnekapı, a central gate in the walls, with the city center. Moreover, the complex was built on the ruins of a famous Byzantine church, the Church of the Holy Apostles. Now Mehmet II added an Ottoman-Muslim layer of meaning to the famous Byzantine site. He chose this particular site to launch his project to revive the city, which contemporaries described as deserted after the fall of Constantinople. Süleyman's hospital is another example: it was included in a complex built on the ruins of the old imperial palace erected by Mehmet II near the bazaar toward the end of the fifteenth century. Hurrem and Nurbanu founded their respective hospitals and complexes in places that at the time were not central, but were an incentive to populate new and important neighborhoods.[24] Ahmet I built his hospital in a complex situated in the central square of Istanbul, Atmeydanı (literally, "The Horses' Square," after the Byzantine hippodrome previously occupying that site). The square is situated opposite the famous imperial mosque of Ayasofya near the main entrance to Topkapı Palace through the Imperial Gate (Bab-ı Hümayun).

The hospital in the Topkapı, the imperial palace in Istanbul, was established in the first court, open to the public. Necipoğlu speculated that the hospital was removed intentionally from the servant dormitories in the private sectors in the palace in order to prevent the spread of disease among courtiers.[25] If fear of contagion was the reason for that decision, it does not seem consistent with the decision to locate a health risk in the first court. The danger there seems greater, as many passersby milled around the hospital and were in direct contact with the patients: they could carry disease with them outside the palace and cause its spread (something that never happened, apparently, or at least the sources are silent about such a case). As is argued below, the notion of contagion and humans as disease carriers were not necessarily prevalent among health-care workers in the early modern Ottoman Empire.

Leprosy, it seems, was regarded differently. The few lazarettos in the empire were situated outside the city walls. Evliya Çelebi devoted an entire volume of his *Book of Travels* (*Seyahatname*) to the description of Istanbul. In it he tells of the leprosarium (*mikinhane*) built on the Asian shore of Istanbul, in Üsküdar. When a leper was discovered within the city limits of Istanbul, he was stripped of his safe-conduct authorization (*aman*), which allowed him to dwell in the city. The leper was then taken to the far-off institution on Asian shores of the city. Evliya explained that since leprosy plagued the regions of Anatolia, cases of leprosy were not ignored. Outside each city there was a special house where the lepers could live their lives comfortably, but apart from the healthy population, with whom they were forbidden to mingle. He said that the situation in the Arab provinces and Egypt was worse: there were many lepers there. Yet in Egypt the attitude toward lepers was different, apparently. Evliya claimed that there were no leper houses there.[26] Both attitudes—namely, the distancing of lazarettos (in contrast to hospitals) as well as accepting lepers wandering on the outskirts of the community on their own—found support in canonical hadith compilations. According to one, Muhammad instructed his followers to "flee from the leper as you flee from the lion"; according to another, the Prophet invited a leper to share his food and eat from his plate.[27]

Being a component in charitable institutions meant that hospitals—and their ill patients—were located very close to mosques. Physical and mental ailments, which regardless of the specific etiological explanation advocated (several coexisted in the Ottoman world, as will be discussed below) were associated with pollution or infection, are combined with purity and holiness. Here is evidence that the dichotomy of holiness and impurity, so fascinating for scholars, was far from being concretely realized in the Ottoman empire.[28] The hospital in the Süleymaniye complex is an example of the close contact between the two types of buildings. The hospital was situated in the far corner of the complex, which included several learning institutions, a soup kitchen, a hostel, a hammam, and so on. Yet the distance from the northwest corner where the hospital was located to the mosque doors did not exceed one hundred meters. Those frequenting the mosque knew what was going on in the hospital. In addition to being in the vicinity of holy mosques, there were prayer halls in the mosques themselves for the benefit of the patients and staff members. Personnel in charge of religious tasks, members of the ulema, were regular staff members in hospitals. In these hospitals, like in the institutions of Beyazid II in Edirne or Nurbanu in Istanbul, a corner in the hospital itself was designated for religious uses. In other cases, hospitals had their mosques in a different building near the main hospital wing. The mosques of the hospitals of Mehmet II and Ahmet I operated in separate buildings adjacent to the hospital.[29]

The Ottomans built on earlier precedents. The thirteenth-century hospital in Akşehir boasted an independent mosque within its precinct, although it is not clear whether it was an original part of the Seljukid building or a later addition.[30] At Divriği, the Il-Khanid hospital and mosque are built back-to-back, sharing a wall. The proximity of ill people and the pure holy places of prayer suggests that the ill were not considered necessarily impure or contaminated by nature.

As hospitals were not considered contaminated or contaminating, they could be located near busy places—for example, places of entertainment. A nineteenth-century English traveler asked why the hospital in the Süleymaniye was situated so close to coffeehouses. He was told that the location was not a coincidence. The sixteenth-century architect wanted to show the patrons of the coffeehouses, institutions described as opium dens, how and where they might end their lives if they continued to consume drugs: they would be locked in the cells for the mad in the hospital. Coffee as a social beverage arrived in Istanbul from the Arab provinces in the middle of the sixteenth century. Under Selim II, claimed one observer, there were no less than six hundred (!) coffeehouses in the capital.[31] The screams of the lunatics behind the hospital walls were supposed to intimidate those who sat in the coffeehouses nearby. Keppel's explanation from the 1830s, which associates coffeehouses with madness, echoes earlier sources. Mustafa Ali, an Ottoman historian and bureaucrat of the sixteenth century, described the coffeehouses in Cairo as full of lunatics spitting saliva. A madman from Aleppo, Aslan Dede, was famous for spending many an hour, both day and night, in the local coffeehouses.[32]

The location of hospitals near other busy social institutions created many opportunities for contact between hospital patients and healthy people. The mingling of ill and healthy also characterized hospitals outside the imperial Ottoman capitals. Leo Africanus (1465-1550), who served as a clerk in a hospital in Fez for several years, described how many people passed by the building. The patients used to engage them in conversation, complaining that they were treated cruelly; they maintained they were in fact healthy and had no business being in a hospital. Those outside who drew near to the hospital later regretted it:

> And hauing thus perswaded the commers-by, approaching neerer and neerer unto them, at length they take hold with one hand on their garments and (like villains) with the other hand they shamefully defile their faces and apparell with dung. And though all of them haue their priuies and close stooles, yet would they be poysoned in their owne filth, if the seuants did not often wash their lodgings: so that their abominable and continuall stinke is the cause why citizens neuer visit them.[33]

In and around hospitals purity and impurity mingled. As we have seen in the previous chapter where we tried to outline the identity of a "regular" patient entitled to hospital care, hospitals also allowed (to some extent) people from different social backgrounds and religious faiths to mingle. A hospital, not unlike a hammam, was a supracommunity institution, where members of different confessional communities could meet.[34]

In the beginning of the seventeenth century there were five functioning hospitals in Istanbul. All five were "general hospitals," and although they varied in size, their staffs had identical medical capabilities. Sixteenth-century London too had five major hospitals, but each had a different purpose.[35] Istanbul hospitals, in contrast, did not develop special medical expertise or social-philanthropic ends to distinguish them from other medical institutions in town, and there was no division of labor among them. The only piece of evidence to the contrary is Evliya's claim about the air in the hospital of Ahmet I. According to him, the hospital excelled in the purity of its air, and therefore treated mostly insane patients who could benefit from it especially.[36]

There were several reasons why the Ottomans attributed such importance to the purity and the beauty of the environment. Disease was associated with dirt and filth, health with cleanliness and harmony.

Hence, there were sweepers and cleaners in each of the hospitals.[37] Several etiological explanations existed in the early modern Middle East, but one medical theory in particular is relevant here. It was very popular among the educated elite in the Ottoman Empire, and it was the one that regulated hospital work. According to Galenic humoralism, the environment—air, climate, and so on—affects one's health. Lack of fresh air can slow recuperation and even damage one's constitution. Egypt, for example, was known as a melancholic place, its dry climate driving locals to insanity sooner or later.[38] Here we meet the ecological aspect of Ottoman integralism. In the second chapter we focused on the conceptualization of the human body as a complex entity of body and soul complementing each other. But in addition to seeking a balance within the body, Ottoman integralism viewed man as one with his world. Illness and health were understood in terms of balance (or lack thereof) with nature.

One translation of the ecological concept was the belief that the changing of seasons (and climates) could also affect one's health. Süleyman I had a medication prepared for him in the beginning of spring, as he was known to suffer annually from the same condition.[39] Two Ottoman medical treatises from the sixteenth century, entitled *Tebi'at-name* (The Book on the Nature of Man) or *'Asa'-yi Piran* (The Walking Stick of the Old Man) and *Der Medh-i Piri* (On Praising Old Age), analyzed the medical influences of the changing seasons. The authors, presumably addressing Süleyman I in his old age, advised the readers, inhabitants of Istanbul, to change their living quarters accordingly. That entailed leaving the city and returning to it whenever it was medically advisable.[40] Some of advice offered to Süleyman clashed, however, with other medical considerations. The two treatises recommended Istanbul for the summer due to the refreshing northern winds from the Black Sea, but pointed out that during the summer the capital was prone to outbreaks of plague.[41] But leaving the capital during the hot summer was well beyond the financial abilities of most Ottomans. As in the case of diet (discussed in the first chapter), following the best learned medicine was only possible for affluent Ottomans.

Ottoman hospitals incorporated ecological concepts as part of the therapeutic process. The Ottomans assigned medical importance to the environment of hospitals. It is true that most imperial hospitals were located at busy sites in the city centers, and surely these cannot claim fame for their cleanliness and fresh air. Evliya's idyllic description of the hospital of Ahmet I and other similar evidence may have been affected by wishful thinking on the part of the observers. But Evliya could rightly claim that hospitals enjoyed tranquility, as even institutions in the heart of towns were surrounded by well-kept gardens. Like preceding Anatolian hospitals,[42] Ottoman hospitals nurtured gardens. The planners of Ottoman hospitals created unique semirural atmosphere for the urban hospitals.

Refined horticulture was a familiar physical aspect of many Muslim societies, including the Ottoman Empire, which was influenced also by Turkish, Persian, Muslim, and Byzantine traditions. Although one study of medieval Arabic poetry suggests that as a generalization many Arab-Muslims were quite indifferent to nature and were not inspired by it,[43] it seems that other discourses present in society (theological, mystical, and so on) were quite conscious of nature. Gardens attest to man's love of nature and considering it as a series of signs from God.[44] These discourses also reveal human desire (and ability) to control and shape nature (plants, animals, and minerals). Gardens were a space where the universe came alive, reconstructed by man. Gardens are thus an artificial creation made of primarily natural materials in an attempt to reproduce the natural while reconstructing it within defined limits.[45]

The most famous and elaborate gardens were the royal gardens, but gardens were not solely for the elite to enjoy. In addition to private gardens there were also public ones, formal or informal, that were open to everyone and could be found everywhere, including around mosques or even in graveyards. Evliya Çelebi's description of Istanbul illustrates the popularity of gardens among early modern Ottomans. Evliya mentions the various neighborhood and villages that composed Istanbul, and his account includes what he took to be important landmarks, like mosques, schools, and other public institutions, in each locality. It is interesting to see that not only did he mention gardens where they existed, but also he elaborated on their shape and size. According to Evliya, his list of gardens in Istanbul was far from exhaustive, as he restricted himself to the more famous ones. However, even with this restriction, one can find references to hundreds of gardens and walks throughout the capital.[46]

Several writers explained the popularity of gardens among Ottomans by going back to the historical origins of both Arabs and Turks. It was thought that their beginning in the desert of Arabia and the plains of central Asia, respectively, where shortage of water was a grim reality, caused both cultures to appreciate water in general, and running water in particular. This type of romantic and essentialist explanation may not be convincing, yet it is true that many Ottomans associated abundance of water and greenery with heaven.

Water symbolized life, and rain was considered one of God's most significant presents to humanity.[47]

To my mind the cultural and social usages of the garden space are the main reasons for the creation of the Ottoman garden culture. In these open spaces one could enjoy tranquility, usually achieved only in another world. Gardens thus became a metaphor for secure private spaces, where people were invited to express their intimate thoughts and feelings—things that could not be exposed to strangers in the public sphere because of a stricter code of conduct. It was a space where public behavior (officially emphasizing discipline, austerity, solemnity, and orthodoxy) could be somewhat relaxed, although it was replaced by another code of conduct of refined and cultured etiquette.[48]

This relaxation could be tied to the fact that Ottoman gardens were characterized by their informality. They were asymmetrical open designs. One scholar has speculated that the Ottomans' origin as nomads or seminomads led them to appreciate nature in its virgin state.[49] Ottoman gardens differed from the rigid structures of Muslim Spain or Persia based on the *chahar-bagh* (literally, "four gardens"), a formal structure that divides garden space into quarters constructed around a central pool/fountain (some scholars see this as a blueprint for "the Muslim garden"). Gardens in the Ottoman Empire also differed from the rigidly laid out formal and monumental gardens of Christian Europe. They seem to fit more with the image of the nongeometrical and hedonistic Egyptian gardens. It is interesting to note the decided difference in the Ottoman garden vocabulary despite shared heritages: Ottomans and Persians relied on Muslim and Persian traditions, while Ottomans and Italians borrowed idioms from classical antiquity and shared the Mediterranean culture, climate, and fauna and flora.[50]

Ottoman horticulture is the context in which to consider the Ottoman medical usages of gardens. Comparison of hopsital gardens to the Ottoman imperial gardens shows that the theme of ecology was common in Ottoman gardens, and at the same time it highlights that seemingly shared features actually set hospital gardens apart from their contemporaries. (The typicality of hospital gardens attests to the fact the gardens in the Ottoman Empire were not composed according to one static model but were created and shaped according to cultural and functional considerations.)

In addition to the noticeable difference in their respective sizes and variety, the palace gardens fulfilled more functions not related directly with health. Palace gardens were a place for leisure and sports (such as javelin, archery, and wrestling) and thus helped the psychological well-being of the dwellers of the palace, especially the sultan. In addition to decoration and leisure, gardens also served political purposes. Some palace gardens were laid down to celebrate a major Ottoman victory and thus symbolize the greatness of the empire and the ruling sultan. Certain ceremonies, like receptions of foreign envoys, meetings with Ottoman bureaucrats, or the launching of the imperial navy, took place in the kiosks and promenades of the Topkapı Palace gardens. Yet another function for imperial gardens was a practical one. There were cultivated areas that supplied flowers, fruit, and vegetables to the palace kitchens and helped to reduce the palace expenditure for foodstuffs; the surplus was sold on the open market, and the gardens were a source of income. The fusion of pleasure, utility, and profit characterized the Ottoman royal gardens, in Topkapı and elsewhere, inherited from Byzantium.[51]

Unlike the palace gardens, the hospital gardens did not contribute to the budget and were not used to grow vegetables and fruits to be converted to foodstuffs or medication for the patients (such gardens could include fruit trees but not for practical reasons). Literary or pictorial sources do not reveal medicinal plants in the gardens in question. Likewise contemporary *materia medica* treatises do not indicate gardens as the usual habitat of the herbs they discuss for drugs. In approximately alphabetical order *materia medica* works provide the reader with information about simples (which included vegetables, animal products, and mineral products). The information comprised a description, alleged healing properties, methods of preparation and adulteration, and sometimes also an illustration. They are silent about gardens. Herbal plants might have existed in gardens, but we have no way of confirming that. Here the Ottoman hospital differed from its counterpart in medieval England. English hospital gardens are known to have supplied fuel, food, and medicinal herbs; they could also provide grazing for the cattle, which supplied the institution with fresh milk, butter, cheese, and meat.[52]

In the Ottoman Middle East, gardens contributed in less obvious or material ways to hospitals: gardens were a central component in the integralistic therapy characteristic of the time. Here it is useful to think of the modern concept of "healing by design," which is gaining more and more weight in contemporary medicine as health-care costs climb and the competition over patients increases. This drives health managers, as well as patients and their families, to consider the role of the designed environment in the healing process.

One aspect of the concept "healing by design" is architecture, as medical care cannot be separated from the buildings in which it is delivered.[53] Another aspect is the natural environment in and around the buildings. After years of preferring medical technology over the mental and the spiritual, there is now recognition that these too have great effect on the healing process and its success.[54] But this new interest in the environment is in fact not new at all, as the use and control of environment in medicine, like gardens, go back to many traditional medical systems, the Ottoman included.

As the theory and practice of "healing by design" gains popularity and experience, it becomes also more elaborate, and today it is customary to differentiate between the general "healing garden" that promotes overall well-being and the more specifically oriented "therapeutic landscape." Although the Ottoman concept of health was integrative by nature, and hence this distinction is anachronistic in regard to the Ottoman period, these terms help us to understand what the roles of gardens in Ottoman space (medical and others) were and were not.

Ottoman hospital gardens provided an environment promoting overall well-being. At the same time, Ottomans believed gardens could provide very effective therapeutics, just like medication, for specific medical problems. In this respect the Ottoman understanding of the healing roles of gardens inside hospitals encompasses the two modern terms. Such gardens usually provide relief from physical symptoms like pain, reduce psychological stress, and strengthen a sense of wellness.

A healing garden can lead the patient to positive responses and stimuli by using a combination of mechanisms wisely, one of them being the aesthetic aspect. Gardens must be beautiful in the eyes of the visitor. (As differences in aesthetic preferences sometimes occur, however, the enforcement of the designer's taste can be counterproductive.) The healing effect is reached by "soft" elements, like greenery, natural light, and shade, or water features (fountains and pools were a popular element inside and outside gardens), rather than elements made of concrete or stone (referred to today as "hardscape")

Ottoman gardens inside and outside hospitals were indeed "soft." They typically included evergreen trees (like cypresses, oaks, mimosa cedars, and pines), fruit trees (citrus like oranges and lemons, but also peaches, apples, figs, olives, cherries, and pomegranate), vegetables, flower beds, flowerpots (of tulips, lilies, jasmines, irises, roses, daffodils, and narcissi), shrubs, and climbers, in addition to a fountain or pool. Sometimes animals provided pleasing noise (like birdsong) and entertainment.[55]

In such a beautiful environment patients need simply to be there, and healing occurs as a result of the direct connection between them and the environment. However, the healing powers of gardens are enhanced by design elements that encourage people to use the garden space in more active ways than simply existing in it. Contemporary sources present us with static gardens. Ottoman gardens were not the dynamic garden we are familiar with from early modern Europe, where visitors walked about the garden on the formal paved paths. Maybe due to a different climate, the Ottoman garden was a place where people sat in the shade and breathed the fresh air, instead of going on extended walks purely for pleasure. Still, elements like pavements, benches, or games encouraged patients to experience nature in other ways than just viewing it and thereby to benefit more from the garden.[56]

Healing gardens are private spaces, set apart from the hustle and bustle of the city outside as well as from the busy life within the institution. Gardens were a space where intrusions from the outside in the form of noise, filth, or the peeking inside of foreigners were minimized. Hospital gardens were inward looking, a distinction they shared with other small gardens. This is where the ill (and maybe staff members as well) could find opportunities for privacy, peace, and quiet, after being cooped up inside the building with dozens of inmates, medical staff, and administration. Gardens in hospitals were a world within a world.

At the same time, gardens were also an extension of the hospital building. It was like another room in the hospital—decidedly a different one, yet not altogether separated. Hospitals shared this feature with many individual private houses in the Ottoman Empire—indeed, throughout the Mediterranean—where the existence of a courtyard allowed privacy and secrecy for family life in a crowded environment.[57] Therefore, the hospital rooms were deliberately built with windows opening onto the gardens, so that these spaces might contribute to the psychological treatment of patients. All of it provided positive distractions from aches and fear. This is how Evliya Çelebi described the hospital in Edirne in 1651: "Each one roars and sleeps like a lion in his lair. Some fix their eyes on the pool and fountain and repeat words like a begging derwish. And some doze in the rose garden, grape orchards and fruit orchards and sing with the unmelodious voices of the mad."[58]

Comparing hospital gardens with other gardens in the Ottoman urban space—public and private, urban and suburban, humble and grand—from the medical point of view reveals the difference between the "healing garden" and "therapeutic landscape." Firstly, the gardens outside hospitals catered for healthy people; the hospital gardens entertained the ill. Secondly, visitors to gardens outside hospitals enjoyed the gardens for rest, sports and play, and social interaction. These activities, combined with the pleasing environment, were means to strengthen overall well-being, which combined the physical and the mental. In hospitals, as we saw, gardens were supposed to have concrete effects, and were not aimed at affording general pleasure.

Another aspect of the hospitals' contribution toward integralistic therapy is a strong belief in the hereafter. This too explains the gardens' central place in the hospital environment. Religious and emotional considerations may have influenced the designers in creating gardens, which would remind the terminally ill of their most desired destination—paradise. Gardens in most cultures are often compared to paradise, and the Ottomans were not unique. Some scholars tend to overemphasize (out of a romantic-orientalistic view?) this aspect in the case of the Muslim ones—including those in the Ottoman Empire. However, the association of gardens with paradise is not just the product of modern scholarly imagination. In many cases Ottomans united gardens and graveyards or even formal mausoleums. Such a synthesis was more than a utilitarian unity. Rather, there were intentional allusions to paradise recreated on earth. Contemporary observers frequently used the metaphor of celestial paradise with reference to worldly gardens.[59]

Evliya Çelebi is just one example of an Ottoman referring regularly to paradise symbolism in relation to several gardens in Istanbul. Writing of the "Arsenal Garden" on the Golden Horn, not far from the neighborhood of Hasköy (known to be a Jewish district, equipped with a large Jewish cemetery), Evliya said the place was patronized first by Mehmet II. It was adorned with kiosks, sofas, dozens of basins, pools, and fountains, and twelve thousand trees of different kinds that kept the sun from beating down. People enjoyed the gardens and played games there, like chess. In addition to supplying worldly pleasures, such a garden evoked images of religious paradise. Indeed, Evliya says, poetically, the perfumed garden conveys an idea of eternal life.[60] Evliya then continued to the village of Beşiktaş down the Bosphorus, today a central neighborhood in Istanbul. Here Evliya commented that there were no less than 160 gardens in that area alone, "every one like a paradise."[61]

Gardens outside the hospital buildings, ulema inside the buildings offering religious services (all hospitals employed them), and the devotion of some of the hospital space to serve as a mosque could all induce the ill to use their time in hospital to contemplate their deeds so far and the unavoidability of death, and to focus on their desire for paradise.

Walls as Barriers and as Connectors: Degrees of Isolation

Although hospitals were not totally removed from the healthy population, and tucked away not to be seen, the patient population of the hospital was not allowed to be fully integrated into the healthy society. Between these two extreme poles—isolation and integration—Ottoman hospitals occupied a position somewhere in the middle. This was another role of gardens in Ottoman hospitals. Thanks to the gardens, hospitals were described by contemporary observers as having an unreal or an unearthly character, despite the fact that hospitals were situated in central places in the cities that were crowded, noisy, and dirty. The gardens were an important component in the healing process taking place in the hospital. They were also a means to separate the hospitals from the city by creating a dividing zone around the hospitals.

Gardens were a "soft" physical barrier; another one was erecting thick and high walls. The importance of walls around hospitals is emphasized in the records of builders employed to repair the walls when necessary.[62] The hospitals also hired doormen twenty-four hours a day. Their job was to prevent outsiders from entering the premises, meeting the ill, and spending the night with them: the doormen locked the hospital doors every night and opened them in the morning. Dozens of hospital budget reports from the sixteenth and seventeenth centuries confirm that such workers were routinely a part of hospital staffs. In Topkapı, the eunuch manager of the hospital stood at the door himself with servants at his beck and call.[63] It is noteworthy that the gatekeepers' duty was to control the entrance of outsiders into the hospitals. But did they forbid the patients from exiting the hospitals? Nothing is said explicitly about that.

Yet sometimes the walls were only partially successful in achieving isolation. Two examples illustrate this. The first is the anecdote about the old *şeyh* from Diyarbakir related in more detail in the previous chapter. The old man preached to a growing audience in Istanbul in the 1650s that the meddling of the sultan's mother in politics was the prime reason for the empire's miseries. After ignoring several warnings from the imperial palace, the *şeyh* was forcibly admitted as a madman into the Süleymaniye hospital. However, he continued his sermons by shouting from his cell to the many admirers who gathered under his window. The vexed authorities finally set him free and sent him back to his hometown in the east.[64]

The second example comes from the description of the pages' hospital in the imperial palace of Topkapı, in Istanbul. An Italian observer claimed that "he [the patient] is look'd unto after the Turkish fashion, and kept so closely, that none may come to the speech of him, except the physician, or apothecary, but with great difficulty."[65]

The pages in the palace lived in the inner court under a strict regimen. They were forbidden to converse in loud voices and in the presence of the sultan communicated silently using hand signs. Every move was watched and scrutinized by their instructors, even social interaction with fellow pages. However, the palace hospital was situated in the first court of the palace, which anyone could enter. Hence the ill had ample opportunity to contact the "outside" world. In fact, the Ottoman historian and bureaucrat Mustafa Ali criticized Süleyman I harshly for founding the hospital in the first court. In allowing the pages easy association with the outside world, claimed Ali, he helped to corrupt them. Other Ottoman observers who were familiar with Topkapı claimed that pages who wanted to talk with friends and family pretended to be ill. When they were wheeled from their private chambers in the inner parts of the palace to the hospital in a cart, they would bribe the cart's drivers to pull the cart ever more slowly so that they could talk with those who were waiting for them. Apparently, for an additional bribe, these "cart talks" could be held in the office of the hospital supervisor himself.[66]

The palace pages in the hospital were also able to smuggle forbidden items into the hospital. Wine, being a medicinal drink, might be consumed within the hospital compound, but the pages always tried to smuggle in more. During the night, cases of wine would be dragged over the hospital walls with ropes behind the backs of the guards patrolling the garden area. The patients even succeeded in smuggling young boys into the hospital dressed up as sellers of sweets (*helvacılar*). Creating an opportunity to fulfill secret sexual desires is mentioned by European observers (who might have been looking for the fantastic Orient) as yet another motivation to be admitted into the hospital. The real sweet sellers earned only a mediocre salary. By loaning their outfits to young boys they could triple their income. The hospital supervisor, a eunuch, and his attendants (a team of five or six men), despite their eagle eyes could not distinguish between the real sellers and the impostors. If the supervisor did suspect foul play, the patients were quick to pacify him with an expensive gift, such as a silk vest. Thus, the smuggling benefited the manager of the hospital as well.[67]

The extensive gardens and high walls around hospitals created for those inside the compound the intimacy and solitude needed for recuperation. These walls granted the ill the quiet and harmonious atmosphere needed to recover, a haven away from (yet physically close to) the busy streets. It is true that there were windows in the Süleymaniye hospital, through which the patients could converse with people outside. Yet they had to *scream* in order to be heard, which suggests some distance between the windows and the street. Although it was possible to smuggle people and wine into the pages' hospital in Topkapı, smuggling—an illegal act—was the only way to do it. Walls and gardens were not described by contemporaries as a means to keep the ill at bay and protect the healthy from physical proximity to the ill (and thus prevent contagion). Rather, they symbolized differentiation and separation of the two social groups.[68]

While there were high walls around hospitals, they could not (and may have not been meant to) prevent all contact between hospital patients and the healthy world outside. The location of hospitals in towns or right next to them allowed the patients and the healthy to stay in constant touch. The closeness between the healthy majority and the ill minority was both physical and emotional, yet their difference was not forgotten. The ill were regarded as different, the "other," yet an integral part of society. The attitude toward them combined curiosity, interest, and compassion with ridicule and fear.[69]

Ottoman and European contemporary sources contain rich references to Ottoman hospitals. Almost all these sources are reports of viewers on the outside looking in; unlike Europeans, Ottomans did not put on paper their personal experiences in hospitals, either as ill patients or as healthy staff members. Very few sources portray hospital life from within the building. It seems that rarely were healthy people allowed to enter hospitals and familiarize themselves with the institution. One such observer was Evliya Çelebi. His first-person description of the hospital in Edirne seemingly attests to his personal familiarity with it. He describes the Mamluk hospital in Cairo as well. In other cases, including for the hospitals in Istanbul, Evliya takes the viewpoint of someone outside the building. Yet, even if his reporting from the hospital building itself is a literary fiction, not a historical reality, it shows that authors were interested in what was happening behind the walls of hospitals and assumed that their readers were as well.

A unique piece of evidence is an early seventeenth-century miniature depicting a scene in a hospital room, part of an album assembled for Ahmet I. The scene shows a hospital room in which three patients are in frenzy. The physicians and attendants (all males) try to take charge of the situation, but they are in physical danger as one unrestrained patient threatens them with a knife, and a second patient has already chained the feet of his physician using a restraining device within the room. All three patients are shackled by their necks to the walls, and two of them have their feet bound in a wood stock. In the back wall of the room there is a window through which three young men are looking in at the scene.

The accessibility of hospitals to the healthy is most interesting in the context of the discussion here. The miniature depicts a scene in a hospital room, based either upon details supplied to the illustrator or according to what he visualized to himself. The picture hints that it was possible—or at least deemed possible—for a healthy person to peep into a hospital building. Hospitals were not institutions sealed off from the world so that people outside them did not and could not know what was going on inside. Yet the three youngsters looking through the rear window are astonished by the scene unfolding before their eyes (they raise their fingers to their mouths—a sign of puzzlement in Muslim painting).[70] Healthy people could see what was going on in the hospital, but they could not necessarily make sense of the behavior of the ill, especially the lunatics among them.

This scene is probably the only Ottoman one to take place in a hospital room. Miniatures that deal with other medical subjects, like hygiene, birth, physicians, the tools of their trade, apprentices, medications, and medical procedures, can be found in abundance in many manuscripts. An Ottoman surgical manual from the fifteenth century includes illustrations of medical procedures that are situated in various environments: inside a private house, outside in a field, by a river, and so on.[71] It does not include a reference to a hospital, although the author, Şerefeddin Sabuncuoğlu, did work as a medical doctor in a hospital. Despite the curiosity about hospitals, this institution apparently was not regarded as an appropriate subject for an illustration.

The attitude of the Edirne population toward the hospital on the outskirts of town also attests to Ottomans' physical and mental access to hospitals. For the people of Edirne, although the hospital was located outside the city and required a walk, it was close physically and mentally: they did not shy away from it. On the contrary, it was exactly its "otherness" that attracted them. The walk to the hospital was a popular diversion in town, especially during the spring. This season was regarded by medical doctors and laymen alike as "the season of madness," during which the number of mad people admitted into the hospital went up. The hospital itself could therefore supply the entertainment of watching the antics of the lunatic patients.[72]

The Marriage of Etiology and Space

The Ottomans paid great attention to the location of hospitals and their surroundings. Ottomans were also particular about hospital interiors, although not necessarily innovative in their choice of architectural plans. In the hospitals of Beyazid I in Bursa, Hafsa Sultan in Manisa, and Ahmet I in Istanbul, as in the Seljuk period, the floor plan resembled the *medrese*: they had a quadrangular hall with a high dome. The hall and several smaller rooms surrounded an inner-court-cum-garden where there was a marble pool whose water made a pleasant background noise. To the sides of the pool there were *eyvan*like raised platforms. The choice of an already familiar floor plan is a plausible explanation as to why some sources identified hospitals wrongly as schools, the more common institution.

Other hospitals did not use what modern architects term a "derived plan"—that is, they did not borrow the configuration of another type of institution.[73] In the hospitals of Mehmet II, Beyazid II, Hurrem, and Süleyman, the architects implemented a "designed plan": new floor plans were laid out primarily for these buildings. Beyazid II and Hurrem's hospitals in Edirne and Istanbul are especially noteworthy in this regard. Their inner spaces were constructed upon a centralized plan (which was adopted in European and later American hospitals, as well). The hexagonal building housing the hospital of Beyazid II reveals its inner centralized space in the external shape of the building.[74] At the same time these innovative hospitals used many familiar aesthetic and functional features from Ottoman-Muslim architecture that can be found in other hospitals, as well as in *medrese*s and private dwellings: features like domed halls, central fountains, *eyvan*like spaces, and colonnades, among others.

The dimensions of the Ottoman hospitals were unassuming in relation to other urban institutions, although some hospitals were grander than others. The hospitals of Mehmet II and Süleyman were part of majestic complexes that adorned the city with their splendor, as one English visitor to the Ottoman capital wrote somewhat poetically.[75] Although Evliya relates that no less than seventy domes made up the roof of Mehmet II's hospital, it seems the hospital itself was more modest (unless Evliya included adjacent buildings that serviced the hospital, like the kitchen and laundry). While this hospital might have not been a huge building, it seems that with the service buildings it created a small yet substantial subcomplex within the bigger mosque complex.[76] The hospital of Ahmet I was described in its endowment deed as a building that would stand for eternity.[77] The author of the deed intended to laud the generous gift of the sultan (a charitable foundation should be eternal and irrevocable), not to praise the physical quality of the building. But surely a solid hospital, which physically stands for ages, is a good monument to the founder's beneficence as well.

The most important space in Ottoman hospitals was designated for the treatment of patients. This area also served as living quarters for the patients. This space differed from other areas in the hospital, such as that of the outpatients, that of rooms where medications were prepared, that of areas used for storage, that of the kitchens, or that of rooms used for administration and a prayer hall.

All patients lived in the same area in the hospital, and there was no division according to type of ailment. Unlike our modern hospitals, in Ottoman hospitals there were no wards. In that regard the Ottomans did not continue the medical tradition established in the Mamluk-period Manṣurī hospital in Cairo, which was divided into separate wards for surgery, ophthalmology, dysentery, fevers, and lunacy, and one that was devoted to women only.[78]

The space of Ottoman hospitals, like their location and environment, was shaped by the medical theories of the times, which guided practice in them. The Ottoman medical system allowed for several types of medical etiology. Ottoman etiologies were the outcome of both personalistic and naturalistic medical systems. A personalistic system is one in which illness is believed to be caused by the active purposeful intervention of a sensate agent who/which may be a supernatural being (a deity or a god), a nonhuman being (such as a ghost, ancestor, or evil spirit), or a human being (a witch or sorcerer). The ill person literally is a victim, the object of aggression or punishment directed specifically against him or her, for reasons that concern him or her alone.[79] In the Ottoman case this took the form of belief in jinns. These spiritlike creatures were sent by God or as a curse by enemies, and they were believed to be able to cause illness. They were composed of vapor or flame, whereas mankind and angels, the other two types of intelligent beings, were created out of clay and light (sura 55/14). Jinns are capable of appearing in different forms, especially in the guise of animals, and they are usually active at night. They can be hostile toward men, if they are irritated, and will then inflict various illnesses, for example hemiplegia.[80]

In the other type of medical system, the naturalistic, illness is explained in impersonal, systematic terms. Naturalistic systems conform to an equilibrium model: health prevails when various elements in the body, like heat, cold, or the humors, are in the balance appropriate to the age and condition of the individual in his or her natural and social environment. When this equilibrium is disturbed, the result is illness.[81] In the Ottoman case, naturalistic etiology resulted in the miasma theory. In this theory, illness was understood to be caused by vapors spread to the air from polluted areas like swamps, burial places, and so on. Another expression of a naturalistic system was a belief in celestial causes: the positions of certain astral bodies in the heavens triggered occurrences in the material world as well, some of which might be auspicious or harmful for mankind.

Personalistic and naturalistic etiological systems are, of course, not mutually exclusive. Yet in spite of much overlap, most people seem committed to one or the other of these explanatory principles to account for most illness. In the Ottoman case the theory that affected hospital construction was that of miasma, a part of medical theory that Islamic (and Ottoman) medicine incorporated from antiquity in general, and from Hippocrates and Galen in particular. It was this type of medicine that the elite patronized, and the elite created these hospitals.

There was no inner division in Ottoman hospitals according to illness: those suffering from different diseases were housed together, usually in pairs in small rooms. Aaron Hill, an English traveler of the seventeenth century, observed, "Infirmaries or Hospitals are commonly *Stone Buildings* of a large *Quadrangular* design, not much unlike *our own*, but that the Beds lie open to each other, no *Apartments* being form'd to keep the *Sick* from the Distemper from *Diseases* of *another* kind, but inconsiderately exposing all to publick View, and dangerous conversations."[82]

This organization of hospital space reflects the belief in miasma as an etiologic agent. According to this belief, there was no reason to keep people who were suffering from different types of illnesses apart from each other, nor for that matter to isolate the ill from the healthy: they could not harm one another. Hence people did not hesitate to purchase the belongings, including the clothes, of people who had just died of a disease. European observers linked this custom with the common belief in predestination: as God decrees one's future well in advance, exposure to illness could not change that future.[83]

Yet the Ottomans could not have been blind to the fact that contagion among animals, as among humans, did occur. Simple experience demonstrated that some diseases were indeed transmissible, and very quickly and easily so. In their everyday life people acted upon this assumption and tried to remove themselves from plague-ridden areas. Even physicians were known to leave such places, in effect deserting their patients.[84] The discussions on this matter should illustrate that Middle Easterners were familiar with contagion, but did not necessarily accept it as their main etiological explanation or elaborate the concept systematically. Moreover, there existed a multitude of discourses, which engaged medical doctors as well as laypersons, like literati and religious scholars. These discourses reveal complex and contradictory opinions (and much confusion), all of which were attempts to explain the mystery of disease in general and the fearsome plague in particular.[85]

Consider the discourses of Evliya Çelebi, the Ottoman literatus and traveler. While discussing a lazaretto in Istanbul, Evliya explains the spread of leprosy in a manner that reminds one of a description of contagion. Evliya did not use the Arabic term *'adwa*, which appears in medieval texts and is translated in English as "contagion," although it has a much broader transitive meaning.[86] However, the term he did use, "sari," echoes something that creeps into things and places, extending and propagating itself, hence contagious and epidemic. Several lines later he goes on to say that leprosy is God's verdict visited on man and continues to the next generations.[87]

This complexity is noted also in the publicly declared positions of religious scholars on this issue. They did not speak with one voice, and their individual positions were usually quite complex (one fourteenth-century physician was outspoken in his condemnation of religious scholars who, according to him, unanimously rejected the possibility of contagion and thus caused Muslims to die unnecessarily).[88] Ebu Su'ud, the *şeyhülislam* and chief mufti of Istanbul and the Ottoman Empire from 1545–1574, claimed that fleeing from a place of illness as well as staying put were both valid actions. On the one hand, he allowed Muslims to send their children and wives to a safe place, including Christian villages. On the other hand, he lamented that at the very first rumor of plague, in Istanbul or elsewhere, holders of religious office ran for their lives, abandoning their flocks just when the latter were most in need of spiritual support. Ebu Su'ud issued *fetvas* ordering that those who fled be punished by dismissal from their posts. He had to issue several orders to this effect, which reveals he had no real results.[89]

Ebu Su'ud's was not a lone voice. Another famous religious figure, Şams al-Din Ahmad b. Süleyman Ibn Kemal Paşa (d. 1534), was more unequivocal. Ibn Kemal Paşa was a Damascene who had studied in Edirne, where he became a judge before his promotion to the position of *şeyhülislam*. In his work *Al-Risāla fī al-tā'ūn wa al-wabā'* (A Treatise on the Plague) he advised his readers to flee from plague-ridden places.[90]

In addition to theoretical comments, famous scholars demonstrated a variety of responses in their behavior to the outbreak of plague. One, Hamid al-Din b. Afdal al-Din al-Hüseyni, an Istanbuli scholar in the days of Mehmet II, took his family away from the city when a plague broke out. He himself, however, returned to his post at a *medrese* in order to continue his classes.[91]

Religious scholars were not different from the other segments of Ottoman society. Whoever could afford it fled a plague-stricken place. The sultans made plans to leave the city for houses prepared for them on the shores of the Black Sea when plagues struck.[92] But as Paul Rycaut, the secretary of the English ambassador in Istanbul and later to be the English consul in Izmir in the 1670s, observed, this pattern of behavior was not restricted to the extremely rich:

> Yet they are councelled not to frequent a contagious habitation, where they have no lawful affair to invite them. But yet I have observed, in the time of an extraordinary Plague, that the *Turks* have not confided so much to the precept of their Prophet, as to have courage enough to withstand the dread and terrour of that sloughter the sickness hath made; but have under other excuses fled to retired and private villages, especially the *Cadees* and men of the Law, who being commonly of more refined wits and judgments then the generality, both by reason and experience have found that a wholesome Air is a preserver of life, and that have lived to return again to their own house in health and strength, when perhaps their next Neighbours have through their brutish ignorance been laid in their Graves.[93]

The bureaucracy of the Ottoman administration, too, was aware of the possibility of transmission of illness and the spread of epidemics. At the very least the imperial administration was aware that some

Ottomans believed so, acted upon this assumption, and ran away. Because of the potential consequences of epidemics for the social, economic, and political order, the central Ottoman administration gathered information on outbreaks of plagues in the provinces. In June 1565 the judicial court in Trabzon on the shores of the Black Sea discussed the flight of one Ibrahim bin Iskender from a village in the district upon the outbreak of plague. The fact that Ibrahim was an Ottoman officer (he was a *sipahi*, a cavalryman who held land in the province for himself and his retinue) made it the business of the authorities, who had to nominate another person for his position within the provincial-military administration.[94] In November 1579 two identical decrees were sent to the Ottoman governor (*beylerbey*) of Basra in Iraq. They dealt with the faltering trade in the area. Merchants were no longer coming to the city, and as a result the income from customs decreased considerably. The decrees blamed twin evils for this state of affairs: the war with Safavid Iran and the plague. In order to compensate for the loss in customs, the *beylerbey* was instructed to impose taxes on dates.[95] In January 1670 the divan, or imperial council, in Istanbul discussed information regarding a small village in northwest Anatolia: the village of Göynük was reported to be empty, save for three people. Everyone else had run away after one villager died from the plague.[96]

The Ottoman authorities could not but be aware of quarantine measures applied by their neighbors in the Mediterranean basin and in the European hinterland, in some cases as early as the 1600s. (The Ottomans first used quarantine on their side of the border only in the nineteenth century.)[97] Italian cities, and some Aegean islands under Italian rule, tried to combat the spread of disease into their territory by instituting quarantine-like policies. The Ottomans, who traded with these places directly, must have been familiar with the relevant procedures. The port inspectors did not allow any ship to dock and unload its goods before the signiors of health released the merchandise. Until the formal release arrived, the ship's crew and goods were put in quarantine, sometimes for as long as forty days (hence the name "quarantine"), on their ship or in a lazaretto nearby. While they were under supervision, a guard stood near the ship to ensure that no direct physical contact took place between the ship and its crew and the people on shore. Even touching the ship's rope was sufficient cause to add a person to the quarantined group. Ships arriving from the Ottoman domains were especially scrutinized. These ships could not present a document from the officials of their point of origin testifying that the port was not plague-ridden. Ships coming from European ports, whose captains could present such a document, were placed under shorter period of quarantine. Sometimes the signiors of health dispensed with a waiting period altogether. But, if during the quarantine one of the ship's crew fell ill, even if from a common illness not related at all to the plague, the quarantine would be prolonged. Such measures naturally had financial outcomes. First, they gave the ships from known ports (usually Italians) an advantage over all the other ships in the Mediterranean. Second, during the waiting period goods could become spoiled.[98]

European observers commented on what they saw as the advantages in not applying quarantine measures. Such measures could and did close trade down and cause severe financial losses to the parties involved. Quarantines also meant strict control over the population, which tried to resist the new policy. This meant more cases of disturbances of order in the attempt to evade restrictions on people's movement.[99]

Yet the same European observers also feared what they believed was a fatalistic approach to disease among the Ottomans. Sir Henry Blount (1602–82), an English knight, attendant to Charles I (reigned 1625–49), member of the Royalist party, and traveler, arrived at Edirne in a carriage from Sarajevo, Belgrade, and Sofia. One Ottoman officer accompanied him and his escort. On the outskirts of Edirne they passed an Ottoman foot soldier lying down, his horse standing beside him. The worn-out soldier tried to persuade the party to let him into their carriage. The Ottoman officer ordered Blount's escort to vacate his seat in the carriage for the soldier and ride his horse following them. When the soldier was laid down and his shirt taken off, the signs of the plague were visible on his body (Blount apparently referred to the swelling of the lymph nodes that characterizes the disease). Blount said that had he known the soldier was ill he would not have allowed him in. But the Ottoman officer calmed the traveler: the ill soldier, he said, posed no danger to them. God had already passed verdict, and their destiny was sealed. If it included the plague, nothing they could do would prevent it. That night the soldier died, but the three travelers came to no harm.[100]

Contagion and the possibility of humans being disease carriers were discussed also in medical and veterinary treatises. An example of this can be found in the writings of Ṣāliḥ b. Naṣrallah Ibn Sallūm (d. 1670), an Arab physician from Aleppo who became the head physician (*hekimbaşı*) of the empire and an intimate of Sultan Mehmet IV.[101] His famous tract on therapy and hygiene was *Ghāyat al-itqān fī tadbīr badan al-insān* (The Greatest Thoroughness in Treatment of the Human Body). Shortly after the appearance of the Arabic work it was translated into Ottoman Turkish by leading Ottoman physicians. Ibn Sallūm's writings enjoyed considerable popularity. Some of his ideas were also translated into Persian,[102] but it is the Ottoman context in which he operated.

Ibn Sallūm incorporated some materials borrowed from the German-speaking physician Paracelsus (Philippus Aureolus Theophrastus Bombastus von Hoenheim, d. 1541) who departed from the common wisdom of his time in criticizing Galen himself. Paracelsus taught that experience, and empiricism, rather than logic and reasoning, produce real and true knowledge in medicine. Moreover, he claimed that the four elements—earth, fire, water, and air—are not the last irreducible elements of matter, but composite bodies in themselves. Each is a mixture of the three principles: sulfur, salt, and mercury, of which all bodies consist. Paracelsus started a reform in medicine (and in theology) in Renaissance Europe during the sixteenth century. The processes in the human body were viewed as chemical in nature, and he was the first to treat his patients with chemical medications that included poisonous ingredients. He is thus seen by his supporters as the founder of chemotherapy and biochemistry.

In his famous encyclopedia, Ibn Sallūm included a discussion of the plague and its causes. He explained that physicians were in disagreement (*ikhtilāf*) about its etiology. Many physicians adopted Galen's position: putridity in the air from the earth—that is, miasma—entered the human body and caused this and other types of illness. (By adopting this concept, this group of doctors categorically denied the possibility of humans infecting each other.) Other physicians, however, claimed that the poisonous disease was restricted to a certain locality, like Istanbul or Egypt, but it extended and propagated itself, and hence was contagious, spreading from one region to another. According to Ibn Sallūm, these doctors believed that it travels first to the heart, then to the soul. Yet another group of doctors maintained that the origins lay with heavenly bodies. He concludes rather diplomatically, without stating his own position, that the origins of this scourge are many, and then combines various etiologies together, some of them not so scientific (celestial influences, miasma, religion, and morality), weaving them together until they complement each other. Ibn Sallūm explains that the plague may originate with moral crimes, like fornication, homosexual acts, rebellions, committing murder, or injustice. It can fall on humanity through the speech of God through his jinns, angels, or stars. There are signs to indicate the nearing visitation of the plague—for example, many stars fall from the sky and beasts and canines in growing numbers roam the land.[103]

At least one reader of Ibn Sallūm agreed with contagion theory and supplied evidence. A remark dated from the year 1770–71, written on the margins of one copy of Ibn Sallūm's manuscript by an anonymous writer, tells the story of a person from Mosul in Iraq who bought his wife a handkerchief in a place where plague had broken out. Soon after he presented his wife with the gift, she developed a high temperature and then her body became covered with inflammations of the skin and boils. She died three days later, her husband and children soon after. From this family the plague passed to others in the city and the villages nearby, killing many of them. Then the plague passed along the Tigris to Baghdad, where it also killed many.[104]

Despite this discussion of contagion, throughout his encyclopedia Ibn Sallūm remained loyal to one etiology, that of miasma. To Ibn Sallūm, like the other authors of Ottoman medical compendia in his day, miasma was still the dominant explanation for the origins of illness, although he acknowledged that, at least in theory, there could be other views on the matter.

In acknowledging several etiological theories Ibn Sallūm was not unique among his peers; in discussing contagion he was. Other seventeenth-century physicians in the Ottoman Empire included in their discussions of the plague only miasma and astral bodies as possible causes for this disease. Emir Çelebi's *Enmüzec-ül-tibb* (A Summary of Medicine), completed in 1625, is an example. Emir Çelebi was an Anatolian physician who had been educated in Cairo, where he stayed on as head physician of the Manṣūrī hospital, before his promotion in Istanbul to the rank of head physician of the empire and to Sultan Murad IV. Emir Çelebi, too, included in his compendium a section on the plague. He opened it by stating that the plague had two etiologies. One set of causes was earthly, among which Emir Çelebi includes miasma; the other set was related to astrology and astronomy.[105] In contrast to Ibn Sallūm, Emir Çelebi did not even entertain the possibility of transmission of illness.

The theory that maladies were transmissible directly from one person to another—namely, the recognition of "contagion," did not gain prominence among doctors in the Ottoman world in the early modern period. Part of the explanation for this lies in the theological consequences attached to contagion, consequences discussed by Lawrence I. Conrad in connection with the early Middle Ages. The discourse was not strictly medical. In a society and a culture dominated by the doctrine of an all-powerful and all-ordaining God, there was no place for a conception of disease causation that allowed for the capricious infection of one individual after another in complete disregard of their good or evil deeds. This denial of contagion was based on considerations far beyond those of medicine or the explanation of epidemic disease. It grew out of the larger moral and theological problem of how a merciful and benevolent God could bring upon mankind a scourge that killed the righteous together with the wicked, the faithful Muslim alongside the unbeliever.[106]

In addition, the theoretical denial that disease was transmissible lies in a tendency observed in Muslim societies to strengthen communal and family ties as a reaction to social disorder. The stimulus for some people to stay put in a place where a plague broke out was also connected to their willingness to stay by the sickbeds of those who otherwise would be left helpless. Disease thus poses social and economic challenges as well as medical and biological ones. The late Michael W. Dols studied the black death of the middle of the fourteenth century. He reached the conclusion that in contrast to Europe, urban communal behavior in the Muslim Middle East during outbreaks of plague generally did not deteriorate into total chaos. The political and social order, and especially family units, continued to function more or less as usual. In Europe, Dols concludes, a Christian responded to the plague as an individual and acted solely in his or her best interests; in the Muslim Middle East, however, people acted both as individuals and as members of a community with responsibilities to the broader social units. Denying the possibility of the transmission of disease gave people the emotional strength to stay put and not flee from the danger.[107] Evidence from the Ottoman period suggests that Dols's argument for the Mamluk period may be valid also for the Ottoman situation.[108]

Clearly, physicians as well as laypersons realized the possibility of the spread of disease among humans as well as animals by way of contagion—namely, by direct contact. There was no single Ottoman position on the matter. Moreover, some Ottomans did act upon the premise that contagion does exist, not just as a theoretical structure but as an actual occurrence. Yet they never developed the idea of contagion into a full theory, and contagion always remained peripheral within the Ottoman medical system. Ottoman hospitals in the early modern period were the product of classical etiological theories that enjoyed a position of hegemony in the medical system at the time. These theories supported the belief in miasma (or vapors) as a cause of illness. Hospitals, which formed part of the "orthodox" medical establishment, were associated closely with the theory of miasma on several levels. This theory shaped the inner space of the hospitals and their very location in the urban space, such as their propinquity to mosques.

CONCLUSION

Ottoman Medicine—Ottoman? Successful?

The four numbered chapters of this book have set out to demonstrate the varieties and complexities within the Ottoman medical system and how they were intimately connected with social realities. Two questions were hinted at in the previous pages, and I discuss them here by reconsidering issues analyzed in the previous chapters as a natural conclusion to the previous discussion. The first question is, How far, and in what ways, was the Ottoman medical system indeed "Ottoman"? The discussion here confronts the question of to what extent medical systems are universal and cosmopolitan entities, or else are embedded in specific social and cultural contexts. The second question is, was the Ottoman medical system at all successful in contemporary eyes? More than the biological efficacy of Ottoman medicine, success in a narrow and material meaning, the question here asks about subtle attitudes toward it. The discussion deals with various images early modern Ottomans held of medicine, both as a body of knowledge and as a profession. Urban Ottomans hoped their physicians, whatever medical tradition they belonged to, were able and caring, but they did not put even their most trusted old doctors on pedestals.

What Is Ottoman in Ottoman Medicine?

The Ottoman medical system we met in previous chapters was very complex. It included three different etiological and therapeutic traditions. Each was a complex world of ideas and techniques of its own. They competed with one another over hegemony, legitimacy, and professional success. At the same time they shared knowledge and skills with one another. They also shared some basic concepts of health and disease. The medical, legal, and theological discussions about basic concepts such as the nature and essence of the human body and its place in this world were complicated and profound. I maintain that this complex medical system was an Ottoman one. Its basic assumptions about humankind and its social organization were owed to Ottoman society and culture, although it drew much from Arab-Muslim medicine, which had evolved from the ninth century onward and was shared by various medical systems within the Muslim world (and to a large extent also by Europe, which also adopted learned, medieval Arab-Muslim medicine). Until now scholars have not commented on the social and intellectual interplay between the Ottoman-specific local medical tradition and the general one. It has been assumed, apparently, that the Ottoman medical system was not autonomous, but simply a local branch of the Arab-Muslim tradition.

Here I should like to emphasize the unique aspects that set the Ottoman medical tradition apart intellectually and socially. I claim that these unique characteristics were the outcome of a process of localization of an Arab-Muslim medical tradition in the Ottoman Empire during the early modern period. Studies on intellectuals, bureaucrats, visual arts, and music in the Ottoman Empire in the early modern period have all shown that important changes in the cultural identity of the elite occurred at this time. Medicine in the Ottoman Empire was part of the wider sociocultural process. Although I would argue that medicine more than the arts has a claim to universality, it is still culturally created.

I do not suggest that Ottoman medicine divorced itself totally from the common Arab-Muslim tradition. The process of localization and Ottomanization of medical knowledge and practices does not mean that such knowledge became totally removed from the medical conceptions common in other Muslim societies. Quite the opposite. Ottoman medicine still claimed to be part of Arab-Muslim tradition, and was right to do so. Ottoman medicine did not become less Arab-Muslim (this is not a case of either/or, a choice of one out of two opposite poles, but a position on a continuum): it became more localized, more Ottoman.

Thus, Cornell H. Fleischer took Mustafa 'Ali, the Ottoman historian and bureaucrat mentioned in the course of this book, as the focus of his biography of a typical Ottoman intellectual of the sixteenth century. Fleischer portrayed 'Ali as 'Ali saw himself: as a product of two cultures and civilizations that he tried to reconcile. The first was regional—the Ottoman tradition. The other, the Islamic one, was universal and cosmopolitan.[1]

Gülru Necipoğlu,[2] a historian of Ottoman art and architecture, has argued that the middle of the sixteenth century marked, from an artistic point of view, a cultural turning point for the Ottomans: the Ottoman court carved out a unique cultural path for itself, different from the shared artistic taste of the broader Turco-Muslim world. In the post-Timurid period there had been an "international" culture that acted as a common link among the Ottomans, the Safavids, and the Moguls of India. The Ottomans developed a unique artistic taste suited to their own values. In support of this, she points out that the drafting technique of Ottoman architects was related to a broader context of Islamic draftsmanship; but at the same time the drawings were also characterized by a unique set of conventions that distinguished them as a group. Before the middle of the sixteenth century, the leading Ottoman master artisans (ceramicists, builders, etc.) were of Iranian origin; they were usually trained in Tabriz or elsewhere in Transoxania. Not surprisingly, in that period Ottoman buildings were decorated with a repertoire technically and stylistically very similar to what can be found in, for example, Khurasan. The repertoire found in later buildings was derived from a different artistic language. These changes in Ottoman architectural taste are important, as architecture, in addition to being an art form, is also a strong indicator of social and political structures.

Walter Feldman, an expert on Ottoman music,[3] has outlined the changes in patterns of professionalism, musical genre, and musical instruments at the Ottoman court between the sixteenth century and the middle of the eighteenth. He concludes that the outcome of these changes was a set of patterns that differed substantially both from patterns known from the Islamic Middle Ages and from what is known in the Persianate world.

Rather than viewing it from the center, Owen Wright studied Ottoman music from the point of view of regional particularism, in this case local Arabic music and its relationships with imperial Ottoman music.[4] Yet Wright arrived at similar conclusions. He commented that before the end of the sixteenth century Istanbul was not a center of a stable tradition in music that could inspire emulation elsewhere. Although links with the Timurid past were preserved and musical contacts with Safavid Isfahan continued, the picture by the end of the seventeenth century is significantly different. Ottoman musicians were clearly in the ascendant. Song texts were no longer in Arabic, but predominantly in Turkish; the modal, rhythmic, and formal underpinnings of the vocal and instrumental repertoire show significant differences from those encountered in treatises and song-text collections of the fifteenth and sixteenth centuries.

The localization and Ottomanization of culture in the early modern period can be applied to the Ottoman medical system in the sixteenth and seventeenth centuries as well. The interplay in the medical scene was not with international Timurid culture, but rather with Arab-Muslim tradition, yet the process is quite the same. It is true that each domain of knowledge and cultural activity balanced the universal and the particular differently. Ottoman medicine shared pivotal characteristics with the general Muslim medical tradition. The Ottomans incorporated Arab-Muslim medical tradition into their own culture and worldview (or perhaps we may say that they were incorporated into this general tradition). At the same time, the Ottomans adapted and adjusted this medical system to their own needs, contributed to it, and for cultural reasons emphasized certain medical issues that were deemed more important. The result of this process was the Ottomanization of Arab-Muslim medicine in the early modern period.

The process of localization of medicine cannot be discerned everywhere in the Ottoman Empire as a whole. The phenomenon of medical Ottomanization occurred essentially in the core area of the Ottoman Empire where "Ottoman-ness" was best noted. In this area a specifically Ottoman culture evolved, distinct from other Islamic and Christian urban traditions. Basing his definition on urban formation, technology, and conceptions of town building, Maurice Cerasi defined the core area as comprising the western parts of the empire—that is, the Balkans and Anatolia as far as the Sivas-Kayseri area.[5] Other areas of the Ottoman Empire cultivated a local culture that went through a process of Ottomanization,[6] but they still retained some local features. The provincial centers resembled the imperial one and modeled themselves upon it, yet were different from it.

Nor can the cultural phenomenon of localization and Ottomanization be discerned throughout Ottoman society as a whole. The only social group that took part in this process was the Ottoman elite. It was concentrated around the major urban centers in western Anatolia and the Balkans.

Two aspects will be discussed here to indicate the unique character of Ottoman medicine. One is the change in the language of medical writing, from Arabic to Ottoman Turkish. Ottoman Turkish did not replace Arabic as a language for medical writing, but joined it, at least in elite circles. Its audience was a growing body of Ottomans who did not necessarily have much, or even any, knowledge of Persian and Arabic, the other two major Muslim languages.

The other aspect is the health system, and here I consider the evolution of hospitals in Ottoman medical systems. The Ottomans inherited hospitals from previous Muslim societies and transformed this medical institution into a bureaucratic and hierarchical institution, similar to other Ottoman institutions.

Ottoman Turkish: From Vernacular to Literary and Scientific Usage

The first element in the process of the evolution of a distinct Ottoman medical system can be seen in the language of medical writing. Here we observe a change, from Arabic to Ottoman Turkish. It is often suggested that the culture of the premodern Islamic world from the Nile to the Oxus was characterized by trilingualism—that is to say, that we have a situation in which three languages (Arabic, Persian, and Turkish) were used alongside each other. There was a certain division of labor among them: Arabic was the language of religion and religious sciences; Persian was used for literature and poetry; and Turkish, from Seljuk times, was the administrative language. Of course, the actual situation cannot have been as neat. For example, many of the non-Muslim groups in the area under consideration will have used one of these three languages as a vernacular but retained other languages (like Syriac, Greek, Hebrew, etc.) for religious and literary expression. Muslim subjects too belonged to many linquistic groups, including—in addition to Turkic dialects—languages like Serbo-Croat, Berber, Kuridish, and many Arabic, and Persian dialects. Overall, however, the elite culture of the dominant majority was the trilingual combination of Arabic, Persian, and Turkish.

With the Ottomans the linguistic division of labor between Arabic, Persian, and Turkish became more complex and ambiguous. Turkish became the primary language in the Ottoman court and thus acquired literary importance. Those who wished to win favor with the Ottoman urban elite groups needed to write in Ottoman Turkish. Their audience consisted of a growing body of Ottomans who did not necessarily have much, or even any, knowledge of Persian and Arabic. These included, for instance, the female members of the Ottoman elite, who were often literate in Ottoman (Turkish) culture, but who lacked education in other Islamic traditions. Translation of medical treatises into Turkish made them accessible to these women as well, and therefore added them to the pool of possible patrons for the authors. Yet another group was professional bureaucrats and merchants.[7]

The linguistic change is apparent in the translation of many medical texts from Arabic (and also from Persian) into Ottoman Turkish in the course of the sixteenth and seventeenth centuries. The change is also apparent in Ottoman subjects whose mother tongue was not Turkish choosing to compose their original medical treatises in Ottoman Turkish, the lingua franca of the empire.

We find a striking example of this in Emir Çelebi, one of the most renowned physicians of the seventeenth century. He was born in Anatolia but studied medicine in Cairo, and he stayed on there as head physician in the Mansurid hospital. He wrote his medical compendium *Enmüzec-ül-tibb* in Ottoman Turkish. A possible explanation of his preference for Ottoman Turkish over Arabic is the fact that he chose to dedicate this text to two Ottoman dignitaries in Istanbul whose patronage he courted: the sultan Murat IV and the admiral Recep Paşa.[8]

One Turkish scholar who claims that medicine had become a Turkish subject estimates that about seventy percent to eighty percent of the medical works written under the Ottomans were composed originally in Turkish.[9] This does not mean that Arabic ceased to be used for medical writing. Far from it, as the vast output in Arabic by Ottomans, even in Istanbul, during this period shows. The use of Ottoman Turkish as a language of medical writing when vying for the patronage of possible patrons was not an absolute rule. One Jewish physician who was educated in Muslim and Christian Spain, was expelled in 1492, and then immigrated to the Ottoman Empire via Naples, dedicated a treatise on the bubonic plague to Selim I. He wrote in Arabic, the scientific language of Iberian Jews.[10]

Some of this vast literature (but by no means all) was later on translated into Ottoman Turkish. One example is the writings of Ibn Sallūm, the Arab physician from Aleppo who became the head physician of the empire and an intimate of Sultan Mehmet IV.[11] For our present purpose, it is worth noting that shortly after the appearance of his Arabic work on therapy and hygiene (*Ghayat al-itqān fi tadbir badan al-insān*) it was translated into Ottoman Turkish by leading Ottoman physicians, hence the existence of *Nuzhat al-abdan fi tarjamat ghayat al-itqan* (The Beauty of the Bodies in the Translation of Ghayat al-itqan) or *Ghayat al-bayan fi tadbir badan al-insan* (The Greatest Explanation in Treatment of the Human Body).[12] Ibn Sallūm presented his works to the sultan, who rewarded him with a fur coat.[13] (It was customary in the Middle East for a ruler to single out a favorite subject and bestow distinction upon him through the presentation of a fine garment.)[14] Ibn Sallūm's writings enjoyed considerable popularity both within the

Ottoman Empire and outside it. His treatises were copied time and again, and many of them still exist in libraries in Turkey and elsewhere. Some of his writings were also translated into Persian.[15]

Another example is the Qayṣūnīzādes, a family of Egyptian physicians whom Selim I (reigned 1512–20) took with him when he returned from Cairo to Istanbul after his conquest of the Mamluk sultanate. The Qayṣūnīzādes were part of a large Cairene convoy leaving with Selim. (It was a deliberate Ottoman policy to tie members of conquered elites to the Ottoman family.) Members of the family served the sultans as their personal doctors till the beginning of the seventeenth century. Muḥammad Badr al-Dīn b. Muḥammad Qayṣūnīzādes (d. 1567/8), a personal physician to Süleyman I, was said to know only poor Turkish. He composed his work in Arabic, and it was later translated into Turkish by others.[16]

In sum, Ottoman Turkish did not replace Arabic but joined it as a language for medical writing, at least in some circles. The use of both Arabic and Ottoman Turkish for medical purposes is another illustration of Ottoman multilingualism. Or to put it differently, Ottoman Turkish added to itself literary and scientific uses.

Hospitals as an Ottoman Institution

Medical treatment was dispensed at various sites: at the private clinic of a physician, at the store in the marketplace, in the house of the patient, in the open air, and *also* at the hospital. Most Ottomans did not receive medical treatment in hospitals (although they could have received other kinds of services from hospitals, as analyzed in the third chapter). The vast majority of physicians practiced their profession outside hospitals and did not seem to consider it as mandatory experience in advancing their careers. In hospitals solely one type of medicine was practiced, although it was the one enjoying elite patronage and the status of "high-learned medicine." As mentioned earlier, the medical treatment practiced in hospitals was humoral, while the Ottoman medical system was composed also of folk medicine and religious medicine ("Prophetic medicine"). Moreover, hospitals practiced curative medicine. The curative characteristic of hospital medicine was the natural outcome of the needs of their customers, who were ill people, not healthy people trying to maintain their health. But Ottoman medicine emphasized another aspect of medicine—namely, preventive measures—just as much, maybe even more so. It also must be kept in mind that there was little in the way of early modern Ottoman medical capabilities that could not be made easily available outside hospitals. Much of household medicine or physician's-shop-cum-clinic medicine was identical with hospital treatment. Illness in itself did not imply hospitalization. All these turned hospitals into marginal medical sites in Ottoman society.

Despite hospitals' marginality in the premodern Middle East, they are nonetheless a very telling institution of the society in which they functioned. Charles E. Rosenberg's observation with regard to the pre–Civil War American hospital is applicable to Ottoman hospitals as well.[17] Hospitals are peculiarly characteristic of their society and are very much a mirror of the society that populates and supports them. They cannot help but reproduce fundamental social relationships and values in microcosm.

The "Ottoman-ness" of hospitals founded by Ottoman elite members could be discerned all over the Ottoman Empire, although the Ottoman Empire was far from being a monolithic entity. Variety was one of the characteristics of early modern Ottoman society and culture. Different cultural, administrative, and medical traditions existed in different places. Istanbul and Cairo, for example, differed in the extent to which Turkish, Anatolian, and Byzantine traditions, on the one hand, and the Arab-Muslim tradition, on the other, influenced local medical institutions. The empire extended over vast territories. Naturally, the great geographical area included different ecological environments. A hospital in Tunisia, for example, took care of medical cases other than those in a hospital in the Anatolian hinterland town of Amasya.

The cultural variety existing in the Ottoman Empire created the Ottoman hospital. The Ottoman medical system, like Ottoman culture as a whole, was the result of combining central Asian, Anatolian, Arab-Muslim, and Byzantine influences. Hospitals were the outcome of the merging of several medical traditions together. For instance, the architecture of Ottoman hospitals that practiced Arab-Muslim medicine was influenced by Seljukid *medrese* and hospital buildings.

The blending of Arab-Muslim and Seljukid medical influences allowed the Ottoman hospital to become the epitome of the basic concept in Ottoman medicine—namely, integralistic medicine. Following integralistic medicine, Ottomans considered quality of life and health, and not just disease; diagnosis and treatment regarded all body parts and mind as meshed into one complex integralistic entity. Hospitals were marginal medical sites in the Ottoman Empire, but they embodied this important medical concept best. Ottomans shared with these two preceding Muslim cultures integralistic perceptions about health and illness and medical treatment. However, it was in the Ottoman hospital that these theoretical conceptions were implemented in an actual course of treatment. Integralism determined the structure of the building, required the nurturing of gardens, and helped to shape the nature of the staff and their duties. Such a comprehensive implementation of integralistic medicine existed only in hospitals, not in private practice. In hospitals general practitioners, ophthalmologists, and surgeons took care of the patients' body; musicians and other personnel took care of the patients' mind and soul. The physicians, the cooks, and other staff members were supposed to treat the patients gently and kindly. In this integralistic course of treatment, hammams occupied an important medical role in hospitals: treatment at the bathhouse was expected to restore the patient's humoral balance and thus his or her physical and mental health. Ornamental fountains and small gardens were active players in creating an integralistic ecology surrounding the ill. They calmed both the temperamental patients and the pressured personnel, and gave them some peace and quiet.

Another characteristic of the hospital reveals an influence from earlier Muslim societies. Hospitals in Ottoman urban centers were all established as charitable institutions (chapter 3). Setting up endowments was the usual legal mechanism for managing and financing charitable activities, including within the medical realm. Like other charitable institutions in the early modern Ottoman Empire, therefore, the hospital was established, and operated, as part of a complex of charities for the community. It was an amalgamation of different institutions, with mosques situated at the very center of the site, offering an urban Ottoman-Muslim community various material and spiritual services. The amalgamation of charitable institutions is what Halil Inalcik has termed the *vakıf-imaret* system, an exclusive feature of the Ottoman Empire.[18]

Hospitals offered multiple services for various social groups (chapter 3). Firstly, they offered medical treatment to ill people. The association of hospitals with (only) ill people was well established in Muslim societies for centuries (unlike in European societies) but the complex admittance policy that balanced various groups was an Ottoman novelty. Patients who were treated at the hospital during their hospitalization were usually foreigners. Other ill people, locals, were treated there as "outpatients" and returned home for the night. In some cases physicians from the hospital even treated at home patients living in the neighborhood of hospitals. Hospitals also served the healthy. In fact, considering the number of healthy people who enjoyed hospitals in some way, it seems that hospitals served mainly the healthy. Hospitals functioned somewhat as a place of internship for medical students. Hospitals employed many people of diverse social and vocational backgrounds. The hospital's inclusive policy, maybe even more so than other institutions, was a means to control society and define its "borders": whoever was entitled to be attached to a hospital, either as a patient or as a staff member, was a member of Ottoman society, even if a marginal one (as in the case of strangers and madmen). Anyone who was not acknowledged as a full member of Ottoman society could not be supported by the hospital at all.

The process of bureaucratization and the co-optation mechanisms into the Ottoman bureaucracy manifested in Ottoman hospitals positioned this medical institution parallel to other Ottoman institutions, like the central administration, the palace harem, and the ulema.[19] Bureaucratization of the hospital came about in two intertwined processes. The first was medical professionalization; the second was evolution of a hierarchy by way of graduating wage levels between hospitals and between staff members. Analysis of physicians' career paths in hospitals attest that hospitals in Istanbul were considered better than those outside it, even the hospitals in previous imperial capitals like Bursa or Edirne. Promotion was always from the provinces into Istanbul. Dozens of annual budget reports from the sixteenth and seventeenth centuries reveal that there was a clear differentiation between medical staff, manual workers, and administration. Within the medical staff it was clear that general-internist physicians belonged to a higher pay rank than ophthalmologists and surgeons, let alone paramedical personnel.

The co-optation of medical doctors to the Ottoman medical system included the selection of physicians belonging to one specific medical tradition (humoral medicine). They received the appropriate medical training; and if they passed the basic requirements (with no formal examination), they entered Ottoman bureaucracy by appointments into hospitals and palaces. They became state employees who drew their salaries from the central treasury. Recruitment of candidates for positions in the hospitals, decisions about appointments, and the supervision of hospitals financially and professionally were all done in an organized manner. The process was a familiar one for the participants, both the supervisors and the supervised.

The dual process of bureaucratization and co-optation brought about three differences between Ottoman hospitals and pre-Ottoman Muslim hospitals. Firstly, Ottoman hospitals employed more staff than had been common in previous periods. Now staff included a couple of dozen people, whereas previous Muslim hospitals usually employed much fewer people. Secondly, the medical staff in Ottoman hospitals was larger, including more physicians, medical specialists, and paramedical professionals. In other words, the increase in the number of employees was not only in (cheap) manual and administrative workers but also in "high-tech" expensive workers. Thirdly, the organization of the Ottoman hospital was more detailed and formal than previously.

Hospitals with such characteristics existed in other societies, but Ottoman hospitals were still a group of their own. While various medical and administrative attributes appeared separately in previous periods, and were not as enhanced or easily noticed, the appearance of all of them at this level of medical and administrative sophistication was a special characteristic of Ottoman imperial hospitals. The fact that hospitals in the Ottoman Empire evolved to be an Ottoman phenomenon was what set them apart from other hospitals in pre-Ottoman Muslim societies and in European societies in the Middle Ages and in the early modern era.

"The sick are cured within three days"

Ottoman medicine emphasized the importance of prevention and constant upkeep of one's health. In the Ottoman case, preventive medicine seems to have been very effective. According to the English traveler Hill, "Turks" were known to live long. He recalled meeting an old man in the meadows by a river in Bulgaria who sang him several songs. His face was wrinkled from old age, but his voice was vibrant and body strong. The man did not know his age, although he recalled his village was burnt down when he was thirty years old. Now, after even his grandchildren had passed away, he was left alone to fend for himself. Locals told Hill that the old man's family had ceased to exist fourteen years earlier when his great-grandchildren (and not his grandchildren), themselves grown-ups, passed away. If indeed he had been thirty when the village caught fire, he was then one hundred sixty-two years old.[20]

The French traveler Thevenot agreed with Hill's claim. He described the "Turks" as blessed with long life during which they rarely suffered from the illnesses that riddled the Christians living by their side. But Thevenot also supplied explanations for this phenomenon. First, Turks were pedantic about their personal hygiene and regular bathing. Second, they practiced moderation in their meals, and their diet was based on a limited number of foodstuffs, in contrast to Christians, whose food was diverse. Third, Turks did not drink large quantities of alcohol, and they exercised.[21] This picture is too simplistic, of course. Early modern Ottoman society was more complex, as we saw in the previous chapter with regard to diet, and earlier in this chapter with regard to alcohol. Yet this was the perception of one Frenchman trying to make sense to himself of what he saw as puzzling: the seemingly continuous health of Ottomans in the middle of the seventeenth century.

However, people did get ill nonetheless. Despite Hill and Thevenot's rosy image of the health conditions of Ottomans, illness and death were common. Prevention did not always work, especially as it demanded resources that were not available for many. How much curative help could Ottoman medicine offer them, then? Did the vast repertoire of medical therapeutics discussed in this book work? The question goes beyond Ottoman medicine biological efficacy (and in the absence of statistics we cannot answer that question, anyway). As one might have suspected, Ottoman responses combined facts and fiction, realities, stereotypes, images, and wishful thinking.

The Ottomans demonstrated a spectrum of responses toward illness and medicine. These ranged from indifference, even fatalism, to pessimism and fear, but most Ottomans demonstrated activity and optimism in the face of illness. As the discussion in previous chapters clearly pointed out, the majority of early modern Middle Easterners did not give up or despair from illness. They did believe in the power of medicine to heal and the ability of most physicians to administer it well, God willing. They were not blind, however, to the moral and professional deficiencies of physicians, and to their limited abilities.

The complex and competitive medical reality explains why no single medical tradition succeeded in securing a monopoly but forever had to compete with other medical traditions. Most Ottomans had a medical preference, but in times of illness many were willing to try other types of healers and therapeutics if their first choice proved lacking. While they favored one medical course or another, it was no blind loyalty. This explains, for example, how the imperial harem was served by the palace medical corps—male physicians working within humoral medicine—as well as by female folk healers.

The complex and competitive medical reality also explains how physicians were portrayed in some sources as the epitome of humanity, goodhearted and doing their utmost for the benefit of their patients, while other sources discuss their vanity and avarice. Patients sought physicians' expertise, relying on their skills, yet were not shy of suing them if the outcome was not the expected one. The relationship was businesslike.

Medical knowledge was esteemed, but not like the knowledge of other branches of high learning. Biographical dictionaries reveal that many learned Ottomans who pursued nonmedical career paths were versed also in humoral medical texts.[22] Medical knowledge was part of the package that made an Ottoman intellectual. Many manuscripts dealing with vast medical interests were to be found in the private libraries of elite Ottomans in Istanbul (now kept at the Süleymaniye Library in Istanbul). They attest that medical knowledge was available in elite circles and that people who acquired manuscripts thought enough of it (as both knowledge and commodity) to invest the money in buying medical ones and reproducing more copies. However, not all Ottoman scholars studied medicine, and it did not seem to harm their prestige as knowledgeable men. Also, those who did study some medicine regarded the medical body of knowledge as of secondary importance in comparison to matters religious. The salaries paid to teachers in a medical school clearly positioned them below their colleagues in the *medreses*. Moreover, the medical school at the Süleymaniye, the only formal one in the Ottoman Empire prior to the nineteenth century, was smaller than the usual imperial *medrese*. A medical career offered students a modest income.

The limited resources directed to medicine in general could be part of the explanation why the foundation hospitals came to a halt in the eighteenth century. The eighteenth century was a period of increased financial pressures in the Ottoman Empire. Hospitals were costly investments. The building hosting a hospital had to be architecturally suited to the unique functions of the institution, and demanded a sewage system, a water system, rooms of various sizes, and so on. The first vast investment was not the end of it. Hospitals demanded a large and expert staff, and constant reequipping of medical devices and medicinal substances. All these resulted in high current expenditures. The high costs involved in the foundation of hospitals and their day-to-day finances may have driven benevolent founders to channel their charitable activity toward cheaper elements, like fountains, hostels, and libraries.[23] Other institutions, like soup kitchens (which were even more costly than hospitals), continued to be founded. Even during periods of more affluence only a limited number of hospitals were founded throughout the empire. Hospitals were deemed useful but not crucial for the community.

Medical practice contained many non-Muslims. Ottoman sources describing the core area, as well as European observers, claimed that many physicians were Jews, Greeks, and Armenians, and they may have outnumbered the Muslims. The number of Turkish Muslims who chose medicine as a profession was quite low. They had more career options on the whole, among which several were considered more profitable and respectable then medicine. Obviously, a career based on Muslim religious education, a venue through which many Ottomans entered state employment, was impossible for non-Muslims. Medicine, however, was a field that allowed non-Muslims to integrate into Muslim society, even to aspire to elite patronage, if they so wished, by treating non-Muslim patients. The void left by Muslim Turks who pursued other career paths was filled by Jews and Christians.[24]

Some Ottomans saw the high percentage of non-Muslims in medicine as a reason for forming a low opinion of the profession. One of them was Muḥammad b. ʿUmar (d. 1647), a *kadi* in Jerusalem, Damascus, and Aleppo. He presented his criticism of his days in Istanbul in the following verse: "Istanbul is one of the wonders of this world, a hospital of this universe; its occupants are ill and crippled, and it is full of lunatics and Jewish physicians."[25] Muḥammad b. ʿUmar's dismal imagery of Istanbul may have something to do with his being an Egyptian. Some Egyptians were critical of Istanbul, regarding it as inferior morally and intellectually, despite—or because of—its being the imperial capital. Whatever his personal reason, it is interesting that Muḥammad b. ʿUmar, who received his medical education in Istanbul, chose to express his opinion of it by associating it with negative images of medicine in general and the Jewish presence in medicine in particular.

Muḥammad b. ʿUmar expressed another common attitude among Ottomans, one that viewed hospitals with contempt, not as a place of health and hope. Although many hospital patients were Ottomans from mainstream social groups, Muḥammad b. ʿUmar associated hospitals with marginal groups. Other Ottomans presented an opposite image. Hospitals were positively associated with medical expertise and cure. The various images Ottomans had of their hospitals reveal complex attitudes and realities.

Hadidi, an early sixteenth-century poet, described the hospital of Mehmet II as a place where the bedridden recover due to the expertise of the physicians there. Hadidi (literally "Pertaining to Iron") made a living as a blacksmith and chose the title of his occupation as his pen name. He is considered a writer of little importance (for instance, he was not granted an audience with the sultan and could not present him with his verse chronicle of the Ottoman dynasty), although İbrahim Peçevi, the important Ottoman historian from the seventeenth century, names him as one of his sources.[26] Evliya Çelebi, a much more central figure, exalted the hospital of Süleyman I in Istanbul as a superb medical institution. He claimed the hospital of

Sultan Süleyman was an establishment so excellent that the ill were generally cured within three days after their admission (with God's help; Evliya hastened to add). The patients in the hospital of Mehmed II in Istanbul were served generous helpings of delicious food twice a day. He went on to say, "[E]ven pheasants, partridges, and other delicate birds are supplied."[27] The French traveler Tavernier described how pages in Topkapı in the late seventeenth century tried to invent valid reasons to be granted admittance into the palace hospital. For them the hospital was a place for rest and recreation.

Various stipulations in the foundation deeds of hospitals make it clear that the patrons expected the patients to recuperate and leave the hospitals. Sometimes things were less rosy. Not all hospital patients entered hospitals of their own free will. Lunatics, for instance, were often admitted into the hospital forcibly. These were madmen who were declared unfit to be outside hospitals and in need of constant medical attention for their own benefit and that of society (the criterion was the extent to which they threatened the public order).

And not all hospital patients were able to leave the institutions. Some died during their stay, when the abilities of the physicians were not enough to help them to recuperate. The founders of the hospitals expected some of their patients would succumb to their illness and stipulated that a portion of the budget should cover burial costs. Patients whom hospitals were not able to help in this world were helped on their way to the hereafter. Special staff members prepared the dead for burial: they ritually cleansed the bodies and wrapped them in shrouds.

A similar complexity existed in contemporary European societies. Some viewed hospitals as a place of hope, where people entered voluntarily of their own accord. They believed they would get better and leave it on their own two feet. Martin Luther (d. 1546), never an admirer of Catholic institutions, was nevertheless impressed with Italian hospitals. He echoes Evliya in his own glowing report: "They are splendidly constructed. . . . The best food and drink are provided, the attendants are extremely diligent, the physicians learned, the beds and coverings very clean, and the bedsteads painted."[28] In Renaissance Florence people indeed entered hospitals voluntarily, expecting to regain their health or at least feel better than when they entered; and their expectations were usually fulfilled.[29]

Other Europeans associated hospitals with desolation and death. Charles E. Rosenberg titled his seminal work on hospitals in the nineteenth-century and twentieth-century United States *The Care of Strangers*. Rosenberg's witty title draws attention to the hospital treatment as a social anomaly. During much of the history of hospitals, recuperating at an institution outside one's home, with no family and friends around seemed almost incomprehensible, unless there was no other viable option. European hospitals were associated for centuries in peoples' minds with a place of death, an option of last resort. Sir Thomas Browne (1605–82), an English intellectual who was also a medical practitioner in London and Norwich, wrote: "For the world, I count it not an Inne, but an Hospital, and a place, not to live but to die in."[30] To a doctor (!) in seventeenth-century England a hospital was a place of death.

Florence Nightingale (1820–1910), the famous nurse, reformed British military and civilian hospital sanitation methods and reconstructed nursing as a modern respectable profession. She started her public campaign by introducing female nurses into the health services for the British wounded in the Crimean War (1854–56) when she headed the nursing staff in the hospital barracks in Üsküdar, the Asian suburb of Istanbul. Nightingale is quoted in popular culture as claiming that the very first requirement in a hospital is that it should do the ill no harm. It was rephrasing of one of the famous dictums in the so-called Hippocratic Corpus, to the effect that a physician should make a habit of two things: to help, or at least to do no harm.

"At least to do no harm"—not an overly optimistic saying—aptly describes the Ottoman reaction to medicine. Ottomans accepted as unavoidable that sometimes physicians and medicine would harm patients (despite the dictum), or at least not be able to offer any real and concrete comfort. This realistic attitude attests that in the Ottoman case, although a negative association of medicine did exist, it seems to be not the prevalent one; at the same time people did not incline to the other extreme, that of naive expectation. Illness and death were regarded with acceptance. Early modern Ottomans lived with them as everyday and normal occurrences.

Illness could be regarded also as an opportunity. Several Ottomans were not shy about notifying the authorities about other people's impeding death and their wish to take their place. Mehmet, son of Şah Çelebi and a client of a *hoca* (chief) of a bureau in the Ottoman bureaucracy, was entitled to a salary of five silver coins from one of the charities (*evkaf*) in Bursa. In the spring of 1571 he was incurably ill, presumably on his deathbed. A person by the name of Kabil sent a letter to Istanbul with these details, asking for himself to be granted three pieces of silver out of the five that were soon to be "free."[31] In Ottoman society, as elsewhere, sickness and death were unfortunate events, but they could open new possibilities for others.

APPENDIX

List of Hospitals Discussed in the Book

Type of Institution	Name of Founder	Location	Period
Hospital	Nūr al-Dīn Maḥmūd (Zangid)	Aleppo	1154
Hospital	Nūr al-Dīn Maḥmūd Zangī	Damascus	circa 1154
Hospital	Nūr al-Dīn Maḥmūd Zangī	Mecca	circa 1154
Hospital	Ṣalāḥ al-Dīn/Saladin al-Ayyūbī	Jerusalem	1187
Hospital and medical school	Gevher Nesibe (Seljukid)	Kayseri	1206
Hospital	I. Izzeddin Keykavus (Seljukid sultan)	Sivas	1217
Hospital	Turan Melik bint Fahreddin Behremşah (Mengüçek princess)	Divriği	1228
Hospital	I. Alaeddin Keykubad (Seljukid sultan)	Konya	circa 1230
Hospital	Qala'un (Mamluk sultan)	Cairo	1284
Hospital	Yıldız Hatun (Il-Khanid)	Amasya	1308
Hospital	I. Yıldırım Sultan Beyazid	Bursa	1400 (date of *vakfiye*)
Hospital	Fatih Sultan Mehmet	Istanbul	circa 1470
Hospital	Topkapı Palace hospital for the pages	Istanbul	circa 1476 (date of palace foundation)
Hospital	II. Sultan Beyazid	Edirne	1493 (date of *vakfiye*)
Hospital	Hafsa Sultan	Manisa	1539
Hospital	Topkapı Palace harem hospital	Istanbul	late sixteenth century
Hospital	Haseki Hurren Sultan	Istanbul	1551 (date of *vakfiye*)
Hospital and medical school	Kanuni Sultan Süleyman	Istanbul	circa 1555
Hospital	Sokullu Mehmet Paşa (grand vizier)	Mecca	1573 (date of *vakfiye*)
Hospital	Nurbanu (Atik-i Valide) Sultan	Istanbul/Üsküdar	1580
Hospital	I. Sultan Ahmet	Istanbul	1613 (date of *vakfiye*)
Hospital	Ḥamūda al-Murādī (the Ottoman provincial governor)	Tunis	1662
Hospital	Gülnüş Sultan	Mecca	1679 (date of *vakfiye*)
Hospital	Bezm-i 'Alem	Istanbul	1845

Notes

Introduction: The Marriage of Medicine and Society

1. Susan Sontag, *Illness as Metaphor* (New York: Farrar, Straus and Giroux, 1978), 3.

2. I follow Maurice Cerasi's definition based on urban formation, technology, and conceptions of town building. Cerasi, "The Many Masters and Artisans of the Ottoman Town's Form and Culture: Chaos out of Order, Syncretism out of Separation—the Eighteenth and Nineteenth Centuries," paper delivered at *Order in Anarchy: The Management of Urban Space and Society in the Islamic World*, the third annual international workshop of the Program for Middle East History at Ben-Gurion University of the Negev, Israel, April 1997; Cerasi, "Open Space, Water and Trees in Ottoman Urban Culture in the XVIIIth–XIXth Centuries," *A.A.R.P. Environmental Design* 2 (1985): 36–49; Cerasi, "The Formation of Ottoman House Types: A Comparative Study in Interaction with Neighboring Cultures," *Muqarnas* 15 (1998): 116–56.

3. Byron J. Good and Mary-Jo Del Vecchio Good, "The Semantics of Medical Discourse," in *Sciences and Cultures: Anthropological and Historical Studies of the Sciences*, ed. Everett Mendelsohn and Yehuda Elkana (Dordrecht: D. Reidel, 1981), 177–212.

4. Two representative examples of Rosen's work are: George Rosen, *A History of Public Health* (New York: MD Publications, 1958); and Rosen, *Madness in Society: Chapters in the Historical Sociology of Mental Illness* (Chicago: University of Chicago Press, 1968).

5. Nancy G. Siraisi, "Some Current Trends in the Study of Renaissance Medicine," *Renaissance Quarterly* 37 (1984): 588–89.

6. Roy Porter, "The Patient's View: Doing Medical History from Below," *Theory and Society* 14 (1985): 175–98.

7. Michel Foucault, *Madness and Civilization: A History of Insanity in the Age of Reason*, trans. Richard Howard (London: Tavistock Publications, 1967); Foucault, *The Archaeology of Knowledge*, trans. A. M. Sheridan Smith (New York: Pantheon Books, 1972); Foucault, *The Birth of the Clinic: An Archaeology of Medical Perception*, trans. A. M. Sheridan (London: Tavistock Publications,

1976); Foucault, *Discipline and Punish: The Birth of the Prison*, trans. A. M. Sheridan (New York: Pantheon Books, 1977).

8. Patrick H. Hutton, "The History of Mentalities: The New Map of Cultural History," *History and Theory* 20 (1981): 237–59; Fedwa Malti-Douglas, "Mentalités and Marginality: Blindness and Mamlûk Civilization," in *The Islamic World from Classical to Modern Times: Essays in Honor of Bernard Lewis*, ed. C. E. Bosworth et al. (Princeton, NJ: Darwin Press, 1989), 211–37.

9. Guenter B. Risse, *Mending Bodies, Saving Souls* (New York: Oxford University Press, 1999). The index bears evidence that (only) a couple of pages address the long history of hospitals in Islam, but the references are to the wrong pages.

10. Sandra Harding, *Is Science Multi-Cultural? Postcolonialisms, Feminisms, and Epistemologies* (Bloomington: Indiana University Press, 1998), 2–4; Robert Figueroa and Sandra Harding, eds., *Science and Other Cultures: Issues in Philosophies of Science and Technology* (New York: Routledge, 2003), 1–3.

11. Emilie Savage-Smith, "Gleanings from an Arabist's Workshop: Current Trends in the Study of Medieval Islamic Science and Medicine," *Isis* 79 (1988): 247.

12. Manfred Ullmann, *Islamic Medicine* (Edinburgh: Edinburgh University Press, 1978).

13. Some of their publications are: Max Meyerhof, *"The Book of the Ten Treatises on the Eye" Ascribed to Hunain ibn Is-haq (809–877 A.D.)* (Cairo: Govt. Press, 1928); Meyerhof, *Sarh Asma' al-Uqqar (Explication des nom de drogues): Un glossaire de matière medicale* (Le Caire: Impr. de l'Institut francais d'archeologie orientale, 1940); Joseph Schacht and Max Meyerhof, *The Medico-Philosophical Controversy between Ibn Butlan of Baghdad and Ibn Ridwan of Cairo: A Contribution to the History of Greek Learning among the Arabs* (Cairo: [n.p.], 1937); Max Meyerhof and Joseph Schacht, *"The Theologus Autodidactus" of Ibn al-Nafis* (Oxford: Clarendon Press, 1968).

14. Peter E. Pormann and Emilie Savage-Smith, *Medieval Islamic Medicine* (Edinburgh: Edinburgh University Press, 2007).

15. Cyril Elgood, *Medicine in Persia* (New York: Hoeber, 1934); Elgood, *A Medical History of Persia and the Eastern Caliphate* (London: Cambridge University Press, 1951); Elgood, *Safavid Medical Practice or the Practice of Medicine, Surgery and Gynaecology in Persia between 1500 A.D. and 1750 A.D* (London: Luzac, 1970).

16. Their publications are too numerous to be mentioned here. The reader is referred to the bibliography for some of Adıvar, Uludağ, and Ünver's representative studies. Other representative works are Mehmet Cevdet, "Sivas Darüşşifası Vakfiyesi ve Tercümesi," *Vakıflar Dergisi* 1 (1938): 35–38; Bedi N. Şehsuvaroğlu, *İstanbul'da 500 Yıllık Sağlık Hayatımız* (İstanbul: İstanbul Fetih Derneği Neşriyati, 1953); Şehsuvaroğlu, Ayşegül Erdemir Demirhan, and Gönül Cantay Güreşsever, *Türk Tıp Tarihi* (Bursa: [n.p.], 1984).

17. Charles E. Rosenberg, *Explaining Epidemics and Other Studies in the History of Medicine* (Cambridge: Cambridge University Press, 1992), 1.

18. See, for example, Franz Rosenthal, "The Physician in Medieval Muslim Society," *Bulletin of the History of Medicine* 52 (1978): 476–91; Rosenthal, *The Herb: Hashish versus Medieval Muslim Society* (Leiden: Brill, 1971).

19. Savage-Smith, "Gleanings from an Arabist's Workshop," 247.

20. Michael W. Dols, "The Plague in Early Islamic History," *Journal of the Economic and Social History of the Orient* 94 (1974): 376–83; Dols, *The Black Death in the Middle East* (Princeton, NJ: Princeton University Press, 1977); Dols, "The Second Plague Pandemic and Its Recurrences in the Middle East: 1347–1894," *Journal of the Economic and Social History of the Orient* 22 (1979): 162–89; Dols, "Leprosy in Medieval Arabic Medicine," *Journal of History of Medicine and Allied Sciences* 34 (1979): 314–33; Dols, "The Leper in Medieval Islamic Society," *Speculum* 58 (1983): 891–916; Dols, "Insanity in Byzantine and Islamic Medicine," *Symposium on Byzantine Medicine, Dumbarton Oaks Papers* 38 (1984): 136–48; Dols, "The Origins of the Islamic Hospital: Myth and Reality," *Bulletin of the History of Medicine* 61 (1987): 367–90; Dols, "Insanity and its Treatment in Islamic Society," *Medical History* 31 (1987): 1–14; Dols, *Majnūn: The Madman in Medieval Islamic Society* (Oxford: Clarendon Press, 1992).

21. Some of Conrad's representative work on plagues is Lawrence I. Conrad, "Arabic Plague Chronologies and Treatises: Social and Historical Factors in the Formation of a Literary Genre," *Studia Islamica* 54 (1981): 51–93; Conrad, "Tā'ūn and Wabā: Conceptions of Plague and Pestilence in Early Islam," *Journal of the Economic and Social History of the Orient* 25 (1982): 268–307; Conrad, "Epidemic Disease in Formal and Popular Thought in Early Islamic Society," in *Epidemics and Ideas: Essays on the Historical Perception of Pestilence*, ed. Terence Ranger and Paul Slack (Cambridge: Cambridge University Press, 1992), 77–99; and Conrad, "A Ninth-Century Muslim Scholar's Discussion of Contagion," in *Contagion: Perspectives from Pre-Modern Societies*, ed. Lawrence I. Conrad and Dominik Wujastyk (Aldershot, UK: Ashgate, 2000), 163–77.

22. Khaled Fahmy, "Law, Medicine and Society in Nineteenth-Century Egypt," *Egypte / Monde Arabe* 24 (1998): 17–51; Fahmy, "Women, Medicine, and Power in Nineteenth-Century Egypt," in *Remaking Women: Feminism and Modernity in the Middle East*, ed. Leila Abu-Lughod (Princeton, NJ: Princeton University Press, 1998), 35–72; Fahmy, "The Anatomy of Justice: Forensic Medicine and Criminal Law in Nineteenth-Century Egypt," *Islamic Law and Society* 6 (1999): 224–71; Fahmy, "Medicine and Power: Towards a Social History of Medicine in Nineteenth-century Egypt," *New Frontiers in the Social History of the Middle East / Cairo Papers in Social Science* 23 (2000): 15–62.

23. Nancy Gallagher, *Medicine and Power in Tunisia, 1780–1900* (Cambridge: Cambridge University Press, 1983); Gallagher, *Egypt's Other Wars: Epidemics and the Politics of Public Health* (New York; Syracuse University Press, 1990); LaVerne Kuhnke, *Lives at Risk: Public Health in Nineteenth Century Egypt* (Berkeley and Los Angeles: University of California Press, 1990); Amira el-Azhary Sonbol, *The Creation of a Medical Profession in Egypt, 1800–1922* (Syracuse, NY: Syracuse University Press, 1991). A recent addition is Sherine F.

Hamdy, "Blinding Ignorance: Medical Science, Diseased Eyes, and Religious Practice in Egypt," *Arab Studies Journal* 13 (2005): 26–45.

24. Compare, for example, Abraham Marcus, *The Middle East on the Eve of Modernity: Aleppo in the Eighteenth Century* (New York: Columbia University Press, 1989), chap. 7 "The Body: Health, Disease and Death," 252–76; Rhoads Murphey, "Ottoman Medicine and Transculturalism from the 16th Century," *Bulletin of the History of Medicine* 66 (1992): 376–403; Sara Scalenghe, "The Deaf in Ottoman Syria, 16th–18th Centuries," *Arab Studies Journal* 13 (2005): 10–25; Mohammad M. I. Ghaly, "Writings on Disability in Islam: The 16th-Century Polemic on Ibn Fahd's al-Nukat al-Ziraf," *Arab Studies Journal* 14 (2006): 9–38; Daniel Panzac, *La peste dans l'Empire Ottoman 1700–1850* (Louvain: Peeters, 1985); Panzac, "Politique sanitaire et fixation des frontièrs: L'example Ottoman (XVIIIe–XIXe Siècles)," *Turcica* 31 (1999):87–108; Panzac, "La peste dans les possessions insulaires du grand seigneur (XVIIe–XIX siècles)," in *Insularités Ottomans*, ed. Nicolas Vatin et Gilles Veinstein (Paris: Maisonneuve & Larose; Institut francais d'etudes anatoliennes, 2004), 223–40.

25. Two noted examples are Arslan Terzioğlu and Nil Sarı. Terzioğlu used his background as an architect to study Ottoman medicine in general and hospitals in particular. Terzioğlu published many studies in German (in addition to Turkish) due to his academic career in Germany. Sarı of the Cerrahpaşa Faculty of Medicine in Istanbul publishes regularly in English, and she is active in international societies for the history of medicine. The reader is referred to the bibliography for their works cited in this book.

26. Ekmeleddin İhsanoğlu, *Science, Technology, and Learning in the Ottoman Empire: Western Influence, Local Institutions, and the Transfer of Knowledge* (Aldershot, UK: Ashgate, 2004).

27. Catherine J. Kudlick, "Disability History: Why We Need Another 'Other,' " *American Historical Review*, 108 (2003): 763–93.

28. Emmanuel Le Roy Ladurie, "Presentation," *Annales: Economies, Sociétés, Civilizations* 29 (1974): 537. See also Alfred W. Crosby, "The Past and Present of Environmental History," *American Historical Review* 100 (1995): 1177–89; Ted Steinberg, "Down to Earth: Nature, Agency and Power in History," *American Historical Review* 107 (2002): 798–820.

29. See the discussion on medical anthropology as a subfield within anthropology in H-MedAnthro, an electronic forum for medical anthropologists, whether they are scholars, practitioners, or activists; http://www.h-net.org/~medanthro/ between February 28 and March 2, 2006.

30. George M. Foster and Barbara Gallatin Anderson, *Medical Anthropology* (New York: J. Wiley, 1978); Sherry B. Ortner, "Theory in Anthropology since the Sixties," *Comparative Studies in Society and History* 26 (1984): 126–66; Donald Joralemon, *Exploring Medical Anthropology*, 2nd ed. (Boston: Allyn & Bacon, 2006).

31. A. Wear, R. K. French, and I. M. Lonie, eds., *The Medical Renaissance of the Sixteenth Century* (Cambridge: Cambridge University Press, 1985), xiv.

32. Charles E. Rosenberg, *The Care of Strangers* (New York: Basic Books, 1997).

33. Mary Lindemann, *Medicine and Society in Early Modern Europe* (Cambridge: Cambridge University Press, 1999), 5.

34. For exposition of the term "early modern Europe" see standard textbooks like H. G. Koenigsberger, *Early Modern Europe, 1500–1789* (London: Longman, 1987); Euan Cameron, ed. *Early Modern Europe* (Oxford: Oxford University Press, 2001); Eugene F. Rice, *The Foundations of Early Modern Europe, 1460–1559,* with Eugene Rice (New York: W. W. Norton, 1994).

35. I outlined some of the changes in the eighteenth and nineteenth centuries in "Old Patterns, New Meaning: The 1845 Hospital of Bezm-i 'Alem in Istanbul," *Dynamis* 25 (2005): 329–50.

Chapter 1: Medical Pluralism, Prevention and Cure

1. Paul U. Unschuld, *Medicine in China: A History of Ideas* (Berkeley and Los Angeles: University of California Press, 1985), 1–15; Lawrence I. Conrad, "Medicine—Traditional Practice," in *The Oxford Encyclopedia of the Modern Islamic World,* 4 vols. (New York: Oxford University Press, 1995), 3:85–88. For a similar description of the early modern English medical system, see Andrew Wear, "Interfaces: Perceptions of Health and Illness in Early Modern England," in *Problems and Methods in the History of Medicine,* ed. Roy Porter and Andrew Wear (London: Croom Helm, 1987), 235, 240–41.

2. Conrad, "Medicine—Traditional Practice," 3:85–88.

3. Cristina Álvarez-Millán, "Graeco-Roman Case Histories and Their Influence on Medieval Islamic Clinical Accounts," *Social History of Medicine* 12 (1999): 19–43; Álvarez-Millán, "Practice versus Theory: Tenth-Century Case Histories from the Islamic Middle East," *Social History of Medicine* 13 (2000): 293–306. For discussion of medicine as literature and social activity in the Muslim Middle Ages, see Lawrence I. Conrad, "Scholarship and Social Context in the Near East," in *Knowledge and the Scholarly Medical Traditions,* ed. Don Bates (Cambridge: Cambridge University Press, 1995), 81–101.

4. Peregrine Horden, "The Millennium Bug: Health and Medicine around the Year 1000," *Social History of Medicine* 13 (2000): 206–7.

5. Foster and Anderson, *Medical Anthropology,* 36

6. For a recent thorough summary of current scholarship in ancient medical studies, see Vivian Nutton, *Ancient Medicine* (London: Routledge, 2004). For a synopsis of Muslim humoral medicine, see Ullmann, *Islamic Medicine,* 55–69; Ali ibn Ali ibn Ja'far Ibn Ridwan, *Medieval Islamic Medicine: Ibn Ridwan's Treatise "On the Prevention of Bodily Ills in Egypt,"* trans. Michael W. Dols, Arabic text edited by Adil S. Gamal (Berkeley and Los Angeles: University of California Press, 1984), 3–24; István Ormos, "The Theory of Humours in Islam (Avicenna)," *Quaderni di Studi Arabi* 5–6 (1987): 601–7.

7. Expiración García Sánchez, "Dietic Aspects of Food in al-Andalus," in *Patterns of Everyday Life,* ed. David Waines (Aldershot, UK: Ashgate, 2002), 276.

8. Ibid., 276.

9. Fazlur Rahman, *Health and Medicine in Islamic Tradition* (New York: ABC International Group, 1989), chap. 3 "The Prophetic Medicine," 41–58, 137–38 (notes); Iremli Perho, *The Prophet's Medicine: A Creation of the Muslim Traditionalist Scholars* (Helsinki: Finnish Oriental Society, 1995), chap. 7 "The reasons for Creating the Prophet's Medicine," 76–83; Uri Rubin, "Muḥammad the Exorcist: Aspects of Islamic-Jewish Polemics," *Jerusalem Studies in Islam* 30 (2005): 94–111; Ekmeleddin İhsanoğlu, "Türkçe Tibb-i Nebevī Yazmaları," *Tıp Tarihi Araştırmaları* 2 (1998): 34–39. It should be noted that "Prophetic medicine" is a term used by Sunni Muslims who regard the Prophet Muhammad as possessing unique therapeutic skills. Shi'ite Muslims, in contrast, take away from the Prophet some of these unique attributes and invest them with the imams. See, for example, E. Kohlberg, "Vision and the Imams," in *Autour de regard: Mélanges Gimaret,* ed. É. Chaumont, D. Aigle, M. A. Amir-Moezzi, and P. Lory, eds. (Louvain: Peeters, 2003), 125–57. However, as Shi'ite religious medicine has been little studied, we still have to guess at its similarities to and differences from Prophetic (Sunni) medicine.

10. *Encyclopaedia of Islam,* 2nd ed., s.v. "Ḳutadgbu Bilig," by A. J. E. Bodrogligeti; O. M. Oztürk and V. Volkan, "The Theory and Practice of Psychiatry in Turkey," in *Psychological Dimensions of Near Eastern Studies,* ed. L. C. Brown and N. Itzkowitz (Princeton, NJ: Darwin Press, 1977), 347; O. M. Oztürk, "Folk Interpretation of Illness in Turkey and Its Psychological Significance," *Turkish Journal of Pediatrics* 7 (1965): 167.

11. Ibn Ridwan, *Medieval Islamic Medicine,* 23.

12. Muḥammad b. Ismā'īl Al-Bukhārī, *Al-Jāmi' al-Ṣaḥīḥ,* 3 vols. ([Cairo:] Dār wa-Maṭābi' al-Sha'b, 1378AH [1958]), al-marḍā /2; Ibn Ḥajar al-'Asqalānī, *Fatḥ al-Bārī bi-Sharḥ al-Bukhārī,* 12 vols. (Miṣr: Maktabat wa-Maṭba'at Muṣṭafā al-Bābī al-Ḥalabī, 1378H/1958), 12:214–15; J. Christoph Bürgel, "Secular and Religious Features of Medieval Medicine," in *Asian Medical Systems: A Comparative Survey,* ed. Charles Leslie (Berkeley and Los Angeles: University of California Press, 1976), 44–62; Lawrence I. Conrad, "Medicine and Martyrdom: Some Discussions of Suffering and Divine Justice in Early Islamic Society," in *Religion, Health and Suffering,* ed. John R. Hinnells and Roy Porter (London: Routledge, 1999), 212–36.

13. Ghada Karmi, "The Colonisation of Traditional Arabic Medicine," in *Patients and Practitioners: Lay Perceptions of Medicine in Pre-Industrial Society,* ed. Roy Porter (Cambridge: Cambridge University Press, 1985), 323–24.

14. Joseph Ziegler, "Religion and Medicine in the Middle Ages," in *Religion and Medicine in the Middle Ages,* ed. Peter Biller and Joseph Ziegler (Rochester, NY: York Medieval Press, 2001), 4.

15. On medical professional ethics in sixteenth-century Istanbul as a by-product of occupational competition, see Miri Shefer, "Medical and Professional Ethics in Sixteenth-Century Istanbul: Towards an Understanding of the Relationships between the Ottoman State and the Medical Guilds," *Medicine and Law* 21 (2002): 307–19.

16. See for example Ṣāliḥ b. Naṣrallah Ibn Sallūm, *Ghāyat al-bayān fī tadbīr badan al-insān*, Ms. Brown P. 27, held at Cambridge University Library), folios 15v–16v.

17. Al-Bukhārī, *Al-Jāmi' al-Ṣaḥīḥ*, ṭibb/item no. 3; Abū 'Abdallah Muḥammad b. Yazīd Ibn Māja, *Ṣaḥīḥ Sunan Ibn Māja*, 2 vols. (Riyadh: Maktab al-Tarbiya al-'Arabī li-Duwal al-Khalīj, 1408H/1988M), tibb / 20–24.

18. Al-Bukhārī, *Al-Jāmi' al-Ṣaḥīḥ*, al-marḍā/item no. 13; al-'Asqalānī, *Fatḥ al-Bārī*, 12:224–25.

19. On the depaganization process of Galenism in Christian Europe, which lasted till the Renaissance, see Vivian Nutton, "God, Galen and the Depaganization of Ancient Medicine," in *Religion and Medicine in the Middle Ages*, ed. Biller and Ziegler (Woodsbridge, UK: York Medieval Press, 2001), 17–32.

20. *Encyclopaedia of Islam*, 2nd ed., s.v. "Al-Suyūṭī Abū al-Faḍl 'Abd al-Raḥmān b. Abū Bakr b. Muḥammad Djalāl al-Dīn"; Marlis J. Saleh, "Al-Suyuti and His Works: Their Place in Islamic Scholarship from Mamluk Times to the Present," *Mamlūk Studies Review* 5 (2001): 73–89.

21. Jalāl al-Dīn al-Suyūṭī, al-Manhaj al-sawī wal-manhal al-rawī fī al-ṭibb al-nabawī, manuscript held at the Wellcome Institute for the History of Medicine Library, Wms.Or.90.

22. Fehmi Edhem Karatay, *Topkapı Sarayı Müzesi Kütüphanesi Arapça Kataloğu* (İstanbul: Topkapı Sarayı Müzesi, 1966), 3:859–60.

23. Perho, *Prophet's Medicine*, 76–110; Emilie Savage-Smith, "Medicine," in *Encyclopedia of the History of Arabic Science*, ed. Roshdi Rashed (3 vols. (London: Routledge, 1996), 3:928.

24. Zeyn al-Din al-Abidin b. Halil, "Shifa'-ı al-feva'id," manuscript help at the Wellcome Institute for the History of Medicine Library, WMs. Turkish 15.

25. For a claim that this is one feature that distinguished hominids from other creatures, see Arthur K. Shapiro and Elaine Shapiro, *The Powerful Placebo: From Ancient Priest to Modern Physician* (Baltimore: Johns Hopkins University Press, 1997), 3.

26. Jack Goody, *Cooking, Cuisine and Class* (Cambridge: Cambridge University Press, 1982), 117; Richard Tapper and Nancy Tapper, " 'Eat This, It'll Do You a Power of Good': Food and Commensality among Durrani Pashtuns," *American Ethnologist* 13 (1986): 62–79.

27. Nil Sarı, "Türk Tıp Tarihinde Yelemk ile Tıp Arasındakı İlışkıye ait Örnekler," in *İkinci Milletarası Yemek Kongresi (3–10 Eylül 1988)*, ed. Feyzi Halıcı (Konya: Türizm Bakanlığı, 1989), 392–402.

28. Cited in Joseph Needham, "Hygiene and Preventive Medicine," with Lu Gwei-Djen, *Journal of the History of Medicine and Allied Sciences* 17 (1962): 448.

29. Otavio Bon, *The Sultan's Seraglio: An Intimate Portrait of Life at the Ottoman Court* (London: Saqi Books, 1996), 35–36, 64, 93–104; C. G. Fisher and A. Fisher, "Topkapi Sarayi in the Mid-Seventeenth Century: Bobovi's Description," *Archivum Ottomanicum* 10 (1985 [1987]): 30–32, 63–64; Metin

And, *Istanbul in the 16th Century: The City, The Palace, Daily Life* (Istanbul: Akbank, 1994), 173–84.

30. Josef W. Meri, trans. *A Lonely Wayfarer's Guide to Pilgrimage: 'Alī ibn Abī Bakr al-Harawī's Kitāb al-Ishārāt ilā Ma'rifat al-Ziyārāt* (Princeton, NJ: Darwin Press, 2004), 96.

31. The Library of Topkapi Palace (Topkapı Sarayı Müzesi Kütüphanesi [TSMK]), defter 8228. See also Necdet Sakaoğlu, "Sources for Our Ancient Culinary Culture," in *The Illuminated Table, The Prosperous House: Food and Shelter in Ottoman Material Culture,* ed. Suraiya Faroqhi and Christoph K. Neumann (Würzburg: Ergon in Kommission, 2003), 34–49.

32. Suraiya Faroqhi, Introduction to *The Illuminated Table, The Prosperous House,* ed. Surayia Faroqhi and Christoph K. Neumann (Würzburg: Ergon in Kommission, 2003), 23.

33. J. Michael Rogers, "The Palace, Potions and the Public: Some Lists of Drugs in Mid-16th Century Ottoman Turkey," in *Studies in Ottoman History in Honour of Professor V. L. Mènage,* ed. Colin Heywood and Colin Imber (Istanbul: Isis Press, 1994), 273–95. On medical diet in the Court of the Abbasid caliphate in Baghdad, see Muhammad Manazir Ahsan, *Social Life under the Abbasids, 170–289 AH, 786–902 AD* (London: Longman, 1979), 117–18, 231.

34. Ömer Lutfi Barkan, "Fatih Cāmi ve İmareti 1489–1490 Yıllarına āit Muhasebe Bilānçoları," *İstanbul Üniversitesi İktisat Fakültesi Macmuası* 23, nos. 1–2 (1962–63): 328–32; Barkan, "Edirne ve Civarındaki Bazı İmāret Tesislerinin Yıllık Muhasebe Bilānçoları," *Belgeler* 1, nos. 1–2 (1964): 278–81.

35. The Archives of Topkapi Palace (Topkapı Sarayı Müzesi Arşivi, Istanbul, [TSMA), evrak 2211/7.

36. Studies on Ottoman food in the context of social and cultural consumption are in their early stages. I rely here mainly on Hedda Reindl-Kiel, "The Chicken of Paradise: Official Meals in the Mid-Seventeeenth Century Ottoman Palace," in *The Illuminated Table, The Prosperous House,* ed. Faroqhi and Neumann (Würzburg: Ergon in Kommission, 2003), 59–88; and Tülay Artan, "Aspects of the Ottoman Elites' Food Consumption: Looking for 'Staples,' 'Luxuries' and 'Delicacies' in a Changing Century," in *Consumption Studies and the History of the Ottoman Empire, 1550–1922,* ed. Donald Quatert (Albany: State University New York Press, 2000), 107–200. See also Nevin Halıcı, "Ottoman Cuisine," in *Culture and Arts,* ed. Kemal Çiçek, vol. 4 of *The Great Ottoman-Turkish Civilization* (Ankara: Yeni Türkiye, 2000), 93–103; Amalia Levanoni, "Food and Cooking during the Mamluk Era: Social and Political Implications," *Mamlūk Studies Review* 9, no. 2 (2005): 201–22.

37. Bon, *Sultan's Seraglio,* 36. Hans Dernschwam, *Tagebuch einer Reise nach der Konstantinopel und Kleinasien (1553–1555)* (Munich: Duncker & Humblot, 1923), 123. See also Ahmet Süheyl Ünver, "Four Medical Vignettes from Turkey," *International Record of Medicine* 171 (1958): 53–54.

38. Amy Singer, *Constructing Ottoman Beneficence: An Imperial Soup Kitchen in Jerusalem* (Albany: State University New York Press, 2002), chap. 2: "A Bowl of Soup and a Loaf of Bread," 58–65; Singer, "Serving up Charity: The Ottoman Public Kitchen," *Journal of Interdisciplinary History* 35 (2005): 485–92;

compare this to E. Ashtor, "The Diet of Salaried Classes in the Medieval Near East," *Journal of Asian History* 4 (1970): 1–24.

39. Nil Sarı and M. Bedizel Zülfikar, "Islâm Tıbbından Osmanlı Tıbbına Kuşlarla Tedavi," in *Dördüncü Milletlerarası Yemek Kongresi, 3–6 Eylül 1992,* ed. Feyzi Halıcı (Konya: Türizm Bakanlığı, 1993), 259–71.

40. Rhoads Murphey, *Ottoman Warfare, 1500–1700* (New Brunswick, NJ: Rutgers University Press, 1999), chap. 5: "Provisioning the Army," pp. 85–103, especially pp. 89–90.

41. Amnon Cohen, Economic Life in Ottoman Jerusalem (Cambridge: Cambridge University Press, 1989), 56.

42. George Sandys, *A Relation of a Journey Begun An. Dom. 1610 Containing a Description of the Turkish Empire . . .*, 6th ed. (London, 1670), 51.

43. Dernschwam, *Tagebuch*, 124.

44. Compare with the Mamluk period, Levanoni, "Food and Cooking during the Mamluk Era," 213–16.

45. Martin Levey, *Early Arabic Pharmacology* (Leiden: Brill, 1973), 70, 83, 87; J. Worth Estes and Laverne Kuhnke, "French Observations of Disease and Drug Use in Late Eighteenth-Century Cairo," *Journal of the History of Medicine and Allied Sciences* 39 (1984): 134–35.

46. See, for example, Gerrit Bos, "Ibn al-Jazzār on Medicine for the Poor and Destitute," *Journal of the American Oriental Society* 118 (1998): 365–75.

47. TSMA, evrak 93/1–2, 2657/1–5, 11942/7–11, 13–16, 18, 25, 28, 30–33, 37, 41, 43–46, 48, 56, 60, 66, 67–69, 71, 73, 75, 78–82, 85, 87–90, 92, 96–98, 102–5, 112, 118, 122–25, 127–28, 131.

48. Sami K. Hamarneh and Henri Amin Awad, "Glass Vessel Stamp Data for Materia Medica," in *Fustat Finds: Beads, Coins, Medical Instruments, Textiles, and Other Artifacts from the Awad Collection,* ed. Jere L. Bacharach (Cairo: American University in Cairo Press, 2002), 167–75.

49. Levey, *Early Arabic Pharmacology*, chap. 4 "Literary Models in Pharmacology," 66–71.

50. Gülbin Özçelikay, Eris Aşıl, Sevgi Şar and Kenan Süveren, "A Study on Prescription Samples Prepared in Ottoman Empire Period," *Hamdard Medicus* 37 (1994): 28–35; Estes and Kuhnke, "French Observations," 132.

51. M. Tayyib Gökbilgin, *XV–XVI Asırlarda Edirne ve Paşa Livāsi* (İstanbul: Üçler Basımevi, 1952), B:158–59, 1666–67. See also Kemāl Edīb Körkçüoğlu, ed., *Süleymaniye Vakfiyesi* (Ankara: Kesimli Posta Matbaası, 1962) B:147–48.

52. Levey, *Early Arabic Pharmacology*, 80.

53. Leslie P. Peirce has encountered in her studies of Aintab (modern Gaziantep, a town in the southeast of Turkey) an interesting reference to *ma'cun* as something drunk rather than eaten. The source differentiated between *macuns* and sherbets by whether they had any medical qualities rather than by their form. In 1541 several locals accused Hussam, a man from Mosul in Iraq who was visiting Aintab, of intoxicating/drugging them. They claimed he did so intentionally: he served them with şerbet he described as *ma'cun*; they drank it without any suspicion but lost consciousness till the morning after! Hussam rejected the accusation. He said he served them with syrup

that was clearly not a *ma'cun*, as it lacked any pharmaceutical attribute. Leslie Peirce, peirce@socrates.berkeley.edu, "re: ma'cunhane," private e-mail message to Miri Shefer, August 5, 1999. This case did not make its way into her book *Morality Tales: Law and Gender in the Ottoman Court of Aintab* (Berkeley and Los Angeles: University of California Press, 2003).

54. Mehmet Süreyya, *Sijill-i Osmanī* (İstanbul: Matba'a-i Amire, 1308 [1890]), 4:363; Nihad Nuri Yürükoğlu, *Manisa Bimarhanesi* (İstanbul: [n.p.], 1948), 25, 51, 57–58; Sadi Bayram, "Sağlık Hizmetlerimiz ve Vakıf Guraba Hastanesi," *Vakıflar Dergisi* 14 (1982): 103.

55. Manuela Marín and David Waines, "The Balanced Way: Food for Pleasure and Health in Medieval Islam," *Manuscripts of the Middle East* 4 (1989): 127–31.

56. For as early as the ninth century, see Selma Tibi, *The Medicinal Use of Opium in Ninth-Century Baghdad* (Leiden: Brill, 2006). For late eighteenth-century Egypt see Estes and Kuhnke, "French Observations," 134–35.

57. Rosenthal, *Herb*, 19, 33; Tibi, *Medicinal Use of Opium in Ninth-Century Baghdad*, xiii, 171–73.

58. Ayşe Saraçgil, "Generi voluttuari e region di stato: Politiche repressive del consumo di vino, caffè e tobacco nell'Impero Ottomano nei secc. XVI e XVII," *Turcica*, 28 (1996): 163–94; James Grehan, "Smoking and 'Early Modern' Sociability: The Great Tobacco Debate in the Ottoman Middle East (Seventeenth to Eighteenth Centuries)," *American Historical Review* 111 (2006): 1352–77.

59. TSMA, evrak, 11942/30, 68; Rogers, "Palace, Potions and the Public," 291.

60. Ayşegül Demirhan, "The Evolution of Opium in the Islamic World and Anatolian Turks," *Studies in History of Medicine* 4 (1980): 73, 76–79.

61. Jean Thevenot, *The Travells of Monsieur de Thevenot into the Levant . . .* (London, 1687), 1:114.

62. Ayşegül Demirhan, *Mısır Çarşısı Drogları* (İstanbul: Sermet Matbaası, 1975), 29–31, 70–71; İsmet Zeki Eyuboğlu, *Anadolu Halk İlaçları* (İstanbul: Hür Yayın ve Ticaret A.Ş, 1977), 51; Nevin Halıcı, "Anadolu Mutfağında Haşhaş," in *İkinci Milletarası Yemek Kongresi*, ed. Halıcı (Konya: Konya Kültür ve Turizm Vakfi, 1989), 170–80.

63. Demirhan, "Evolution of Opium," 73, 76, 78. Cannabis and hemp, likewise, were popular agricultural products. Hemp also was used by the thriving Anatolian textile industry: the cortical fiber of this plant was used for making cordage, and woven into stout fabrics. See Suraiya Faroqhi, *Towns and Townsmen of Ottoman Anatolia: Trade, Crafts and Food Production in an Urban Setting, 1520–1650* (Cambridge: Cambridge University Press, 1984), chap. 5, "Textile Manufacture: Geographical Distribution and Historical Development," 125–55.

64. Frank Dikötter, Lars Laamann, and Zhou Xun, *Narcotic Culture: A History of Drugs in China* (Chicago: University of Chicago Press), 17.

65. Nev'izade Ata'i, *Hada'iq al-Ḥaqa'iq fi Takmilat al-Shaqa'iq*, 2 vols. (İstanbul: Matbaa-i Amire, 1268 [1851]) 1:196–97. See the discussion by Uriel Heyd, "Moses Hamon, Chief Jewish Physician to Sultan Suleyman the Magnificent," *Oriens* 16 (1963): 161–63; *Encyclopaedia of Islam*, 2nd ed., s.v. " 'Aṭā'ī," by J.

Walsh. On the political factions at court during Süleyman's reign, see Leslie Peirce, "The Family as Factions: Dynastic Politics in the Reign of Süleymân," in *Soliman le Magnifique et son temps*, ed. Gilles Veinstein (Paris: Documentation française, 1992), 105–6. See also Rudolf Veselý, "Neues zur Familie al-Qūṣūnī: Ein Beitrag zue Genealogie einer Ägyptischen Ärzte- und Gelehrtenfamilie," *Oriens* 33 (1992): 437–44.

66. Muḥammad Amīn b. Faḍlallah al-Muḥibbī, *Tarīkh Khulaṣat al-Athr fī A'yān al-Qarn al-Ḥādī Ashar*, 4 vols. (Beirut: Maktabat Khayyāṭ, n.d.), 1:296–97. For another biography of Ibn al- Munqār that repeats the main story, see Najm al-Dīn Muḥammad b. Muḥammad al-Ghazzī (d. 1651), *Luṭf al-Samr wa-Qaṭf al-Thamr* (Dimashq: Wizārat al-Thaqāfa wal-Irshād al-Qawmī, 1981), 1:284–85.

67. Demirhan, "Evolution of Opium," 79.

68. Nicolas de Nicolay, *The Navigations, Peregrinations, and Voyages, Made into Turkie by Nicolas de Nicolay. . . .*, trans. T. Washington (London, 1593 [1585]), f. 91; Aaron Hill, *A Full and Just Account of the Present State of the Ottoman Empire . . .* (London, 1709), 123–24; Sandys, *Relation of a Journey*, 44, 51–52. See also Fernand Braudel, *Civilization and Capitalism, 15th–18th Century*, vol. 1: *The Structures of Everyday Life: The Limits of the Possible* (New York: Harper & Row, 1985), 260–65.

69. Dikötter, Laamann, and Xun, *Narcotic Culture*, 19–20.

70. Dernschwam, *Tagebuch*, 52–54, 105.

71. M. Nihat and Baha Dörder, *Türk Tiatrosu Ansiklopedisi* (İstanbul: [n.p.], 1967), 210, 244–45.

72. Felix Klein-Franke, "No Smoking in Paradise: The Habit of Tobacco Smoking Judged by Muslim Law," *Le Muséon* 106 (1993): 155–83; Li Guo. "Paradise Lost: Ibn Dāniyāl's Response to Baybars' Campaign against Vice in Cairo," *Journal of the American Oriental Society* 121 (2001): 219–35.

73. Muhammad b. Mustafa Rashed, *Ta'rih-i Rashed*, 6 vols. (İstanbul: Matbaa-i Amire, 1282), 1:250.

74. Paul Rycaut, *The History of the Turkish Empire from the Year 1623 to the Year 1677 . . .* (London, 1680), 2:255.

75. Ibid., 1:43, 59.

76. Ahmet Altınay Refik, *Onuncu Asr-i Hicrī'de İstanbul Hayatı* (İstanbul: Enderun Kitabevi, 1988), 141–42, 146–47.

77. Ahmet Altınay Refik, *Onikinci Asr-i Hicrī'de İstanbul Hayatı* (İstanbul: Enderun Kitabevi, 1988), 83–84.

78. Sami Hamarneh, "Pharmacy in Medieval Islam and the History of Drug Addiction," *Medical History* 16 (1972): 226–37.

79. Douglas Scott Brookes, "Table of Delicacies Concerning the Rules of Social Gatherings: An Annotated Translation of Gelibolulu Mustafa Âli's *Mevâ'idü'n-Nefâ'is fi Kavâ'idi'l-Mecâlis*," PhD diss., University of California, Berkeley, 1998), chap. 17 "Excessive Recourse to Narcotics," 106–11, chap. 54 "Wine Gatherings," 233–35.

80. Evliya Çelebi, *Seyahatname*, 10 vols. (İstanbul: Matbaa-i Amire, 1314AH/1894), 1:383; Evliya Çelebi, *The "Seyahatname" of Evliya Çelebi: Facsimile*

of Topkapı Sarayı Bağdat 304 (Cambridge, MA: Harvard University Press, 1993), 1b:231; Evliya Efendi, *Narrative of Travels in Europe, Asia, and Africa in the Seventeenth Century*, trans. Ritter Joseph von Hammer (London, 1834), 1b:26.

81. Nicolay, *Navigations, Peregrinations, and Voyages, Made into Turkie*, 92a.

82. Miri Shefer, "Insanity and the Insane in the Ottoman Empire," in *Minorities, Foreigners and Marginals*, ed. Shulamit Volkov (Jerusalem: Merkaz Zalman Shazar, 2000), 191–204 (in Hebrew); Michael W. Dols, *Majnūn*; Boaz Shoshan, "The State and Madness in Medieval Islam," *International Journal of Middle East Studies* 35 (2003): 329–40.

83. İbrahim Peçevi, *Tarih-i Peçevi*, 2 vols. (İstanbul: Matbaa-i Amire, 1283 [1867]), 1:363–66. See also E. Birnbaum, "Vice Triumphant: The Spread of Coffee and Tobacco in Turkey," *Durham University Journal* 49, n.s. 18, (1956–57): 21–27.

84. M. Ertuğrul Düzdağ, *Şeyhülislâm Ebussu'ûd Efendi'nin Fatvalarına Göre Kanunī Devrinde Osmanlı Hayatı* (İstanbul: Şûle Yayınları, 1998), nos. 261–62 (pp. 108–9); 699–701 (p. 230), 724 (pp. 235–36).

85. Sami K. Hamarneh and Henri Amin Awad, "Medical Instruments," in *Fustat Finds*, ed. Jere L. Bacharach (Cairo: American University in Cairo Press, 2002), 176–89.

86. Emilie Savage-Smith, "Attitudes toward Dissection in Medieval Islam," *Journal of the History of Medicine and Allied Sciences* 50 (1995): 67–110; Savage-Smith, "The Practice of Surgery in Islamic Lands: Myth and Reality," *Social History of Medicine* 13 (2000): 307–21.

87. *Encyclopaedia of Islam*, 2nd ed., s.v. "Tashrīḥ," by Emilie Savage-Smith.

88. Hajji Khalifa, *Kashf al-Ẓunūn an Asāmī al-Kutūb wal-Funūn*, 2 vols. (Istanbul, 1360AH/1941), 1:409. On Katip Çelebi see Gottfried Hagen, *Ein Osmanischer Geograph bei der Arbeit Entstehung und Gedankenwelt von Kātib Čelebis Ǧihānnümā* (Berlin: Klaus Schwartz Verlag, 2003), 7–78; *Encyclopaedia of Islam*, 2nd ed., s.v. "Ḳātib Çelebi" by Orhan Şaık Gökyay; Eleazar Birnbaum, "The Questing Mind: Kātib Chelebi, 1609–1657," in *Corolla Torontonesis: Studies in Honour of Ronald Morton Smith* (Toronto: TSAR, 1994), 133–58.

89. Nil Sarı and Ali H. Bayat, "The Medical Organization at the Ottoman Court," *Studies in History of Medicine and Science*, n.s. 16 (1999–2000): 41.

90. Esin Kâhya, "One of the Samples of the Influences of Avicenna on the Ottoman Medicine, Shams al-Din Itaqi," *Belleten*, 64, no. 4 (2000): 66–67. On Ibn al-Nafīs see *Encyclopaedia of Islam*, 2nd ed., s.v., "Ibn al-Nafīs," by Max Meyerhof and J. Schacht.

91. Esin Kâhya, *Şemseddîn-I İtâkî'nin Resimli Anatomi Kitabı* (Ankara: Atatürk Kültür Merkezi Yayını, 1996), esp. 255–358 for reproduction of the drawings from Itaki and Vesalius; Gül Russell, " 'The Owl and the Pussycat': The Process of Cultural Transmission in Anatomical Illustration," in *Transfer of Modern Science and Technology to the Muslim World*, ed. Ekmeleddin Ihsanoğlu (Istanbul: Research Centre for Islamic History, Art and Culture, 1992), 191–95; Adnan Abdülhāk Adıvar, *Osmanlı Türklerinde İlim*, 5. printing (İstanbul: Remzi

Kitabevi, 1991), 129–30; Esin Kâhya and Aysegül D. Erdemir, *Bilimin Işığında Osmanlıdan Cumhuriyete Tıp ve Sağlık Kurumları* (Ankara: Türkiye Diyanet Vakfı Yayınları, 2000), 177–79; Kâhya, "Shams al-Din Itaqi," 67–68; Savage-Smith, "Tashrīh" 355.

92. Sura 17/al-Isra, The Night Journey, 22; English translation from Arthur J. Arberry, *The Koran Interpreted* (London: G. Allen & Unwin, 1955).

93. Şerefeddin Sabuncuoğlu, *Cerrahiyyetü'l-Hāniyye*, trans. and ed. İlter Uzel, 2 vols. (Ankara: Türk Tarih Kurumu, 1992), 1:7–10 (Turkish), 43–46 (English); Ahmet Süheyl Ünver, "XVinci Asırda Türkiyede Tecrubi Tababete ait İki Misal," *İstanbul Üniversitesi Tıp Fakültesi Mecmuası* 3 (1949): 1–4.

94. Emir Çelebi, "Enmüzec-ül-Tibb," manuscript held at the British Library, OIOC, Or. 7282, f. 8r.

95. *Encyclopaedia of Islam*, 2nd ed., s.v. "Al-Zahrāwī, Abū al-Ḳāsim Khalaf b. al-'Abbās," by Emilie Savage-Smith; Sami Khalaf Hamarneh, *Drawings and Pharmacy in al-Zahrawi's 10th century Surgical Treatise* (Washington, DC: Smithsonian Institution, 1961); M. S. Spink and G. L. Lewis, *Albucasis on Surgery and Instruments* (London: Wellcome Institute of the History of Medicine, 1973), introduction, vii–xii.

96. I consulted the facsimile edition published as volume 2 in Sabuncuoğlu, *Cerrahiyyetü'l-Haniyye*. It is the manuscript held at the Bibliothèque National, Paris, with additions from the copy kept at the Fatih Millet Library in Istanbul.

97. Gönül Güreşsever, "Kitab al-Cerrahiyet al-Hāniye (İstanbul Tıp Tarihi Enstitüsü Nüshası) Minyatürler," in *I. Milletarası Türkoloji Kongresi. Tebliğler*; 3 vols. (İstanbul: [n.p.], 1979), 3:775.

98. Evliya's account of the seven hospitals in Vienna is to be found in *Seyahatname*, vol. 7 (Istanbul: Matbaari 'Amire, 1928), 277–85. See also J. W. Livingston, "Evliya Çelebi on Surgical Operation in Vienna," *Al-Abhāth*, 23 (1970): 223–45; Arslan Terzioğlu, "Evliya Çelebi's Beschreibung der Südosteuropäischen Hospitäler und Heilbäder des 17. Jahrhunderts und ihre Kulturgeschichtliche Bedeutung," *Revue des Études Sud-Est Européennes* 13 (1975): 429–42.

99. Gottfried Hagen, "Some Considerations on the Study of Ottoman Geographical Writing," *Archivum Ottomanicum* 18 (2000):192–93; Robert Dankoff, *An Ottoman Mentality: The World of Evliya Çelebi* (Leiden: Brill, 2004).

100. Evliya Çelebi, *Seyahatname*, 7:277–80; Livingston, "Evliya Çelebi on Surgical Operation in Vienna," 225–29, 230–32, 238–40. Livingston is skeptical about whether St. Stephan had a hospital (p. 229), but other secondary sources reaffirm that one did exist. See Terzioğlu, "Evliya Çelebi's Beschreibung der Südosteuropäischen Hospitäler," 431. Livingston errs in some dates (Marcello Malpighi died in 1694, not in 1661, p. 226), but this does not affect Livingston's basic thesis about Evliya's accurate description.

101. Roy Porter, *The Greatest Benefit to Mankind* (London: Harper Collins, 1997), chap. 8 "Renaissance," 163–200, chap. 9 "The New Science," 201–44; Harold Ellis, *A History of Surgery* (London: Greenwich Medical Media, 2001), 38–52.

102. Andrea Carlino, " 'Know Thyself": Anatomical Figures in Early Modern Europe," *Res* 27 (1995): 52–69.

103. Andrew Cunningham, *The Anatomical Renaissance: The Resurrection of Anatomical Projects of the Ancients* (Aldershot, UK: Scolar Press, 1997).

104. Raphael Mordekhai Malki, *Ma'amarin bi-Refu'a le-Rabi Refa'el Mordekhai Malki*, ed. Meir Benayahu (Jerusalem: Yad ha-Rav Nissim, 1986), 42, 84, 149–50 (in Hebrew). See al-Bukhārī, *Al-Jāmi' al-Ṣaḥīḥ*, ṭibb/item no. 3, 10–14, 16; al-'Asqalānī, *Fatḥ al-Bārī*, 12:242–44, 254–60 for references to Muhammad.

105. Thevenot, *Travells*, 1:37–38. For more cases of bloodletting as a routine medical procedure, see Amnon Cohen, Elisheva Ben-Shimon-Pikali and Eyal Ginio, *Jews in the Moslem Religious Court, the XIX Century* (Jerusalem: Yad Ben-Zvi, 2003), 209–10 (doc. 104).

106. Sabuncuoğlu, *Cerrahiyyet-ü'l-Haniyye*, 2:17r ff. for treating headaches (23r for melancholy), 121r ff. for treating fistulas and hemorrhoids, with miniatures of treating a boy's rump, and elsewhere in the treatise; Sadettin Özçelik, "Bāsur Hastalığı ve Tedavisiyle İlgili 15. Yüzyılda ait bir Metin," *Yeni Tıp Tarihi Araştıtmaları* 4 (1998): 207–24; Karmi, "Colonisation of Traditional Arabic Medicine," 319.

107. Thevenot, *Travells*, 1:42.

108. Rycaut, *The State of the Ottoman Empire* (London, 1668), 157; Gül A. Russell, "Physicians at the Ottoman Court," *Medical History* 34 (1990): 247, 260.

109. *The Complete Letters of Lady Mary Wortley Montagu*; ed. R. Halsbad, 3 vols. (Oxford: Clarendon Press, 1965–67), 1:337–40.

110. See several typical cases from the Muslim court archives in Jerusalem: Amnon Cohen, Elisheva Simon-Pikali and Ovadia Salama, *Jews in the Moslem Religious Court: Society, Economy and Communal Organization in the XVIII Century; Documents from Ottoman Jerusalem* (Jerusalem: Yad Ben-Zvi, 1996), docs. 324 (pp. 324–25), 282–83 (p. 327), 286 (p. 328), 287 (pp. 329–30); *Jews in the Moslem Religious Court . . . the XIX Century*, 209–10 (doc. 104).

111. Malki, *Ma'amarin bi-Refu'a le-Rabi Refa'el Mordekhai Malki*, 43–44, 106–7.

112. Mustafā Ālī, *Muṣṭafā 'Ālī's Counsel for Sultans of 1581*, ed. and trans. Andreas Tietze, 2 vols. (Vienna: Verlag der Osterreichischen Akademie der Wissenschaften, 1979–82), 2:46, 171–72.

113. C. Bryce, "Sketch of the State and Practice of Medicine at Constantinople," *Edinburgh Medical and Surgical Journal* 35 (1831): 11.

114. Halil Sahillioğlu, "Üsküdar'ın Mamure (Cedide) Mahallesi Fıtık Cerrahları," *Yeni Tıp Tarihi Araştıtmaları* 4 (1998): 59–66.

Chapter 2: "In health and in sickness": The Integrative Body

1. Christopher Lawrence and George Weisz, eds. *Greater than the Parts: Holism in Biomedicine, 1920–1950* (New York: Oxford University Press, 1998), vii.

2. S. Nomanul Haq, "Islam," in *A Companion to Environmental Philosophy*, ed. Dale Jamieson (Oxford: Blackwell, 2001), 111–29; Haq, "Islam and Ecology: Toward Retrieval and Reconstruction," *Daedalus* 130, no. 4 (Fall 2001): 141–78; Federico Peirone, "Islam and Ecology in the Mediterranean Muslim *Kulturkreise*," *Hamdard Islamicus* 5, no. 2 (1981): 3–31; Richard C. Foltz, *Animals in Islamic Tradition and Muslim Cultures* (Oxford: Oneworld, 2006).

3. J. C. Smuts, *Holism and Evolution* (London: Macmillan, 1926), 99, 127.

4. J. C. Smuts, "Some Recent Scientific Advances in Their Bearing on Philosophy," in *Our Changing World-View* (Johannesburg: University of the Witwatersrand Press, 1932), 12.

5. Ken Wilber, *The Marriage of Sense and Soul: Integrating Science and Religion* (Dublin: Gateway, 1998).

6. Charles E. Rosenberg, "Holism in Twentieth-Century Medicine," in Lawrence and Weisz, *Greater than the Parts*, 335–55.

7. Michael W. Dols, "Islam and Medicine," *History of Science* 26 (1988): 419.

8. Charles E. Rosenberg, "Body and Mind in Nineteenth-Century Medicine: Some Clinical Origins of the Neurosis Construct," in *Explaining Epidemics and Other Studies in the History of Medicine* (Cambridge: Cambridge University Press, 1992), 74.

9. Adıvar, *Osmanlı Türklerinde İlim*, 27–28.

10. Dimitri Gutas, "Philopenus and Avicenna on the Separability of the Intellect: A Case of Orthodox Christian-Muslim Agreement," *Greek Orthodox Theological Review* 31 (1986): 121–29; Michael Marmura, "Avicenna's 'Flying Man' in Context," *Monist*, 69 (1986): 383–95; Thérèse-Anne Druart, "The Human Soul's Individuation and Its Survival after the Body's Death: Avicenna on the Causal Relation between Body and Soul," *Arabic Sciences and Philosophy* 10 (2000): 259–73; Peter Adamson, *The Arabic Plotinus: A Philosophical Study of the Theology of Aristotle* (London: Duckworth, 2002); Deborah L. Black, "Psychology: Soul and Intellect," in *The Cambridge Companion to Arabic Philosophy*, ed. Peter Adamson and Richard C. Taylor (Cambridge: Cambridge University Press, 2005), 308–26.

11. Saadia Khawar Chishti, "*Fitra*: An Islamic Model for Humans and the Environment," in *Islam and Ecology: A Bestowed Trust*, ed. Richard C. Foltz, Frederick M. Denny and Azizan Baharuddin (Cambridge, MA: Center for the Study of World Religions, Harvard Divinity School; distributed by Harvard University Press, 2003), 67.

12. Robert G. Morrison, "The Portrayal of Nature in a Medieval Qur'an Commentary," *Studia Islamica* 94 (2002): 115–37; Morrison, "Reasons for a Scientific Portrayal of Nature in Medieval Commentaries on the Qur'ān," *Arabica* 52 (2005): 182–203.

13. Perho, "Prophet's Medicine," 78–82, 130–43.

14. Peregrine Horden, "Ritual and Public Health in the Early Medieval City," in *Body and City: Histories of Urban Public Health*, ed. Sally Sheard and Helen Power (Aldershot, UK: Ashgate, 2000), 17.

15. W. F. Bynum and Roy Porter, eds. *Medicine and the Five Senses* (Cambridge: Cambridge University Press, 1993), 1–6.

16. Osman Sevki [Uludağ], *Beş Büçük Asırlık Türk Ṭebābeti Ta'rihi* (İstanbul: Matbaa-i Amire, 1341H/1925), 118–24; Rahmi Oruç Güvenç, "The Tradition of Turkish Music Therapy," in Çiçek, *Culture and Arts*, 652–54; J. Ch. Bürgel, "Psychosomatic Methods of Cures in the Islamic Middle Ages," *Humaniora Islamica* 1 (1973): 163.

17. Jean-Claude Chabrier, "Musical Science," in Rashed, *Encyclopedia of the History of Arabic Science*, 2:581; Recep Uslu, "Musicians in the Ottoman Empire and Central Asia in the 15th Century According to an Unknown Work of Aydınlı Şemseddin Nahifi," in Çiçek, *Culture and Arts*, 548–55.

18. Amnon Shiloah, *The Theory of Music in Arabic Writings (c. 900—1900)* (Munich: G. Henle, 1979), 1–9; Johann Cristoph Bürgel, *The Feather of Simurgh: The "Licit Magic" of the Arts in Medieval Islam* (New York: New York University Press, 1988), 92–97; Charles Barnett, " 'Spiritual Medicine': Music and Healing in Islam and Its Influence in Western Medicine," in *Musical Healing in Cultural Contexts*, ed. Penelope Gouk (Aldershot, UK: Ashgate, 2000), 85–91; Jamie Croy Kassler, "Apollo and Dionysus: Music Theory and the Western Tradition of Epistemology," in *Music and Civilization: Essays in Honor of Paul Henry Lang*, ed. Edmond Strainchamps and Maria Rika Maniates (New York: W.W. Norton, 1984), 457–71; Kassler, "Man—A Musical Instrument: Models of the Brain and Mental Functions before the Computer," *History of Science* 22 (1984): 59–92.

19. Amnon Shiloah, "Musical Modes and the Medical Dimension: The Arabic Sources," in *Metaphor: A Musical Dimension*, ed. Jamie C. Kassler (Sydney: Currency Press, 1991), 153–56; Kassler, *Music in the World of Islam: A Socio-Cultural Study*, ed. Jamie C. Kassler (Detroit: Wayne State University Press, 1995), 52. See also the tables in Fadlou Shehadi, *Philosophies of Music in Medieval Islam* (Leiden: Brill, 1995), 163–64 and Bürgel, *Feather of Simurgh*, 94–96.

20. Peregrine Horden, "Religion as Medicine: Music in Medieval Hospitals," in *Religion and Medicine in the Middle Ages*, ed. Peter Biller and Joseph Ziegler (Rochester, NY: York Medieval Press, 2001), 135–53.

21. Reynold A. Nicholson, ed., *The Kashf al-Mahjūb: The Oldest Persian Treatise on Sufism*, new ed. (London: Printed for the Trustees of the "E. J. W. Gibb Memorial" and published by Luzac, 1976), 407; *Encyclopaedia of Islam*, 2nd ed., s.v. "al-Hudjwīrī" by Hidayet Hosain.

22. Barnett, " 'Spiritual Medicine,' " 89. See also the outdated but informative Henry George Farmer, *A History of Arabian Music to the XIIIth Century* (London: Luzac, 1929).

23. Sevki, *Beş Büçük Asırlık Türk Ṭebābeti Ta'rihi*, 120; See also Henry George Farmer, ed. and trans., *Turkish Instruments of Music in the Seventeenth Century as Described in the Siyāḥat nāma of Ewliyā Chelebi*, (1937 rpt., Portland, ME: Longwood Press, 1976), 7.

24. Evliya Çelebi, *Seyahatname*, 1:620–25; Evliya Çelebi, *Seyahatname of Evliya Çelebi: Facsimile of Topkapı Sarayı Bağdat 304*, 1b:407–10.

25. Evliya Çelebi, *Seyahatname*, 1:321, 3:470; Evliya Çelebi, *Seyahatname of Evliya Çelebi: Facsimile of Topkapı Sarayı Bağdat 304*, 1a:189. See also Farmer, *Turkish Instruments of Music*, 8–45; Ünver, "Four Medical Vignettes from Turkey," 52. On Ottoman instrumental repertoire and musical conventions, see Walter Feldman, *Music of the Ottoman Court: Makam, Composition and the Early Ottoman Instrumental Repertoire* (Berlin: VWB-Verlag für Wissenschaft und Bildung, 1996). See also various articles in Çiçek, *Culture and Arts*, 533–656.

26. Güvenç, "Tradition of Turkish Music Therapy," 654–55.

27. Penelope Gouk, introduction to *Musical Healing in Cultural Contexts*, ed. Penelope Gouk (Aldershot, UK: Ashgate, 2000), 8.

28. Muṣṭafā 'Ālī, *Muṣṭafā 'Ālī's Description of Cairo of 1599*, ed. and trans. Andreas Tietze (Vienna: Verlag der Osterreichischen Akademie der Wissenschaften, 1975), 38, 109.

29. John Ray, ed. *A Collection of Curious Travels and Voyages* (Istanbul, 1693), 1:308.

30. Jerome W. Clinton, "Madness and Cure in the 1001 Nights," *Studia Islamica* 61 (1985): 107–25.

31. Ahmad 'Īsā, *Ta'rīkh al-Bīmāristānāt fī al-Islām*, 2nd ed. (Bayrūt: Dār al-Rā'īd al-'Arabī, 1401 [1981]), 102.

32. West, *Music in Greek Life*, 32; Leaman, *Islamic Aesthetics*, 109–13.

33. Brookes, "Table of Delicacies Concerning the Rules of Social Gatherings," 97–106, esp. 98 n. 258, 102.

34. Nicholson, *Kashf al-Mahjūb* , 407.

35. Martin West, *Music in Greek Life* (Oxford: Oxford University Press, 1992), 31–32; West, "Music Therapy in Antiquity," in *Music as Medicine: The History of Music Therapy since Antiquity*, ed. Peregrine Horden (Aldershot, UK: Ashgate, 2000), 51–68. Amnon Shiloah believes that music was indeed a highly regarded regular practice in Muslim hospitals and Muslim medicine at large, at least in the Abbasid period. Amnon Shiloah, "Jewish and Muslim Tradition of Music Therapy," in Horden, *Music as Medicine*, 69–83.

36. Shehadi, *Philosophies of Music in Medieval Islam*, 95–162; Bürgel, *Feather of Simurgh*, chap. 4, "Music: Nourishment of the Soul," 89–118; Oliver Leaman, *Islamic Aesthetics: An Introduction* (Edinburgh: Edinburgh University Press, 2004), 105–9, 118–19. See also James Robson, ed. and trans., *Tracts on Listening to Music* (London, 1938), 1–13, reprinted in Hiroyuki Mashita, ed. *Theology, Ethics and Metaphysics: Royal Asiatic Society Classics of Islam* (London: RoutledgeCurzon, 2003).

37. Katip Çelebi, "Mizan al-hakk fi ikhtiyar al-ahakk," manuscript held at the Cambridge University Library, Add. 442), f. 36r–37r; *The Balance of the Truth*; trans. G. L. Lewis (London: G. Allen and Unwin, 1957), 12, 38–41; Eleazar Birnbaum, "Questing Mind," 133–58.

38. Düzdağ, *Şeyhülislâm Ebussu'ûd Efendi'nin Fatvalarına Göre Kanunī Devrinde Osmanlı Hayatı*, nr. 341 (pp. 131–32), 344 (pp. 132–33), 348–52 (pp. 134–37), 648 (p. 215).

39. And, *Istanbul in the 16th Century*, 242, 250–51.

40. This was the impression of foreign travelers. Sandys, *Relation of a Journey*, 45, 56; Thevenot, *Travells*, 1:50; And, *Istanbul in the 16th Century*, 242.

41. Thevenot, *Travells*, 1:47.

42. Sally Sheard and Helen Power, "Body and City: Medical and Urban Histories of Public Health," in *Body and City: Histories of Urban Public Health*, ed. Sally Sheard and Helen Power (Aldershot, UK: Ashgate, 2000), 1.

43. *Oxford English Dictionary*, s.v. "Privacy." Second edition, online.

44. Abraham Marcus, "Privacy in Eighteenth-Century Aleppo: The Limits of Cultural Ideals," *International Journal of Middle East Studies* 18 (1986): 165–83; Marcus, *Middle East on the Eve of Modernity*, 322–24, 384 (notes).

45. Janet Abu-Lughod, "The Islamic City—Historic Myth, Islamic Essence, and Contemporary Relevance," *International Journal of Middle East Studies* 19 (1987): 167–69.

46. Dror Ze'evi, "The Ottoman Century: The Sancak of Jerusalem in 17th Century," (PhD diss., Tel Aviv University, 1991), 320–24. This section is not included in the book based on this dissertation, *An Ottoman Century: The District of Jerusalem in the 1600s* (Albany: State University New York Press, 1996).

47. Eli Alshech, " 'Do Not Enter Houses Other than Your Own': The Evolution of the Notion of a Private Domestic Sphere in Early Sunnī Islamic Thought," *Islamic Law and Society* 11 (2004): 292–332.

48. Paulina B. Lewicka, "Restaurants, Inns and Taverns that Never Eere: Some Reflections on Public Consumption in Medieval Cairo," *Journal of the Economic and Social History of the Orient* 48 (2005): 40–91.

49. Iris Agmon, *Family and Court: Legal Culture and Modernity in Late Ottoman Palestine* (Syracuse, NY: Syracuse University Press, 2005), 209.

50. Sandys, *Relation of a Journey*, 54; Luigi Bassano, *Costumi et i modi particolari della vita de'turchi, Roma 1545* (Monaco di Baviera: M. Huber, 1963), 5–6 (the original pagination), 17–19 (modern pagination); Salomon Schweigger, *Ein Newe Reyssbeschreibung auss Teutschland nach Constantinopel und Jerusalem* (Graz: Akademische Druck-u. Verlagsanstalt, 1964), 116; Thevenot, *Travells*, 1:31–32; Hill, *Full and Just Account of the Present State of the Ottoman Empire*, 50; Nicolay, *Navigations, Peregrinations, and Voyages, Made into Turkie*, 59a–59b, 61a; Tho. Thomas, *An Account of the City of Prusa in Bythinia, and a Continuation of the Historical Observation Relating to Constantinople . . .* in *A Collection of Curious Travels and Voyages*, ed. John Ray (London, 1693), 69; Süheyl Ünver, "Türk Hamamları," *Türk Dünyası* 5 (1950): 198–203.

51. Schweigger , *Ein Newe Reyssbeschreibung auss Teutschland nach Constantinopel und Jerusalem*, 112, 114.

52. *Encyclopaedia of Islam*, 2nd ed., s.v. "Ḥammām," by A. L. Louis.

53. Al-Bukhārī, *Al-Jāmi' al-Ṣaḥīḥ*, ṭibb/item #28; al-'Asqalānī, *Fatḥ al-Bārī*, 12:282–86.

54. *Süleymaniye Vakfiyesi*, B:150; The Archives of the General Directorate for Charitable Institutions (Vakıflar Genel Müdürlüğü, Ankara [VGM]), defter 608/23, 231; VGM, dolap 1550, 36 (71).

55. Gökbilgin, *XV–XVI Asırlarda Edirne ve Paşa Livāsi*, B:164–65; *Süleymaniye Vakfiyesi*, B:150; VGM, defter 608/23, 231; TSMA, defter 1781, 3v; VGM, dolap 1550, 36 (71); TSMA, evrak 2211/7; Barkan, "Edirne ve Civarındaki Bazı İmāret Tesislerinin Yıllık Muhasebe Bilançoları," 280.

56. TSMA, defter 7017/1, 15v. On the duties of the washers of the dead, see Savage-Smith, "Attitudes toward Dissection in Medieval Islam," 78–79; *Encyclopaedia of Islam*, 2nd ed., s.v. "Djanāza," by A. S. Tritton; *Encyclopaedia of Islam*, 2nd ed., suppl., s.v. "Ghassāl," by M. A. J. Beg; *Encyclopaedia of Islam*, 2nd ed., s.v. "Ḥināṭa," by A. S. Tritton.

57. *Fatih Mehmet II Vakfiyeleri* (Ankara: n.p., 1938), 279–80, Gökbilgin, *XV–XVI Asırlarda Edirne ve Paşa Livāsi*, B:160–61; *Süleymaniye Vakfiyesi*, B:149, VGM, defter 608/23 231; TSMA, defter 7017/1, 15v; VGM, dolap 1550, 36 (71).

58. *Fatih Mehmet II Vakfiyeleri*, 280.

59. Refik, *Onuncu Asr-ı Hicri'de İstanbul Hayatı*, 63.

60. Evliya Çelebi, *Seyahatname*, 1:398, 403, 414; 3:399–400 (on Sophia); Evliya Çelebi, *Seyahatname of Evliya Çelebi: Facsimile of Topkapı Sarayı Bağdat 304*, 1b:243, 246, 252; A. Süheyl Ünver, "İstanbul'un Bazı Acı ve Tatlı Sularının Halkça Maruf Şifa Hassaları Hakkında," *Türk T Tarihi Arkivi* 5, no. 18 (1940): 90–96. For the popularity of the hot springs of Tiberias in the sixteenth century among the local Muslim, Christian, and Jewish communities, see Uriel Heyd, "Turkish Documents about Building Tiberias in the Sixteenth Century," *Sephunot* 10 (1966): 202 (in Hebrew).

61. Evliya Çelebi, *Seyahatname* 3:21–25.

62. Thevenot, *Travells*, 1:88–89.

63. Ibid., 2:42.

64. M. A. S. Abdel Haleem, "Medical Ethics in Islam," in *Choices and Decisions in Health Care*, ed. Andrew Grubb (Chichester, UK: J. Wiley, 1993), 2.

65. Michael Winter, "Islamic Attitudes toward the Human Body," in *Religious Reflections on the Human Body*, ed. Jane Marie Law (Bloomington: Indiana University Press, 1995), 40; Fuad I. Khouri, *The Body in Islamic Culture* (London: Saqi Books, 2001), esp. part 1 "Body Ideology," 15–86.

66. Arthur K. Shapiro and Elaine Shapiro, "The Placebo Effect: Is It Much Ado about Nothing?" in *The Placebo Effect*, ed. Anne Harrington (Cambridge, MA: Harvard University Press, 1997), 12–36; Shapiro and Shapiro, *The Powerful Placebo*, chaps. 1, 2, and 3.

67. Marín and Waines, "Balanced Way," 127.

68. Another example is *laban*, cultured milk, mentioned in prophetic sayings. See al-Bukhārī, *Al-Jāmi' al-Ṣaḥīḥ*, ṭibb/item #5–6; al-'Asqalānī, *Fatḥ al-Bārī*, 12:247–48. The Abbasids associated seafood with aphrodisiacs and the ability to bolster sexual potency. Ahsan, *Social Life under the Abbasids*, 85.

69. Sandys, *Relation of a Journey*, 51–52; Thevenot, *Travells*, 1:33.

70. In addition to Thevenot and Sandys quoted above, see also William Lithgow, *The Total Discourse of the Rare Adventures and Painful Peregrinations of Long Nineteen Yeares Traveyles from Scotland to the Most Famous Kingdoms in Europe, Asia and Africa* (London, 1632), 58–59. The description of Pietro Della

Valle who visited Istanbul in 1615 is cited in Reay Tannahill, *Food in History*, 2nd and rev. ed. (Harmondsworth, UK: Penguin, 1988), 275. Robert Burton's impressions of coffee in Istanbul in 1621 are brought together in Bernard Lewis, *A Middle East Mosaic: Fragments of Life, Letters and History* (New York: Random House, 2000), 393.

71. Ahmet Süheyl Ünver, "Eski Evlerimizde Mualece Dolapları, Sandıkları ve İhtiva Ettigi İlāçlara Ait Bir Misal," *Türk Tıb Tarihi Arşivi*, 15 (1940): 121.

72. Shapiro and Shapiro, *Powerful Placebo*, 59–60.

73. Howard Brody, "The Doctor as Therapeutic Agent: A Placebo Effect Research Agenda," in *The Placebo Effect*, ed. Anne Harrington (Cambridge, MA: Harvard University Press, 1997), 77–92.

74. See several receipts from Topkapı, TSMA, evrak 11942/32, 48, 56, 80, 81, 104, 122, 125, 127, 131.

75. Geroge E. White, "Evil Spirits and the Evil Eye in Turkish Lore," *Moslem World* 9 (1919): 179–86.

76. Rubin, "Muḥammad the Exorcist," 103–9.

77. Esin Atıl, *The Age of Sultan Süleyman the Magnificent* (Washington, DC: National Gallery of Art, 1987), 196–98 for images of talismanic shirts handmade for the sultans. Birgit Krawietz. "Islamic Conception of the Evil Eye," *Medicine and Law* 21 (2002): 339–55.

78. Thevenot, *Travells*, 1:43.

79. "*Book of Prayers*," manuscript held at the Wellcome Library for the History of Medicine, WMS.Turkish.25; Thomas, *Account of the City of Prusa in Bythinia*, 71; Bryce, "Sketch of the State and Practice of Medicine at Constantinople," 4–5.

80. Muṣṭafā ʿĀlī, *Muṣṭafā ʿĀlī's Counsel for Sultans of 1581*, 2:78–81, 178–93; Brookes, "Table of Delicacies," 233–35; 73 "Wine Taverns," 272–74; and 74, "*Boza* Taverns," 274–75; Dernschwam, *Tagebuch*, 47, 84–85, 96, 102, 104, 135; Nicholay, *Navigations, Peregrinations, and Voyages*, 91b; François Georgeon, "Ottomans and Drinkers: The Consumption of Alcohol in the Nineteenth Century," in *Outside In: On the Margins of the Modern Middle East*, ed. Eugene Rogan (London: I. B. Tauris, 2001), 7–30; Elyse Semerdjian, "Sinful Professions: Illegal Occupations of Women in Ottoman Aleppo, Syria," *Hawwa* 1 (2003): 78–81.

81. *Encyclopaedia of Islam*, 2nd ed., s.v. "Khamr," by J. Sadan; *Encyclopaedia of Islam*, 2nd ed., s.v., "Mashrūbāt," by J. Sadan; *Encyclopaedia of Islam*, 2nd ed., s.v. "Nabīdh," by P. Heine; David Waines, "Abū Zayd al-Balkhī on the Nature of Forbidden Drink: A Medieval Islamic Controversy," in *La alimentación en las culturas islámicas*, ed. Manuela Marín and David Waines (Madrid: Agenica Española de Cooperacion International, 1994), 111–26; Nurdeen Deursaeh, "Is Imbibing al-Khamr (Intoxicating Drink) for Medical Purposes Permissible by Islamic Law?" *Arab Law Quarterly* 18 (2003): 355–60.

82. Deursaeh, "Is Imbibing al-Khamr . . . Permissible?" 360–64.

83. Dā'ūd al-Anṭākī, "Tadhkirat ūlā al-albāb wal-jamī' al-mu'jab al-a'jāb" (Ms. Add. 3510 (11) held at Cambridge University Library), f. 227.

84. For the use of Christian religious chants in medieval European hospitals, mainly the Byzantine Empire, see Horden, "Religion as Medicine," 135–53.

85. Foster and Anderson, *Medical Anthropology*, 40.

86. As appears in the forward to the constitution of the WHO, published in the *Chronicle of the World Health Organization* 1 (1947): 29 (discussion of this point and the first article dealing with the objective of the organization appears on p. 13).

87. Helen King, "Introduction: What is Health?" in *Health in Antiquity*, ed. Helen King (London: Routledge, 2005), 2–5; Arthur Kleinman, "The Meaning Context of Illness and Care: Reflection on a Central Theme in the Anthropology of Medicine," in *Sciences and Cultures: Anthropological and Historical Studies of the Sciences*, ed. Everett Mendelsohn and Yehuda Elkana (Dordrecht: D. Reidel, 1981), 168.

88. The mutual influence of illness and poverty has caught the interest of several historians. See for example, Katherine Park, "Healing the Poor: Hospitals and Medical Assistance in Renaissance Florence," in *Medicine and Charity before the Welfare State*, ed. Jonathan Barry and Colin Jones (London: Routledge, 1991), 27; Michel Mollat, *The Poor in the Middle Ages: An Essay in Social History* (New Haven, CT: Yale University Press, 1986), 5–7; Miri Rubin, *Charity and Community in Medieval Cambridge* (Cambridge: Cambridge University Press, 1987), 7–8.

89. Felix Klein-Franke, "Health and Healing in Medieval Muslim Palestine," in *Health and Disease in the Holy Land*, ed. Manfred Wassermann and Samuel S. Kottek (Lewiston, NY: E. Mellen Press, 1996), 106.

90. Abdel Haleem, "Medical Ethics in Islam," 10.

91. Muṣṭafā ʿĀlī, *Muṣṭafā ʿĀlī's Counsel for Sultans of 1581*, 2:45, 170.

92. Robert Hoyland, "Physiognomy in Islam," *Jerusalem Studies in Arabic and Islam* 30 (2005): 361–402.

93. Hajji Khalifa, *Kashf al-Ẓunūn*, 2:1241.

94. Seyyid Lokman Çelebi, *Kiyâfetü'l-İnsâniyye fî Şemâili'l-ʿOsmâniyye* (İstanbul: The Historical Research Foundation, Istanbul Research Center, 1987), 10–12; Ingomar Weiler, "Inverted *Kalokagathia*," in *Representing the Body of the Slave*, ed. Thomas Wiedemann and Jane Gardner (London: Frank Cass, 2002), 11–28. On *qiyafa* and *firasa* in medieval Arabic Muslim culture, see *Encyclopaedia of Islam*, 2nd ed., s.v., "Firāsa," by T. Fahd; *Encyclopaedia of Islam*, 2nd ed., s.v., "Ḳiyāfa," by T. Fahd.

95. On physiognomy in Europe, see Danielle Jacquart, "La physiognomonie à l'époque de Frédéric II: Le traité de Michel Scot," *Micrologus* 2 (1994): 19–37; Ludmilla Jordanova, "The Art and Science of Seeing in Medicine: Physiognomy 1780–1820," in *Medicine and the Five Senses*, ed. W. F. Bynum and Roy Porter (Cambridge: Cambridge University Press, 1993), 122–33, 297–98 (notes).

96. Hoyland, "Physiognomy in Islam," 392–96. See also Cambridge University Library MS Qq. 184 which contains two treatises on physiognomy in Arabic (folios 1–23 and 24–43). They do not include a date, but apparently

are from the twelfth or thirteenth century: Edward G. Browne, *A Hand-list of the Muhammadan Manuscripts including all those Written in the Arabic Character Preserved in the Library of the University of Cambridge* (Cambridge: Cambridge University Press, 1900), 87–88, 199–200.

97. Russell, "Physicians at the Ottoman Court," 251–52. Most recently Dror Ze'evi has dealt with Ottoman physiognomy, but his book reached me too late to be thoroughly incorporated into my own narrative. Dror Ze'evi, *Producing Desire: Changing Sexual Discourse in the Ottoman Middle East, 1500–1900* (Berkeley and Los Angeles: University of California Press, 2006), chap. 1 "Medicine and Physiognomy," 1–16.

98. Amnon Cohen and Elisheva Simon-Pikali, *Jews in the Moslem Religious Court: Society, Economy and Communal Organization in the XVIth Century; Documents from Ottoman Jerusalem* (Jerusalem: Yad Ben-Zvi, 1993), doc. 303 (pp. 269–70).

99. Wms.Turkish.19 (manuscript held at the Wellcome Institute for the History of Medicine Library), f.2r.

100. Russell, "Physicians at the Ottoman Court," 251–52.

101. Brookes, "Table of Delicacies," 347–51; Russell, "Physicians at the Ottoman Court," 251.

102. Ogier Ghislain de Busbecq, *The Turkish Letters of Ogier Ghiselin de Busbecq*, translated from the Latin of the Elzevir edition of 1633 by Edward Seymour Forster (Oxford: Clarendon Press, 1968), 59–61.

103. Hoyland, "Physiognomy in Islam," 390–91.

104. Stephen O. Murray, quoting Busbecq, sees in the application of physiognomy in the Ottoman court a case of homosexual nepotism, a move from beauty to sexuality. He suggests that criteria such as bodily perfection might have a sexual attraction as well as an aesthetic or functional motivation. See his "Homosexuality among Slave Elites in Ottoman Turkey," in *Islamic Homosexualities: Culture, History, and Literature*, ed. Stephen O. Murray and Will Roscoe (New York: New York University Press, 1997), 175–77.

105. Rycaut, *The Present State of the Ottoman Empire . . .*, 25–26.

106. Bryce, "Sketch of the State and Practice of Medicine at Constantinople," 5.

107. Estes and Kuhnke, "French Observations," 134–35.

108. Başbakanlık Osmanlı Arşivi [The Archives of the Ottoman Prime Ministry, Istanbul, hereafter BOA], mühimme defteri 6, p. 527, item #1147.

109. BOA, mühimme defteri 13, p. 26, item #171 (April 1571).

110. BOA, mühimme defteri 15, p. 23, item #169.

111. On the dependence of officeholders in the Ottoman provincial bureaucracy on their source of income, see I. Metin Kunt, *The Sultan's Servants: The Transformation of Ottoman Provincial Government, 1550–1650* (New York: Columbia University Press, 1983), in particular p. 77.

112. BOA, mühimme defteri 2, p. 33, item #302 (March 1556); mühimme defteri 4, p. 4, item #24 (January 1560); mühimme defteri 13, p. 61, item #460 (May 1571); mühimme defteri 24, p. 322, item #877 (May 1574).

113. J. B. Tavernier, *A New Relation of the Inner-Part of the Grand Seraglio* (London, 1677), 22–23; Gülru Necipoğlu, *Architecture, Ceremonial, and Power: The Topkapi Palace in the Fifteenth and Sixteenth Centuries* (Cambridge, MA: MIT Press, 1991), 49.

114. As cited in Aḥmad al-Aybash and D. Qutayba al-Shihābī, eds., *Dimashq al-Shām fī Nuṣūs al-Raḥāllīn wal-Jughrāfiyyin wal-Buldāniyyin al-'Arab wal-Muslimīn min al-Qarn al-Thālith ilā al-Qarn al-Thālith 'Ashr lil-Hijra* (Dimashq: Wizārat al-Thaqāfa, 1998), 2:617

Chapter 3: "Feed the hungry, visit the sick and set those who suffer free": Medical Benevolence and Social Order

1. Singer, *Constructing Ottoman Beneficence*; Singer, "Serving up Charity: The Ottoman Public Kitchen," 481–500; Michael Bonner, Mine Ener, and Amy Singer, eds., *Poverty and Charity in Middle Eastern Contexts* (Albany: State University New York Press, 2003). See also Shirine Hamadeh, "Splash and Spectacle: The Obsession with Fountains in Eighteenth-Century Istanbul," *Muqarnas* 19 (2002): 125–26.

2. Marcel Mauss, *The Gift: Forms and Functions of Exchange in Archaic Societies*, trans. Ian Cunnison (London: Cohen & West, 1954).

3. Roy Porter, "The Gift Relation: Philanthropy and Provincial Hospitals in Eighteenth-Century England," in *The Hospital in History*, ed. Lindsay Granshaw and Roy Porter (London: Routledge, 1989), 149–78; Mayfair Mei-Hui Yang, *Gifts, Favors, and Banquets: The Art of Social Relationships in China* (Ithaca, NY: Cornell University Press, 1994); Yun-xiang Yan, *The Flow of Gifts: Reciprocity and Social Networks in a Chinese Village* (Stanford, CA: Stanford University Press, 1996); Nadir Özbek, "The Politics of Poor Relief in the Late Ottoman Empire, 1876–1914," *New Perspectives on Turkey* 21 (1999): 1–33; Özbek, "Imperial Gifts and Sultanic Legitimation during the Late Ottoman Empire, 1876–1909," in *Poverty and Charity in Middle Eastern Contexts*, ed. Michael Bonner, Mine Ener, and Amy Singer (Albany: State University of New York Press, 2003), 203–20.

4. Donald Quataert, "The Social History of Labor in the Ottoman Empire: 1800–1914," in *The Social History of Labor in the Middle East*, ed. Ellis Jay Goldberg (Boulder, CO: Westview Press, 1996), 28.

5. Marco H. D. van Leeuwen, "Logic of Charity: Poor Relief in Pre-Industrial Europe," *Journal of Interdisciplinary History* 24 (1994): 589–613; Leeuwen, "Histories of Risk and Welfare in Europe during the 18th and 19th Centuries," in *Health Care and Poor Relief in 18th and 19th Century Northern Europe*, ed. Ole Peter Grell, Andrew Cunningham, and Robert Jütte (Aldershot, UK: Ashgate, 2002), 32–66. Foucault's relevant studies are cited in the introduction, note 7.

6. Ole Peter Grell, "The Protestant Imperative of Christian Care and Neighbourly Love," in *Health Care and Poor Relief in Protestant Europe, 1500–1700,* ed. Ole Peter Grell and Andrew Cunningham (London: Routledge, 1997), 45.

7. *Encyclopaedia of Islam,* 2nd ed., s.v. "al-Bukhārī, Muḥammad b. Ismā'īl," by J. Robson; *Encyclopaedia of Islam,* 2nd ed., s.v., "Muslim b. al-Ḥadjdjādj," by G. H. A. Juynboll.

8. See, for example, the stipulation regarding the *dar-ül-hadīth* included in the complex around the Istanbul mosque of Sultan Ahmet I in the beginning of the seventeenth century: VGM, defter 574, 82.

9. Al-Bukhārī, *Al-Jāmi' al-Ṣaḥīḥ,* al-marḍā/item #5; al-'Asqalānī's commentary to "The Book of the Sick" is included in his *Fatḥ al-Bārī,* 12:206–38.

10. A reference to Qur'an, "Repentance," 9:60, which specifies the categories of uses for the *zakat.* Among these categories is "those whose hearts are brought together," referring to Muhammad allowing the booty from his campaigns to be given to new converts to Islam, thus convincing them to maintain their allegiance to the new religion and to Muhammad.

11. Al-'Asqalānī, *Fatḥ al-Bārī,* 12:223–34. Al-'Asqalānī cites al-Māwārdī in his discussion of section 11—visiting a sick *mushrik*—in "The Book of the Sick."

12. Al-Bukhārī, *Al-Jāmi' al-Ṣaḥīḥ,* al-marḍā/item #8.

13. Al-Bukhārī, *Al-Jāmi' al-Ṣaḥīḥ,* al-marḍā/items #4–5, 8–11; al-'Asqalānī, *Fatḥ al-Bārī,* 12:217. The text and commentary do not elaborate whether men should visit sick women too.

14. John Hardwig, "What about the Family," *Hastings Center Report,* 20, no. 2 (March/April 1990): 5–10; Hilde Lindemann Nelson and James Lindemann Nelson, *The Patient in the Family: An Ethics of Medicine and Families* (New York: Routledge, 1995).

15. On the medieval period see Franz Rosenthal, "The Defence of Medicine in the Medieval Muslim World," *Bulletin of the History of Medicine* 43 (1969): 519–32; H. H. Biesterfeldt, "Some Opinions on the Physician's Remuneration in Medieval Islam," *Bulletin of the History of Medicine* 58 (1984): 16–27; Peter E. Pormann, "The Physician and the Other: Images of the Charlatan in Medieval Islam," *Bulletin of the History of Medicine* 79 (2005): 189–227.

16. Harl. 5500 (Ms held at the British Library, OIOC collections), f.40r; Titley, *Miniatures from Turkish Manuscripts,* 30–31.

17. Baydabā, *Kalīla wa Dimna* (Beirut: Dār al-Kutub al-'Āmiya, 1970), 86. This saying is attributed first to Barzoe, the famous Persian physician who was sent to India by the Sassanids to bring a legendary book of wisdom. He translated it to Pahlavi Persian and later it came to be known in Arabic as *Kalīla wa Dimna.*

18. The basic concepts are discussed in some detail in *Encyclopaedia of Islam,* 2nd ed., s.v., "Sadaḳa," by T. H. Weir and A. Zysow; *Encyclopaedia of Islam,* 2nd ed., s.v., "Zakāt," by A. Zysow. The bibliography on *zakāt* and *ṣadaḳa,* including *vakıf,* is too vast to be mentioned here. In recent years many

scholars have been attracted to this topic. I base myself mainly on Amy Singer's pioneering work on Ottoman charity (see n. 1 above).

19. Norman A. Stillman, "Charity and Social Service in Medieval Islam," *Societas* 5 (1975): 105–15.

20. Ibid., 112.

21. Roy H. Elling, "The Hospital-Support Game in Urban Centers," in *The Hospital in Modern Society,* ed. Eliot Freidson (New York: Free Press of Glencoe, 1963), 73–111.

22. Livingston, "Evliya Çelebi on Surgical Operations in Vienna," 236, 244.

23. VGM, defter 608/22, 79–82; defter 990, 167–70.

24. VGM, defter 575, 82–106; defter 613, 27–50; *Fatih Mehmet II Vakfiyeleri* (n.p.); A. Süheyl Ünver, "Fatih Külliyesinin Ilk Vakfiyesine Göre Fatih Darüşşifası," *Türk Tıb Tarihi Arşivi* 17 (1940): 13–17.

25. VGM, defter 613, 65–70.

26. *Süleymaniye Vakfiyesi.*

27. VGM, defter 608/23, 222–35.

28. VGM, dolap 1550, 51–94.

29. VGM, defter 574, 80–86.

30. VGM, kasa 58; İbrahim Hakki Konyalı, "Kanunī Sultan Süleyman'in Annesi Hafsa Sultan'ın Vakfiyyesi ve Manisa'daki Hayir Eserleri," *Vakıflar Dergisi* 8 (1969): 47–56; TSMA, defter 7017/1.

31. VGM, dolap 1550, 207–32.

32. VGM, defter 2138, 1–7.

33. Gallagher, *Medicine and Power in Tunisia, 1780–1900,* 102–5.

34. Arslan Terzioğlu, *Die Hofspitäler und undere Gesundheitseinrichtungen der Osmanischen Palastbauten unter Berücksichtigung der Ursprungsfrage sowie Ihre Beziehungen zu den Abendländischen Hofspitälern* (Munich: Dr. Rudolf Trofenik, 1979).

35. Loqman, an official court historian, wrote a Turkish work in prose in two volumes describing the appearance, the qualities, and the virtues of the Ottoman sultans as far as Süleyman I. Franz Babinger, *Die Geschichtsschreiber des Osmanen und ihre Werke* (Leipzig: Otto Harrassowitz, 1927), 164–67; *Encyclopaedia of Islam,* 2nd ed., s.v., "Luḳmān b. Sayyid Ḥusayn," by H. Sohrweide.

36. Necipoğlu, *Architecture, Ceremonial, and Power,* 43 (for Loqman's *Hünername,* 1:15r); Barnette Miller, *Beyond the Sublime Porte* (New Haven, CT: Yale University Press, 1931), 167.

37. Tavernier, *New Relation of the Inner-Part of the Grand Seignior's Seraglio,* 22–23.

38. Said Amir Arjomand, "Philanthropy, the Law, and Public Policy in the Islamic World before the Modern Era," in *Philanthropy in the World's Traditions,* ed. Warren F. Ilchman, Stanley N. Katz and Edward L. Queen II (Bloomington: Indiana University Press, 1998), 109.

39. Gallagher, *Medicine and Power in Tunisia, 1780–1900,* 102.

40. TSMA, defter 7017/1, 8r.

41. On the distinction between collective and private interests, see Leeuwen, "Logic of Charity," 589–613.

42. *Encyclopaedia of Islam,* 2nd ed., s.v., "Istanbul," by H. Inalcik.

43. Dols, "Second Plague Pandemic," 162–89; N. N. Ambraseys & C. F. Finkel, *The Seismicity of Turkey and Adjacent Areas: A Historical Review, 1500–1800* (Istanbul: Eren, 1995); A. D. Ibrāhīm Khalīl Ahmad, "Al-Amrāḍ wal-Awbī'a win'ikasātuhā 'alā Mujtama' al-Mawṣil ibbānā al-Ahd al-'Uthmānī," *Arab Historical Review for Ottoman Studies/Al-Majalla al-Ta'rīkhiyya al-'Arabiyya lil-Dirāsāt al-'Uthmāniyya* 17, no. 8 (1998): 19–26; Hüseyin Arslan, *16yy. Osmanlı Toplumunda Yönetim, Nüfus, İskân, Göç ve Sürgün* (İstanbul: Kaknüs Yayınları, 2001), 213–15; Marcus, *Middle East on the Eve of Modernity,* 256.

44. TSMA, defter 7017/1, 11v–12r. This is the formula used to explain the addition of another *medrese* to the complex.

45. Çağatay Uluçay, "Kanunī Sultan Süleyman ve Ailesi ile İlgili Bazi Notlar ve Vesikalar," *Kanuni Armağani* (Ankara: Türk Tarih Kurumum 1970), 230.

46. Al-Maqrīzī, *Al-Mawāi'ẓ wal-I'tibar fi Dhikr al-Khiṭaṭ wal-Athar* (2 vols., Beirut: Dār Ṣādir, 1960), 2:406. Interestingly, Ibn Iyās, a Mamluk historian of a later generation, related a different story, a much less flattering one, although citing al-Maqrīzī as his source. He claims that Qala'ūn massacred some commoners who quarreled with his mamluks and stoned them. After three days of slaughter on the streets the sultan wanted to atone for his abominable behavior and chose to establish a hospital after several judges advised him to undertake an act of piety. The sultan hoped this good deed would outweigh his sins. Ibn Iyās, *Badā'i' al-Zuhūr fī Waqā'i' al-Duhūr,* ed. Muḥammad Mustafā (al-Q Qāhira: al-Hay'a al-Miṣriyya al-'Āmma lil-kitāb, 1403A.H./1982), 1(i) 354. 'Īsā, *Ta'rīkh al-Bīmāristānāt fī al-Islām,* 91–92; Adam A. Sabra, *Poverty and Charity in Medieval Islam: Mamluk Egypt, 1250–1517* (Cambridge: Cambridge University Press, 2000), 76.

47. Birnbaum, "Questing Mind," 139.

48. Leslie Peirce, *The Imperial Harem: Women and Sovereignty in the Ottoman Empire* (New York: Oxford University Press, 1993).

49. Ole Peter Grell and Andrew Cunningham, "The Reformation and Changes in Welfare Provision in Early Modern Northern Europe," in *Health Care and Poor Relief in Protestant Europe, 1500–1700,* ed. Ole Peter Grell and Andrew Cunningham (London: Routledge, 1997), 1; Ole Peter Grell and Andrew Cunningham, "The Counter-Reformation and Welfare Provision in Southern Europe," in *Health Care and Poor Relief in Counter-Reformation Europe,* Ole Peter Grell and Andrew Cunningham (London: Routledge, 1999), 1; Ole Peter Grell and Andrew Cunningham, "Health Care and Poor Relief in 18th and 19th Century Northern Europe," in *Health Care and Poor Relief in 18th and 19th Century Northern Europe,* ed. Ole Peter Grell, Andrew Cunningham and Robert Jütte (Aldershot, UK: Ashgate, 2002), 5–6.

50. David Rosner, "Social Control and Social Service: The Changing Use of Space in Charity Hospitals," *Radical History Review* 21 (1979): 195.

51. Evliya Çelebi, *The Intimate Life of an Ottoman Statesman: Melek Ahmed Paşa (1588–1662)*; trans. and ed. R. Dankoff (Albany: State University of New York Press, 1991), 207–14. Evliya also related stories about other cases of illness and other sick people. See, for example, 99–104 (a plague that also infected Melek Ahmet Paşa), 108–10 (the fatal illness of the grand vizier, despite the various treatments of many learned physicians), 231 (death in childbirth of Kaya Sultan, Melek Ahmet Paşa'a wife), 263–64 (Melek Ahmet Paşa's death after consuming too large a meal in the imperial palace, a meal that included beverages of unknown origin). In all these cases the sick were treated—although not necessarily with great success—at home by private physicians, and not in hospitals.

52. I am influenced here by Ingrid Mattson, "Status-Based Definitions of Need in Early Islamic *Zakat* and Maintenance Laws," in *Poverty and Charity in Middle Eastern Contexts*, ed. Michael Bonner, Mine Ener, and Amy Singer (Albany: State University New York Press, 2003), 31–51.

53. Singer, "Serving Up Charity," 486–87.

54. *Süleymaniye Vakfiyesi*, B:145–46.

55. Ibid., 151.

56. Al-Muḥibbī, *Tarīkh Khulaṣat al-Athr*, 1:296–97; al-Ghazzī, *Luṭf al-Samr wa-Qaṭf al-Thamr*, 1:284–85.

57. For a similar situation in the ancient world, see Peregrine Horden, "The Earliest Hospitals in Byzantium, Western Europe, and Islam," *Journal of Interdisciplinary History* 35 (2005): 362.

58. Hardwig, "What about the Family?" 5–10.

59. Peregrine Horden, "A Discipline of Relevance: The Historiography of the Later Medieval Hospital," *Social History of Medicine* 1 (1988): 373 n. 47; Nelson and Nelson, *Patient in the Family*.

60. Evliya Çelebi, *Seyahatname*, 3:321.

61. Sandys, *Relation of a Journey*, 45.

62. Said Öztürk, *Askeri Kassama ait Onyedinci Asır İstanbul Tereke Defterleri (Sosyo-Ekonomik Tahlil)* (İstanbul: OSAV, 1995), 135–37, 327, 360, 369, 377, 442, 462, 466.

63. Ibid., 301, 310, 311.

64. BOA, mühimme, defter 73, page 242/item 564 (20 Ramazan 1003 [29 May 1595]).

65. Suraiya Faroqhi, *Pilgrims & Sultans: The Hajj under the Ottomans* (London: I. B. Tauris, 1990), 122.

66. BOA, mühimme 7, 365/item 1057 (14 Ramazan 975 [13 March 1568]), 402/item 1154 (28 Ramazan 975 [27 March 1568]).

67. Tavernier, *New Relation of the Inner-Part of the Grand Seignior's Seraglio*, 22–23; Thevenot, *Travells*, 1:23–24; Bon, *Sultan's Seraglio*, 27, 108.

68. Cited in Ismail Baykal, "Yeni Sarayda 'Enderun Hastahanesi,' " *Türk Tıb Tarihi Arkivi* 17 (1940): 37. On the author see Babinger, *Die Geschichtsschreiber des Osmanen und ihre Werke*, 232; Terzioğlu, *Die Hofspitäler*, 119, 137, 139, 142.

69. Franz Rosenthal, "The Stranger in Medieval Islam," *Arabica* 44 (1997): 43. See also the section "Dislocation and Nostalgia: *Al-ḥanīn ilā l-awṭān*," in

Myths, Historical Archetypes, and Symbolic Figures in Arabic Literature: Towards a New Hermeneutic Approach, ed. Angelika Neuwirth et al. (Beirut: In Kommission bei Franz Steiner Verlag, 1999), with articles on medieval literature by Wadad al-Qadi ("Expressions of Alienation in Early Arabic Literature," 3–31); Kathrine Müller ("*Al-ḥanīn ilā l-awṭān* in Early *Adab* Literature," 33–58); and Susanne Enderwitz ("Homesickness and Love in Arabic Poetry," 59–70).

70. Patricia Crone and Shmuel Moreh, trans., *The Book of Strangers: The Medieval Arabic Graffiti on the Theme of Nostalgia* (Princeton, NJ: M. Wiener Publishers, 2000).

71. Mark R. Cohen, "The Foreign Jewish Poor in Medieval Egypt," in Bonner, Ener, and Singer. *Poverty and Charity in Middle Eastern Contexts*, 53–72; Cohen, *Poverty and Charity in the Jewish Community of Medieval Egypt* (Princeton, NJ: Princeton University Press, 2005), chap. 2 "The Foreign Poor," 72–108.

72. See, for instance, Sami Hamarneh, "Development of Hospitals in Islam," *Journal of the History of Medicine and Allied Sciences* 17 (1962): 377–80.

73. VGM, defter 575, 43–44.

74. Gökbilgin, *XV–XVI Asırlarda Edirne ve Paşa Livāsi*, B:150–51, 168–71.

75. For Jerusalem see Cohen, *Jews in the Moslem Religious Court—Society, Economy and Commercial Organisation in the XVIth Century*, docs. 366 (p. 321), 382 (p. 339), (in Hebrew). A summary of the documents from the sixteenth century was published accompanied by facsimile copies in Amnon Cohen, *A World Within: Jewish Life as Reflected in Muslim Court Documents from the Sijill of Jerusalem (XVIth Century)* (Philadelphia: Center for Judaic Studies, University of Pennsylvania, 1984), 163 [F/297], 165 [F/299]. For the eighteenth century, see Cohen, *Jews in the Moslem Religious Court—the XVIIIth Century, Documents from Ottoman Jerusalem*, docs. 138 (p. 172), 142 (p. 176 n. 3), 278 (p. 319) (in Hebrew).

76. Evliya Çelebi, *Seyahatname*, 1:321; Evliya Çelebi, *Seyahatname of Evliya Çelebi: Facsimile of Topkapı Sarayı Bağdat 304*, 1a:189. It is not certain to what institution and building Evliya was referring here.

77. Cohen, *Jews in the Moslem Religious Court—the XVIth Century*, 163, 165.

78. S. D. Goitein, *A Mediterranean Society: The Jewish Communities of the Arab World as Portrayed in the Documents of the Cairo Geniza* (Berkeley and Los Angeles: University of California Press, 1967–88), 2:251.

79. See Joshua Prawer "The Jewish Community in Jerusalem in the Crusader Period," in *The History of Jerusalem: Crusaders and Ayyubids (1099–1250)*, ed. Joshua Prawer and Haggai Ben-Shammai (Jerusalem: Yad Ben-Zvi, 1991), 194–212 (in Hebrew).

80. B. Z. Kedar, "News from the Hospital," *'Et-mol*, 5, no. 145 (July 1999): 6–9 (in Hebrew).

81. Cohen et al., *Jews in the Moslem Religious Court—the XVIIIth Century*, doc. 279 (pp. 324–25), 282 (p. 327), 283 (p. 327), 285 (p. 328), 286 (p. 328), 287 (pp. 329–30).

82. Miller, *Beyond the Sublime Porte*, 166.

83. Evliya Çelebi, *Seyahatname*, 1:321; Evliya Çelebi, *Seyahatname of Evliya Çelebi: Facsimile of Topkapı Sarayı Bağdat 304*, 1a:189.

84. Evliya Çelebi, *Seyahatname*, 10:264; Gary Leiser and Michael Dols, "Evliya Chelebi's Description of Medicine in Seventeenth-Century Egypt; Part II: Text," *Sudhoff's Archiv* 72 (1988): 55.

85. Monica H. Green, "Women's Medical Practice and Health Care in Medieval Europe," in *Sisters and Workers in the Middle Ages*, ed. J. Bennet et al. (Chicago: Chicago University Press, 1989), 39–78.

86. Joseph Schacht, *An Introduction to Islamic Law* (Oxford: Clarendon Press, 1964), 162 and passim.

87. Ian C. Dengler, "Turkish Women in the Ottoman Empire: The Classical Age," in *Women in the Muslim World*, ed. Lois Beck and Nikki Keddie (Cambridge, MA: Harvard University Press, 1978), 232, 237.

88. Bon, *Sultan's Seraglio*, 146 n. 14. And see also Tavernier, *A New Relation of the Inner-Part of the Grand Seignior's Seraglio*, 22–23.

89. Bon, *Sultan's Seraglio*, 89–90.

90. Uluçay, "Kanunī Sultan Süleyman ve Ailesi," 245.

91. Susan A. Skilliter, "Three Letters from Ottoman 'Sultana' Safiye to Queen Elizabeth I," in *Documents from Islamic Chanceries*, ed. S. M. Stern (Oxford: B. Cassirer, 1965), 144; Bernard Lewis, *The Jews of Islam* (Princeton, NJ: Princeton University Press, 1984), 144; and the relevant entries in Leslie Peirce, *The Imperial Harem: Women and Sovereignty in the Ottoman Empire* (New York: Oxford University Press, 1993).

92. This consistent Ottoman policy differed from that of the previous occupants of Istanbul, the Byzantine emperors of Constantinople. An imperial Byzantine hospital founded by Constantine IX in the middle of the eleventh century in Constantinople was meant specifically to serve members of the top social and political echelon of Byzantine society, including royalty. Constantine himself was hospitalized there when on his deathbed. Seventy years later, Alexius I was transported to this hospital by his physicians, who wanted to treat his fatal disease in this fine institution. Timothy S. Miller, *The Birth of the Hospital in the Byzantine Empire*, rev. ed. (Baltimore: Johns Hopkins University Press, 1997), 149.

93. ʿĪsā, *Taʾrīkh al-Bīmāristānāt fī al-Islām*, 138.

94. *Süleymaniye Vakfiyesi*, B:150.

95. TSMK, B. 408. During my work in the library access to this manuscript was restricted. The miniature was published and discussed by Ahmet Süheyl Ünver in his "L'album d'Ahmed Ier," *Annali dell'Istituto Universitario Orientale di Napoli* 13 (1963): 137–38, 161–62 and Dols, *Majnūn*, 130–31.

96. Evliya Çelebi, *Seyahatname*, 3:469.

97. Ibid., 10:264; Leiser and Dols, "Evliya Chelebi's Description of Medicine, part II," 55.

98. Schacht, *Introduction to Islamic Law*, 124.

99. Ali Raza Naqvi, "Adoption in Muslim Law," *Muslim Studies* 19 (1980): 283–302; Amira al-Azhary Sonbol, "Adoption in Islamic Society: A Historical Survey," in *Children in the Muslim Middle East*, ed. Elizabeth Warnock Fernea

(Austin: University of Texas Press, 1995), 45–67; Andrea B. Rugh, "Orphanages in Egypt: Contradiction or Affirmation in a Family-Oriented Society," *Children in the Muslim Middle East*, 124–41; Mahmoud Yazbak, "Muslim Orphans and the *Sharī'a* in Ottoman Palestine according to *Sijill* Records," *Journal of the Economic and Social History of the Orient* 44 (2001): 123–40; M. S. Sujimon, "The Treatment of the Foundling (*al-laqīṭ*) according to the Ḥanafīs," *Islamic Law and Society* 9 (2002): 358–85; Ella Landau-Tessaron, "Adoption, Paternity and False Genealogical Claims," *Bulletin of the School of Oriental and African Studies* 66 (2003): 169–92; *Encyclopaedia of Islam*, 2nd ed., s.v. "Laḳīṭ," by A.-M. Delcambre; *Encyclopaedia of Islam*, 2nd ed., s.v. "Tabann^{in}," by E. Chaumont; *Encyclopaedia of Islam*, 2nd ed., s.v. "Yatīm," by E. Chaumont and R. Shaham.

100. From the *vakfiye* of Ahmet I. VGM, defter 574, 83.

101. Al-Aybash and al-Shihābī, eds., *Dimashq al-Shām fī Nuṣūṣ al-Raḥāllīn wal-Jughrāfiyyin wal-Buldāniyyin al-'Arab*, 2:617.

102. *Süleymaniye Vakfiyes*, B:148–49.

103. Many travelers included anecdotes about the Ottoman lunatics they saw. Evliya Çelebi's description of the mad is especially famous. In his description of the guilds' procession in Istanbul Evliya included a section on the keepers from the hospitals for the mad who led a couple of hundreds of screaming lunatics in the streets for the crowds' amusement (Evliya Çelebi, *Seyahatname*, 1:530–31). Also known is his description of the hospital of Sultan Bayezid II in Edirne (ibid., 3:468–70). European travelers too were not indifferent to the Ottoman madmen. See, for example, Thevenot, *Travell*, 1:143, on the lunatics of Cairo.

104. Evliya Çelebi, *Seyahatname*, 9:542.

105. Kāmil Jamīl al-'Asalī, *Muqaddama fī Ta'rīkh al-Ṭibb fī al-Quds* (Ammān: al-Jāmi'a al-Urduniyya, 1994), 166.

106. Evliya Çelebi, *Seyahatname*, 10:264; Leiser and Dols, "Evliya Chelebi's Description of Medicine, part II," 55.

107. Thevenot, *Travells*, 1:143.

108. In addition to Dols's important book on madmen in medieval Islamic society, other works of his are cited in the bibliography to the present work.

109. See, for example, Nicolay, *Navigations, Peregrinations, and Voyages*, 57b; and Ahmet Süheyl Ünver, "Anadolu ve İstanbulda İmaretlerin Aşhane, Tabhane ve Misafirhanelerine ve Müessislerinin Ruhī Kemallerine dair," *İstanbul Üniversitesi Tıb Fakültesi Mecmuası* 4, no. 18 (1941): 2390–410. Ünver discusses pre-Ottoman institutions in Anatolia as well, and points out that the three-day limit was not necessarily practiced in all the institutions (p. 2392).

110. Park, "Healing the Poor," 34–36.

111. Here I reverse my own presentation of Ottoman hospitals in the early modern period as put forward in Miri Shefer, "Charity and Hospitals in the Ottoman Empire in the Early Modern Period," in *Poverty and Charity in Middle Eastern Contexts*, ed. Michael Bonner, Mine Ener, and Amy Singer (Albany: State University New York Press, 2003), 121–43.

112. Park, "Healing the Poor," 33; Miri Rubin, "Development and Change in English Hospitals, 1100–1500," in *The Hospital in History*, ed. Lindsay Granshaw and Roy Porter (London: Routledge, 1989), 48; Horden, "Earliest Hospitals in Byzantium, Western Europe, and Islam," 384.

113. Foucault, *Madness and Civilization*; Foucault, *Archaeology of Knowledge*; Foucault, *Birth of the Clinic: An Archaeology of Medical Perception*; Foucault, *Discipline and Punish: The Birth of the Prison*.

114. See for example Peter Sedgwick, "Michel Foucault: The Anti-History of Psychiatry," *Psychological Medicine* 11 (1981): 235–48.

115. Margaret Pelling, "Healing the Sick Poor: Social Policy and Disability in Norwich, 1550–1640," *Medical History* 29 (1985): 115–37; Pelling, "Illness among the Poor in an Early Modern English Town: The Norwich Census of 1570," *Continuity and Change* 3 (1988): 273–90; Marjorie K. McIntosh, "Local Responses to the Poor in Late Medieval and Tudor England," *Continuity and Change* 3 (1988): 209–45; Brian Pullan, "Support and Redeem: Charity and Poor Relief in Italian Cities from the Fourteenth to the Seventeenth Century," *Continuity and Change* 3 (1988): 177–208; Park, "Healing the Poor," 37–38.

116. Rosner, "Social Control and Social Service," 183–97; Rosenberg, *Care of Strangers*.

117. Boaz Shoshan, "The State and Madness in Medieval Islam," *IJMES* 35 (2003): 329–40.

118. Evliya Çelebi, *Seyahatname*, 1:381–87; 3:468–70; Evliya Çelebi, *The Seyahatname of Evliya Çelebi: Facsimile of Topkapı Sarayı Bağdat 304*, 1b:230–34; Evliya Efendi, *Narrative of Travels in Europe, Asia, and Africa in the Seventeenth Century*, 1b:25–29. See also several cases from Jerusalem where similar patterns of behaviour were treated differently: Cohen, *Jews in the Moslem Religious Court—the XVIth Century*, doc. 173 (p. 168), 178 (178); Cohen, *World Within*, 49 [F/57], 160 [F/292]; Cohen, Elisheva Simon-Pikali and Ovadia Salama, *Jews in the Moslem Religious Court—the XVIIIth Century*, docs. 276–78 (pp. 318–39).

119. VGM, defter 575, 106; Ünver, "Fatih Külliyesinin İlk Vakfiyesine Göre Fatih Darüşşifası," 16; *Fatih Mehmet II Vakfiyeleri*, 275.

120. VGM, defter 608/23, 231.

121. *Fatih Mehmet II Vakfiyeleri*, 281–82.

122. The recipe was entered into the Manisa *sijill* in the year 959 [1551–52] Yürükoğlu, *Manisa Bimarhanesi*, 51.

123. Ünver, "Büyük Selçuklu İmperatorluğu Zamanında Vakıf Hastanelerin Bir Kısmına Dair," 17–20, 23.

124. Gary Leiser, "Medical Education in Islamic Lands from the Seventeenth to the Fourteenth Century," *Journal of History of Medicine and Allied Sciences* 38 (1983): 49–53; Goitein, *Mediterranean Society*, 2:249–50.

125. Ahmet Süheyl Ünver, "Fatih Külliyesine ait Diğer Mühim bir Vakfiye," *Vakfılar Dergisi* 1 (1938): 43; Ünver, "İstanbul'un Zabtından Sonra Türklerde Tibbī Tekāmüle Bir Bakış," *Vakfılar Dergisi* 1 (1938): 75; Ünver, "Fatih Külliyesinin İlk Vakfiyesine Göre Fatih Darüşşifası," 17; Nil Sarı (Akdeniz), "Educating the Ottoman Physician," *Tıp Tarihi Araştırmaları* 2 (1988): 40–64;

Ayten Altıntaş, "Fatih Darüşşifası Tıp Eğitim Yapılıyor Muydu?" *Tarih ve Toplum,* 27, no. 161 (May 1997): 291–95.

126. BOA, ev.hmh 153, p.11; MAD 5019, p. 51; Ibnülemin, Sihiyye / 29v; Ali Emiri, Mehmet IV / 4419; Mühimme 25, p. 83 / item 929, p. 111 / item 1226.

127. Ünver, "Fatih Külliyesinin İlk Vakfiyesine Göre Fatih Darüşşifası," 17.

128. Ibid., 14; *Fatih Mehmet II Vakfiyeleri,* 271–72, 273–75; VGM, defter 575, 105; Gökbilgin, *XV–XVI Asırlarda Edirne ve Paşa Livāsi* B:150–55; *Süleymaniye Vakfiyesi,* B:139–43; VGM, defter 608/23, 230–31; TSMA, defter 7017/1, 14r–15v; VGM, dolap 1550, 36 (70–71); Nil Sarı, "Osmanlı Darüşşifalarına Tayin Edilecek Görevlilerde Aranan Nitlikler," *Yeni Tıp Tarihi Araştırmaları* 1 (1995): 11–54.

129. VGM, defter 575, 105; *Fatih Mehmet II Vakfiyeleri,* 271, 277–78, 279–80; Gökbilgin, *XV–XVI Asırlarda Edirne ve Paşa Livāsi* B:156–57, 160–61, 164–65, 1666–69; *Süleymaniye Vakfiyesi,* B:145, 149–51; VGM, defter 608/23, 231; TSMA, defter 7017/1, 15v; VGM, dolap 1550, 36 (71).

130. Evliya Çelebi, *Seyahatname,* 1:534; Evliya Çelebi, *Seyahatname of Evliya Çelebi: Facsimile of Topkapı Sarayı Bağdat 304,* 1b:320.

131. BOA, Ali Emiri, Ahmet I / 851/1.

132. BOA, Ibnül Emin / Sihiyye, 29v.

133. BOA, mühimme, 25, p. 223, item 2092.

134. Based on Gabriel Baer, "Patrons and Clients in Ottoman Cairo," in *Mèmorial Ömer Lütfi Barkan* (Paris: Adrien Maisonneave, 1980), 11–18; and, following the description of food distribution in Ottoman elite kitchens, *Encyclopaedia of Islam,* 2nd ed., s.v. ""Maṭbakh," by Halil Inalcik.

Chapter 4: Spaces of Disease, Disease in Space

1. Stanley Ireland and William Bechhoefer, ed. *The Ottoman House: Papers from the Amasya Symposium, 24–27 September 1996* (London: British Institute of Archaeology at Ankara, 1998), 1; Nimrod Luz, "Urban Residential Houses in Mamluk Syria: Forms, Characteristics and the Impact of Socio-Cultural Forces," in *The Mamluks in Egyptian and Syrian Politics and Society,* ed. Michael Winter and Amalia Levanoni (Leiden: Brill, 2004), 339.

2. Jonathan Hughes, "The 'Matchbox on a Muffin': The Design of Hospitals in the Early NHS," *Medical History* 44 (2000): 21.

3. Rosner, "Social Control and Social Service," 183–97; Lindsay Prior, "The Architecture of the Hospital: A Study of Spatial Organization and Medical Knowledge," *British Journal of Sociology,* 39 (1988): 86–94; Prior, "The Local Space of Medical Discourse: Disease, Illness and Hospital Architecture," in *The Social Construction of Illness,* ed. Jens Lachmund and Gunner Stollberg (Stuttgart: Robert Bosch Stiftung, 1992), 67–84; Jeane Kisacky, "Restructuring Isolation: Hospital Architecture, Medicine, and Disease Prevention," *Bulletin of the History of Medicine* 79 (2005): 1–49.

4. Rubin, "Development and Change in English Hospitals," 42.

5. Sally Sheard and Helen Power, "Body and City," in Sheard and Power, *Body and City*, 1.

6. Peter Mandler "Poverty and Charity in the Nineteenth-Century Metropolis: An Introduction," in *The Uses of Charity: The Poor on Relief in the Nineteenth-Century Metropolis*, ed. Peter Mandler (Philadelphia: University of Pennsylvania Press, 1990), 1–6.

7. Horden, "Earliest Hospitals in Byzantium, Western Europe, and Islam," 363, 367.

8. Ibid., 371.

9. Klein-Franke, "Health and Healing in Medieval Muslim Palestine," 121–22. For Saladin's many Christian physicians, see Samira Jadon, "The Physicians of Syria during the Reign of Ṣalāḥ al-Dīn, 570–598 A.H. 1174–1193 A.D.," *Journal of the History of Medicine and Allied Science* 25 (1970): 323–40.

10. Faroqhi, *Pilgrims & Sultans*, 122.

11. Marina Tolmacheva, "Female Piety and Patronage in the Medieval 'Ḫajj,' " in *Women in the Medieval Islamic World*, ed. Gavin R. G. Hambly (New York: St. Martin's Press, 1998), 165.

12. Çiğdem Kafesçioğlu, "The Ottoman Capital in the Making: The Reconstruction of Constantinople in the Fifteenth Century" (PhD diss., Harvard University, 1996); Gülru Necipoğlu-Kafadar, "The Süleymaniye Complex in Istanbul: An Interpretation," *Muqarnas* 7 (1996): 92–117.

13. Arslan Terzioğlu, "15. ve 16. Yüzyılda Türk-İslam Hastane Yapıları ve Bunların Dünya Çapındaki Önemi," in *II. Ulusarası Türk-Islam Bilim ve Teknoloji Tarihi Kongresi (I.T.Ü 28 Nisan–2 Mayıs 1986)* (İstanbul: [n.p.], 1987), 3:160.

14. Sandys, *Relation of a Journey*, 58. For discussion of Sandys's description see Peirce, *Imperial Harem*, 61–63.

15. Peirce, *Imperial Harem*, chap. 7 ("The Display of Sovereign Prerogative"), 186–218, especially pp. 200–202.

16. Gülru Necipoğlu, "A Ḳānūn for the State, a Canon for the Arts: Conceptualizing the Classical Synthesis of Ottoman Arts and Architecture," in *Soleiman le Magnifique et son temps*, ed. Gilles Veinstein (Paris: Documentation française, 1992), 208–9.

17. Barkan, "Fatih Câmi ve İmareti Tesîslerini 1489–1490 Yıllarına âit Muhasebe Bilânçoları," 330.

18. Peter Ian Kuniholm, "Dendochronologically Dated Ottoman Monuments," in *A Historical Archaeology of the Ottoman Empire*, ed. Uzi Baram and Lynda Carroll (New York: Kluwer Academic/Plenum Publishers, 2000), 120–21; Godfrey Goodwin, *A History of Ottoman Architecture* (London: Thames and Hudson, 1971), 50.

19. See J. M. Rogers, "Innovation and Continuity in Islamic Urbanism," in *The Arab City: Its Characteristics and Islamic Cultural Heritage*, ed. Ismail Serageldin and Samir El-Sadek (Riyadh: Arab Urban Development Institute, 1982), 55–57 for a different view. Rogers claims that the vast water systems in Istanbul evolved only toward the end of the sixteenth century. He regards this as evidence that previous complexes were not considered by their founders

important or prestigious enough to invest in these systems. If this is indeed so, water was not a major factor in decisions about the location of the first hospitals in Istanbul.

20. Compare with considerations of this matter in medieval Europe in James William Brodman, *Charity and Welfare: Hospitals and the Poor in Medieval Catalonia* (Philadelphia: University of Pennsylvania Press, 1998), 61–62.

21. Aptullah Kuran, *The Mosque in Early Ottoman Architecture* (Chicago: University of Chicago Press, 1968), 111; Kuran, "A Spatial Study of Three Ottoman Capitals: Bursa, Edirne and Istanbul," *Muqarnas* 13 (1996): 114–18.

22. Ulya Vogt-Göknil, *Living Architecture: Ottoman*, photography by Edward Widmer (London: Grosset & Dunlap, 1966), 19.

23. Evliya Çelebi, *Seyahatname*, 3:469; Goodwin, *History of Ottoman Architecture*, 143. In January 1998 and May 2000 I followed Edirne people and walked from the city center (the Mosque of the Three Galleries, the Üç Şerefeli Camii) to the complex of Beyazid II across the river. One can negotiate the distance in twenty-five minutes of easy walking.

24. Halil Inalcik, "Istanbul: An Islamic City," *Journal of Islamic Studies* 1 (1990): 1–23.

25. Necipoğlu, *Architecture, Ceremonial, and Power*, 49.

26. Evliya Çelebi, *Seyahatname of Evliya Çelebi: Facsimile of Topkapı Sarayı Bağdat 304*, 1b:288–89; Evliya Çelebi, *Seyahatname*, 1:475, 10:516–17; Gönül Cantay [Güreşsever], *Anadolu Selçuklu ve Osmanlı Darüşşifaları* (Ankara: Atatürk Kültür Merkezi Yayını, 1992), 7–8; Gary Leiser and Michael Dols, "Evliya Chelebi's Description of Medicine in Seventeenth Century Egypt; Part I: Introduction," *Sudhoffs Archiv* 71 (1987): 205.

27. Al-Bukhārī, *Al-Jāmi' al-Ṣaḥīḥ*, ṭibb/item no. 19; al-'Asqalānī, *Fatḥ al-Bārī*, 12:264–78.

28. J. P. Goubert, "Twenty Years on: Problems of Historical Methodology in the History of Health," in *Problems and Methods in the History of Medicine*, ed. Roy Porter and Andrew Wear (London: Croom Helm, 1987), 48.

29. Hafiz Hüseyn b. al-Haj Ismail Ayvanseray, *Hadiqat-ül-Jamai'*, 2 vols. (Istanbul: Matbaa-i Amire, 1281 [1865]), 1:8, 108, 110–11, 115; Aptullah Kuran, *Sinan: The Grand Old Master of Ottoman Architecture* (Washington, DC: Institute of Turkish Studies; Istanbul: Ada Press Publishers, 1985), 189.

30. Ahmet Süheyl Ünver, "Büyük Selçuklu İmperatorluğu Zamanında Vakıf Hastanelerin Bir Kismına Dair," *Vakıflar Dergisi* 1 (1938): 22 (a 1483 Ottoman document).

31. George Keppel, *Narrative of a Journey Across the Balcan* (London, 1831), 1:75–76; Ralph S. Hattox, *Coffee and Coffeehouses: The Origins of a Social Beverage in the Medieval Near East* (Seattle: University of Washington Press, 1988), chap. 6 ("Taverns without Wine: The Rise of the Coffeehouse"), 72–91. For the spread of coffeehouses in Jerusalem see Amnon Cohen, "Coffee and Coffeehouses in Jerusalem," in *Studies in the History of Muslim Peoples: Papers Presented at a Conference in Memory of David Ayalon, 9 June 1999* (Jerusalem: Israel Academy of Sciences and Humanities, 2006), 103–12. (in Hebrew).

32. Musṭafā 'Ālī, *Musṭafā 'Ālī's Description of Cairo of 1599*, 38, 109; al-Muḥibbī, *Tarīkh Khulasat al-Athr*, 1:419–22.

33. Leo Africanus, *The History and Description of Africa and the Notable Things Therein Contained*, 3 vols. (New York: B. Franklin, 1960), 2:426.

34. Kafesçioğlu, "Ottoman Capital in the Making," 117–18.

35. Paul Slack, "Hospitals, Workhouses and the Relief of the Poor in Early Modern London," in *Health Care and Poor Relief in Protestant Europe 1500–1700*, ed. Ole Peter Grell and Andrew Cunningham (London: Routledge, 1997), 236.

36. Evliya Çelebi, *Seyahatname*, 1:322; Evliya Çelebi, *Seyahatname of Evliya Çelebi: Facsimile of Topkapı Sarayı Bağdat 304*, 1a:189; Evliya Efendi, *Narrative of Travels in Europe, Asia, and Africa*, 1a:175.

37. *Fatih Mehmet II Vakfiyeleri*, 279–80; Gökbilgin, *XV–XVI Asırlarda Edirne ve Paşa Livāsi*, B:160–61; *Süleymaniye Vakfiyesi*, B:149; VGM, defter 608/23, 231; TSMA, defter 7017/1, 15v; VGM, dolap 1550, 36 (71).

38. Evliya Çelebi, *Seyahatname*, 10:263; Leiser and Dols, "Evliya Chelebi's Description of Medicine, part II," 53; Sandys, *Relation of a Journey*, 29–30; Jean Thevenot, *Travells*, 1:128.

39. A. Süheyl Ünver, "Kanunī Süleyman'a İlkbaharda İlāç Yapılması," *Türk Tıp Tarihi Arkivi* 14, no. 4 (1939): 83–85.

40. Uriel Heyd, "An Unknown Turkish Treatise by a Jewish Physician under Suleyman the Magnificent," *Eretz Israel* 7 (1964): 48*–50*.

41. Paul Rycaut, *The History of the Turkish Empire from the Year 1623 to the Year 1677* . . . (London, 1680), 2:81. See also Jason Goodwin, *Lords of the Horizons* (London: Vintage, 1998), 252; Henry Blount, *A Voyage into the Levant* (London, 1636), 44; Evliya Çelebi, *Seyahatname*, 10:515–16; Leiser and Dols, "Evliya Chelebi's Description of Medicine, part I," 203–4; Thevenot, *Travells*, 2:53–54.

42. On the size of gardens in pre-Ottoman hospitals in Anatolia see Ünver, "Büyük Selçuklu İmperatorluğu Zamanında Vakıf Hastanelerin Bir Kısmına Dair," 20; Erdal Sargutan, "Selçuklular'da Tıb ve Tıb Kuruluşları," *Vakıflar Dergisi* 11 (1976): 318. The Manṣūrī hospital in Cairo from Mamluk times, for example, lacked a garden but used big fans to clear the air inside the building; branches and leaves from fragrant trees like mastics and pomegranates were spread on the floor to enhance the sweet smells. 'Īsā, *Ta'rīkh al-Bīmāristānāt fī al-Islām*, 102–3.

43. Gustave E. von Grunebaum, "The Response to Nature in Arabic Poetry," *Journal of Near Eastern Studies* 4 (1945): 137–51.

44. Shah-Khan, "The Song of Creation: Sufi Themes on Nature," *Sufi* (London) 18 (Summer 1993): 27–30; İbrahim Özdemir, "Toward an Understanding of Environmental Ethics from a Qur'anic Perspective," in *Islam and Ecology: A Bestowed Trust*, ed. Richard C. Foltz, Frederick M. Denny and Azizan Baharuddin (Cambridge, MA: Center for the Study of World Religions, Harvard Divinity School; distributed by Harvard University Press, 2003), 3–37. See also other articles in *Islam and Ecology*.

45. Leaman, *Islamic Aesthetics*, 125; Yasin Çağatay Seçkin, "Gardens of the Ninteenth-Century Imperial Palaces in Istanbul," *Studies in the History of Gardens and Designed Landscape* 23 (2003): 72.

46. Evliya Çelebi, *Seyahatname of Evliya Çelebi*, 1b:237–309; Evliya Çelebi, *Seyahatname*, 1:391–487; Evliya Efendi, *Narrative of Travels in Europe, Asia, and Africa*, 1b:33–34, 40–42, 46, 59–60, 62–63, 64, 82, 84–86.

47. Vogt-Göknil, *Living Architecture*, 20; Mine F. Thompson, "Turkey," in *Encyclopedia of Gardens: History and Design* (Chicago: Fitzroy Dearborn Publishers, 2001), 3:1333.

48. Bon, *Sultan's Seraglio*, 25–26; Necipoğlu, *Architecture, Ceremonial, and Power*, chaps. 9 ("The Hanging Garden of the 3rd Court, Its Pavilions, and the Outer Garden"), and 10 ("The Pavilions of the Outer Garden"), 184–241; Richard Ettinghausen, introduction to Elisabeth B. MacDougall and Richard Ettinghausen, eds., *The Islamic Garden* (Washington, DC: Dumbarton Oaks, Trustees for Harvard University, 1976), 3–10; Godfrey Goodwin, "Sinan and City Planning," *Environmental Design* 5, nos. 5–6 (1987): 15; James Dickie (Yaqub Zaki), "Garden and Cemetery in Sinan's Istanbul," *Environmental Design* 5, nos. 5–6 (1987): 72.

49. Thompson, "Turkey," 1333.

50. Gülru Necipoğlu, "The Suburban Landscape of Sixteenth-Century Istanbul as a Mirror of Classical Ottoman Garden Culture," in *Gardens in the Time of the Great Muslim Empires*, ed. Attilio Petruccioli (Leiden: Brill, 1997), 44–45; Doris Behren-Abouseif, "Gardens in Islamic Egypt," *Der Islam* 69 (1992): 302–12.

51. Nılgün Ergun and Özge İskender, "Gardens of the Topkapi Palace: An Example of Turkish Garden Art," *Studies in the History of Gardens and Designed Landscape* 23 (2003): 57–71; Necipoğlu, "Suburban Landscape of Sixteenth-Century Istanbul," 34.

52. Carole Rawcliffe, "Hospital Nurses and Their Work," in *Daily Life in the Late Middle Ages*, ed. Richard Britnell (Stroud, UK: Sutton Pub., 1998), 58–61; Carmélia Opsomer-Halleux, "The Medieval Garden and Its Role in Medicine," in *Medieval Gardens*, ed. Elisabth B. MacDougall (Washington, DC: Dumbarton Oaks Research Library and Collection, 1986), 95–113.

53. C. Robert Horsburgh, Jr., "Healing by Design," *New England Journal of Medicine* 333 (1995): 735–40 and subsequent correspondence between author and readers in 334 (1996): 334–36.

54. The following discussion on gardens and the healing process is based on Clare Cooper Marcus and Marni Barnes, eds., *Healing Gardens: Therapeutic Benefits and Design Recommendations* (New York: J. Wiley, 1999); Jean Larson and Mary Jo Kreitzer, "Healing by Design: Healing Gardens and Therapeutic Landscapes," *Implications* 2, no. 10 (a newsletter by InformeDesign, a Web site for design and human behavior research at the University of Minnesota), http://www.informedesign.umn.edu/_news/nov_v02-p.pdf; Roger S. Ulrich, "Health Benefits of Gardens in Hospitals," paper delivered at *Plants for People*, International Exhibition Floriade 2002, http://www.planterra.com/SymposiumUlrich.pdf.

55. Nicholas Stavroulakis, "The Flora of Ottoman Gardens: I. Trees," *Mediterranean Garden* 10 (1997): 7–16; Stavroulakis, "The Flora of Ottoman Gardens: II. Flowering Plants," *Mediterranean Garden* 11 (1997–98): 11–20;

Norah Titley and Frances Wood, *Oriental Gardens: An Illustrated History* (San Francisco: Chronicle Books, 1992), 11–23; Thompson, "Turkey," 1334.

56. Necipoğlu, "Suburban Landscape of Sixteenth-Century Istanbul," 42; Emma Clark, *The Art of the Islamic Garden* (Ramsbury, UK: Crowood Press, 2004), 13–14.

57. Thompson, "Turkey," 1334; Luz, "Urban Residential Houses in Mamluk Syria," 344–45, 352–53.

58. Evliya Çelebi, *Seyahatname,* 3:469. The English translation is taken from Dols, *Majnūn,* 172.

59. The Ottomans were not unique in using motifs of life and paradise in their gardens. See, for example, D. Fairchild Ruggles, "Humayun's Tomb and Garden," in *Gardens in the Time of the Great Muslim Empires,* ed. Attilio Petruccioli (Leiden: Brill, 1997), 173–86; Ruggles, *Gardens, Landscape, and Vision in the Palaces of Islamic Spain* (University Park: Pennsylvania State University Press, 2000), chap. 9 "Illusion and Paradise," 209–22; 248–50 (notes).

60. Evliya Çelebi, *Seyahatname of Evliya Çelebi,* 1b:252; Evliya Çelebi, *Seyahatname,* 1:414–15; Evliya Efendi, *Narrative of Travels in Europe, Asia, and Africa,* 1b:42. See also Attilio Petruccioli, "Nature in Islamic Urbanism: The Garden in Practice and in Metaphor," in *Islam and Ecology: A Bestowed Trust,* ed. Richard C. Foltz, Frederick M. Denny, and Azizan Baharuddin (Cambridge, MA: Center for the Study of World Religions, Harvard Divinity School; distributed by Harvard University Press, 2003), 499–510; James L. Jr. Westcoat, "From the Gardens of the Qur'an to the 'Gardens' of Lahore," in *Islam and Ecology: A Bestowed Trust,* ed. Richard C. Foltz, Frederick M. Denny, and Azizan Baharuddin (Cambridge, MA: Center for the Study of World Religions, Harvard Divinity School; distributed by Harvard University Press, 2003), 511–26.

61. Evliya Çelebi, *Seyahatname of Evliya Çelebi,* 1b:274; Evliya Çelebi, *Seyahatname,* 1:449; Evliya Efendi, *Narrative of Travels in Europe, Asia, and Africa,* 1b:64.

62. *Fatih Mehmet II Vakfiyeleri,* 280.

63. *Fatih Mehmet II Vakfiyeleri,* 278; Gökbilgin, *XV–XVI Asırlarda Edirne ve Paşa Livāsi,* B:164–65; TSMA, defter 7017/1, 15b; Bon, *Sultan's Seraglio,* 108; Tavernier, *New Relation of the Inner-Part of the Grand Seraglio,* 22; Hill, *Full and Just Account of the Present State of the Ottoman Empire,* 132. Hospital budget reports are found mainly in the Prime Ministry Ottoman Archive (BOA) in the *maliyyeden müdevver* classification.

64. Mustafa Na'ima, *Tarih-i Naima: Rawdat al-Husayn fi Khulasat Akhbar al-Khafiqin;* 6 vols. (İstanbul: Matbaa-i Amire, 1281AH), 5:320–21.

65. Bon, *Sultan's Seraglio,* 108.

66. Fisher and Fisher, "Topkapi Sarayi in the Mid-Seventeenth Century," 76; Gülru Necipoğlu, *Architecture, Ceremonial, and Power,* 49.

67. Tavernier, *New Relation of the Inner-Part of the Grand Seraglio,* 22–23; Fisher and Fisher, "Topkapi Sarayi in the Mid-Seventeenth Century," 49–50; Paul Rycaut, *Present State of the Ottoman Empire . . .* (London, 1668), 33–34.

68. It is interesting to compare hospital walls with the walls around mosques, which have been explained as a means for separating the holy from

the profane. Augusto Romano Burelli, "Visions and Representation of Urban Space," *Environmental Design*, 5, nos. 5–6 (1987): 42, 46.

69. For minority groups on a sociomedical basis in the Muslim Middle Ages see Dols's pioneering work *Majnūn*. For attitudes toward madness in modern Turkey, see O. M. Öztürk, "Folk Interpretation of Illness in Turkey and Its Psychiatry Significance," *Turkish Journal of Pediatrics* 7 (1965): 165–79; Öztürk, "Folk Treatment of Mental Illness in Turkey," in *Magic, Faith and Healings*, ed. A. Kiev (New York: Free Press of Glencoe, 1964), 343–63; O. M. Öztürk and V. Volkan, "The Theory and Practice of Psychiatry in Turkey," in *Psychological Dimensions of Near Eastern Studies*, ed. L. C. Brown and N. Itzkowitz (Princeton, NJ: Darwin Press, 1977), 330–61.

70. Dols, *Majnūn*, 130–31.

71. Gönül Güreşsever, "Kitab al-Cerahiyet al-Hāniye (Istanbul Tıp Tarihi Enstitüsü Nüshası) Minyatürler," *I. Milletarası Türkoloji Kongresi. Tebliğler* (İstanbul: n.p., 1979), 3:771–86.

72. Visiting hospitals as an entertainment is a familiar theme in Muslim literature dating back to the *Thousand and One Nights*. See Dols, *Majnūn*, 129 n. 4. See also one of the *maqāmāt* of al-Hamadhani (d. 1008) entitled "Al-Maqāma al-Maristāniyya," quoted in Muḥammad Muḥī al-Dīn 'Abd al-Ḥamīd, *Sharḥ Maqāmāt Badī' al-Zamān al-Hamādhānī* (Mişr: Maktaka ve Maṭba'at Muḥammad 'Alī Ṣabīh, 1902/1381 AH), 150–61.

73. John A. Thompson and Grace Goldin, *The Hospital: A Social and Architectural History* (New Haven, CT: Yale University Press, 1975), xxvii.

74. Cantay, *Anadolu Selçuklu ve Osmanlı Darüşşifaları*, 9–14; Osman Şevki Uludağ, "Haseki Darüşşifası," *Tıb Dünyası* 9 (1938): 3728–29; Terzioğlu, "15. ve 16. Yüzyılda Türk-İslam Hastane Yapıları," 155–97.

75. Sandys, *Relation of a Journey*, 45. For the size of Seljuk hospitals, see Ünver, "Büyük Selçuklu İmperatorloğu Zamanında Vakıf Hastanelerin bir kısmına dair," 19–20; and Sargutan, "Selçuklular'da Tıb ve Tıb Kuruluşları," 318.

76. Ahmet Süheyl Ünver, *İstanbul Üniversitesi Tarihi Baslangiç, Fatih Külliyesi ve Zamanı Hayatı* (Istanbul: n.p., 1946), 243; Ahmet Süheyl Ünver, "Fatih Darüşşifası Plâni," *Türk Tıp Tarihi Arkivi* 21, no. 2 (1943): 23–28.

77. VGM, defter 574, 83.

78. Evliya Çelebi, *Seyahatname*, 10:263; Leiser and Dols, "Evliya Chelebi's Description of Medicine, part II," 52–53; 'Īsā, *Ta'rīkh al-Bīmāristānat fī al-Islām*, 87, 101, 152–53.

79. Foster and Anderson, *Medical Anthropology*, 53.

80. On jinns see *Encyclopaedia of Islam*, 2nd ed., s.v. "Djinn," by H. Massé.

81. Foster and Anderson, *Medical Anthropology*, 53.

82. Hill, *Full and Just Account of the Present State of the Ottoman Empire*, 132.

83. Bon, *Sultan's Seraglio*, 86; Blount, *Voyage into the Levant*, 86; Rycaut, *Present State of the Ottoman Empire*, 116.

84. John Ray, ed. *A Collection of Curious Travels*... (London, 1693), 1:219.

85. For the European case see Owsei Temkin, "An Historical Analysis of the Concept of Infection," in *Studies in Intellectual History* (Baltimore: Johns Hopkins Press, 1953), 123–47.

86. Conrad, "Ninth-Century Muslim Scholar's Discussion of Contagion," 163–64.

87. Evliya Çelebi, *Seyahatname*, 1:475; Evliya Çelebi, *Seyahatname of Evliya Çelebi: Facsimile of Topkapı Sarayı Bağdat 304*, 1b:288–89.

88. Lisan al-Din Ibn al-Khatib, "A Very Useful Inquiry into the Horrible Sickness," an excerpt included in John Aberth, ed. *The Black Death: The Great Mortality of 1348–1350: A Brief History with Documents* (Boston: Bedford/St. Martin's, 2005), 114–16.

89. M. Ertuğrul Düzdağ, *Kanunī Devrinde Osmanlı Hayatı* (İstanbul, 1998), 148 (item 395), 282 (item 888), 290 (item 913).

90. A manuscript held at the British Library, Or. 9009; Sami K. Hamarneh, *Catalogue of Arabic Manuscripts on Medicine and Pharmacy at the British Library* (Cairo: [n.p.], 1975), 226–27.

91. Ahmad b. Mustafa Tashköprüzade, "Al-Shaqā'īq al-Nu'māniyya," manuscript held at the Süleymaniye Library, Esad Ef. 2308, f. 82.

92. And, *Istanbul in the 16th Century*, 93.

93. Rycaut, *Present State of the Ottoman Empire*, 116–17. On Palestine in 1688 see William Daniel, *A Journal or Account of William Daniel: His Late Expedition or Undertaking to go from London to Surrat in India*... (London, 1702), 64.

94. Ronald Jennings, "The Society and Economy of Maçuka in the Ottoman Judicial Registers of Trabzon, 1560–1640," in *Continuity and Change in Late Byzantine and Early Ottoman Society*, ed. Anthony Bryer and Heath Lowry (Birmingham: Centre for Byzantine Studies and Modern Greek, University of Birmingham, 1986), 135–36.

95. BOA, *mühimme defteri*, 40, p. 289, item 662 and p. 291, item 669 (27 Ramazan 987 [November 17th, 1579]).

96. BOA, *Cevdet/Sihiyye*, 1204 (21 Sha'ban 1080 [January 14, 1670]). See also *mühimme defteri*, 3, p. 346, item 1022 (27 Rajab 967 [April 23, 1560]); 5, p. 600, item 1660 (end of Shawwal 973 [middle of May 1566]); 35, p. 184, item 467 (Jumada al-Akhira 986 [August–September 1578]); 48, p. 5, item 12 (beginning of Rajab 990? [end of July 1582?]).

97. John Baldry, "The Ottoman Quarantine Station on Karaman Island, 1881–1914," *Studies in History of Medicine* 2 (1978): 3–138; Panzac, "Politique sanitaire et fixation des frontiéres," 87–108.

98. Sandys, *Relation of a Journey*, 5–6. See also C. M. Cipolla, *Public Health and the Medical Profession in the Renaissance* (Cambridge: Cambridge University Press, 1976), 11–66.

99. Blount, *Voyage into the Levant*, 86. See the Egyptian case in the nineteenth century, discussed in LaVerne Kuhnke, *Lives at Risk: Public Health in*

Nineteenth Century Egypt (Berkeley and Los Angeles: University of California Press, 1990). See also Nancy E. Gallagher, "Contagion and Quarantine in Tunis and Cairo, 1800–1870," *Maghreb Review* 7 (1982): 108–11.

100. Blount, *Voyage into the Levant*, 86; Kenneth Parker, ed. *Early Modern Tales of Orient: A Critical Anthology* (London: Routledge, 1999), 175–76. See also And, *Istanbul*, 93–94 for more Europeans reporting what they regarded as Ottoman disregard for the dangers of epidemics.

101. Al-Muḥibbī, *Tarīkh Khulaṣat al-Athr*, 2:240–42; Mustafa Rashed, *Tarih-i Rashed*, 1:96; Adıvar, *Osmanlı Türklerinde İlim*, 131–32; Kâhya and Erdemir, *Bılımın Işığında Osmanlıdan Cumhuriyete Tıp ve Sağlık Kurumları*, 179–84.

102. See, for example, two manuscripts in the Cambridge University Library from the first half of the nineteenth century. See the entires in Edward G. Browne, *A Supplementary Hand-List of the Muhammadan Manuscripts including all those Written in the Arabic Character, Preserved in the Libraries of the University and Colleges of Cambridge* (Cambridge: Cambridge University Press, 1922), 169.

103. "Ghāyat al-bayān fī tadbīr badan al-insān," manuscript held at the Cambridge University Library, P.27 Brown, f. 99v.

104. "Ghāyat al-bayān fī tadbīr badan al-insān," manuscript held at the Cambridge University Library, Add. 3532, f. 218v–219r.

105. Emir Çelebi, "Enmüzec-ül-Tibb," manuscript held at the British Library, Or. 7282, f. 121.

106. Conrad, "Epidemic Diseases in Formal and Popular Thought in Early Islamic Society," 77–99; Conrad, "A Ninth-Century Muslim Scholar's Discussion of Contagion," 163–77.

107. Dols, *Black Death in the Middle East*, chaps. 4, 6, 8.

108. See, for example, the response of two Mosul quarters in face of the civil war and plague devastating the city in the eighteenth century: Dina Rizk Khoury, "Slippers at the Entrance or Behind Closed Doors: Domestic and Public Spaces for Mosuli Women," in *Women in the Ottoman Empire: Middle Eastern Women in the Early Modern Era*, ed. Madeline C. Zilfi (Leiden: Brill, 1997), 122. The studies on the social and cultural responses of Ottomans to natural disasters, including the plague, are scarce, as the few scholars who were interested in the matter focused on demography.

Conclusion: Ottoman Medicine—Ottoman? Successful?

1. Cornell H. Fleischer, *Bureaucrat and Intellectual in the Ottoman Empire: The Historian Mustafa Âli (1541–1600)* (Princeton, NJ: Princeton University Press, 1986).

2. Gülru Necipoğlu, "Plans and Models in 15th- and 16th-Century Ottoman Architectural Practice," *Journal of the Society of Architectural Historians*, 45 (1986): 224–43; Necipoğlu, "From International Timurid to Ottoman: A Change of Taste in Sixteenth-Century Ceramic Tiles," *Muqarnas* 7 (1990):

136–70; Necipoğlu, "A Ḳānūn for the State, A Canon for the Arts," 195–216; Necipoğlu, "Framing the Gaze in Ottoman, Safavid, and Mughal Palaces," *Ars Orientalis* 34 (1993): 303–42.

3. Feldman, *Music of the Ottoman Court.*

4. O. Wright, "Under the Influence? Preliminary Reflections on Arab Music during the Ottoman Period," in *The Balance of Truth: Essays in Honour of Professor Geoffrey Lewis,* ed. Çiğdem Balim-Harding and Colin Imber (İstanbul: Isis Press, 2000), 407–29. Wright's previous studies of early Ottoman musicology agree with his views here. See his "*Çargâh* in Turkish Classical Music versus Theory," *Bulletin of the School of Oriental and African Studies* 53 (1990): 224–44; Wright, *Words without Songs: A Musicological Study of an Early Ottoman Anthology and Its Precursors* (London: School of Oriental and African Studies, University of London, 1992); Wright, "On the Influence of a 'Timurid Music,' " *Oriente Moderno,* n.s., 15 (1996): 665–81.

5. Cerasi, "Many Masters and Artisans,"; Cerasi, "The Deeper Structures of Ottoman Urban Housing Fabric: Conservation of Space and Forms through Basic Parameters," in *The Ottoman House: Papers from the Amasya Symposium, 24–27 September 1996,* ed. Stanley Ireland and William Bechhoefer (London: British Institute of Archaeology at Ankara, 19987), 9–15; Cerasi, "Open Space, Water and Trees in Ottoman Urban Culture," 2:36–49; Cerasi, "Formation of Ottoman House Types," 116–56.

6. Ehud Toledano, "The Emergence of Ottoman-Local Elites (1700–1800): A Framework for Research," in *Middle Eastern Politics and Ideas: A History from Within,* ed. I. Pappe and M. Ma'oz (London: Tauris Academic Studies, 1997), 145–62.

7. Fleischer, *Bureaucrat and Intellectual in the Ottoman Empire,* 247. Fleischer contrasted these groups with ulema and educated statesmen whom he believes to have been literate also in Arabic and Persian. One can at least wonder what the actual degree of fluency was in languages other than Turkish of (some? most?) members of these classes.

8. Emir Çelebi, "Enmüzec-ül-Tibb," manuscript held at the British Library, Or. 7282, fol. 8; Adıvar, *Osmanlı Türklerinde İlim,* 128–29; Kâhya and Erdemir, *Osmanlıdan Cumhuriyete Tıp ve Sağlık Kurumları,* 173–74.

9. Cevat İzgi, *Osmanlı Medreselerinde İlim,* 2 vols. (İstanbul: İz Yayıncılık, 1997), 2:42–43.

10. Ron Barkai, "Between East and West: A Jewish Doctor from Spain," in *Intercultural Contacts in the Medieval Mediterranean,* ed. Benjamin Arbel (London: F. Cass, 1996), 49–63.

11. Al-Muḥibbī, *Tarīkh Khulaṣat al-Athr,* 2:240–42; Rashed, *Tarih-i Rashed,* 1:96; Adıvar, *Osmanlı Türklerinde İlim,* 122–23, 131–32; Kâhya and Erdemir, *Osmanlıdan Cumhuriyete Tıp ve Sağlık Kurumları,* 179–84.

12. This is the title of the Ottoman translation according to Sami Hamarneh, in his British Library catalogue. An Ottoman manuscript kept at the Cambridge University Library bears a slightly different title: "Ghāyat al-bayān fī tadbīr badan al-insān," Browne P.27, f.4b. For the original Arabic work, see MSS Reşid Efendi 698 and Şehid Ali Paşa 2062 held in the

Süleymaniye Library and Add. 3532 held in the Cambridge University Library. For the Turkish translation, see manuscripts held at the Cambridge University Library, Browne P. 27 and the Princeton University Library Garret 1181H and New Series 998.

13. Rashed, *Tarih-i Rashed,* 1:96.

14. *Encyclopaedia of Islam,* 2nd ed., s.v. "Khil'a," by N. A. Stillman.

15. See, again, the two manuscripts in Cambridge University Library from the first half of the nineteenth century, reproduced in Browne, *Supplementary Hand-List of the Muhammadan Manuscripts,* 169.

16. Najm al-Dīn Muḥammad b. Muḥammad al-Ghazzī, "Al-kawākib al-sā'ira fī a'yān al-mi'ā al-'āshira," manuscript held at the Süleymaniye Library, H. Hüsnü Paşa 876, 225b. See also Adıvar, *Osmanlı Türklerinde İlim,* 115–16; Kâhya and Erdemir, *Osmanlıdan Cumhuriyete Tıp ve Sağlık Kurumları,* 162; and Heyd, "Moses Hamon," 152–70 who discusses Qayṣūnīzāde's rivalry with a Jewish physician in Süleyman's court.

17. Rosenberg, *Care of Strangers.*

18. Inalcik, "Istanbul: An Islamic City," 1–23.

19. Miri Shefer, "Hospitals in the Three Ottoman Capitals: Bursa, Edirne & Istanbul in the Sixteenth and Seventeenth Centuries" (PhD diss., Tel Aviv University, 2001), chap. 2 "The Hospital Staff," 72–133 (in Hebrew).

20. Hill, *Full and Just Account of the Present State of the Ottoman Empire,* 57.

21. Thevenot, *Travells,* 1:37.

22. Doris Behrens-Abouseif, "The Image of the Physician, Arab Biographies of the Post-Classical Age," *Der Islam* 66 (1989): 331–43.

23. *Encyclopaedia of Islam,* 2nd ed., s.v. "Istanbul," by Halil Inalcik.

24. A similar explanation for the increase of non-Muslim physicians in the Mamluk sultanate appears in Doris Behrens-Abouseif, *Fatḥ Allāh and Abū Zakariyya: Physicians under the Mamluks* (Cairo: Institut Francais d'Archeologie Orientale, 1987), 12.

25. Al-Muḥibbī, *Tarīkh Khulaṣat al-Athr,* 4:82–89.

26. Ahmet Süheyl Ünver, *İstanbul Üniversitesi Tarihi Baslangıç, Fatih Külliyesi ve Zamanı Hayatı* (İstanbul: [n.p.], 1946), 244; *Encyclopaedia of Islam,* 2nd ed., s.v. "Ḥadīdī," by V. L. Ménage.

27. Evliya Çelebi, *Seyahatname,* 1:321; Evliya Efendi, 1:174; Evliya Çelebi, *Seyahatname of Evliya Çelebi: Facsimile of Topkapı Sarayı Bağdat 304,* 1a:189.

28. Katherine Park and John Henderson, " 'The First Hospital among Christians': The Opsedale di Santa Maria Nuova in Early Sixteenth-Century Florence," *Medical History* 35 (1991): 164.

29. Katherine Park, "Healing the Poor," 36.

30. *OED,* s.v. "hospital." Second edition, online.

31. BOA, mühimme defteri, 15, p. 152, item #1294.

Bibliography

Primary Sources

Archives

Başbakanlık Osmanlı Arşivi [Archives of the Ottoman Prime Ministry, Istanbul]:
Mühimme Defterleri: 1–7, 13–15, 23, 25, 31, 33, 35, 40, 45, 48, 53, 62, 70, 73, 80, 105, 111
Nezaret Öncesi Evkaf Defteleri (EV.HMH): 55, 153, 258, 271
Ali Emiri: Selim I/15, Mehmet III/6, Ahmet I/762, 851, Murad IV/364, 559, 656, 671, Mehmet IV/54, 433, 968–71, 973, 975, 1010, 1177–78, 1462–63, 1949, 3109–12, 4419, 5115, 5141, 5460, 5604, 5609, 5611, 8021, 8661, 10704, 11055, Süleyman II/1782, 2986, Ahmet II/1075, 1812, Mustafa II/474, 2008
Ibnülemin: Sihhiye/1, 3–9, 13, 16–18, 24, 28–29, 33, 34, 41, 43, 66, 80, 94, 98–99, 117–18, Vakıf/854, 935
Maliyeden Müdevver (MAD): 111, 471, 986, 989, 990, 1151, 1672, 1684, 1686, 1757, 1805, 1913, 2094, 2096, 2097, 2102, 2104, 2105, 2239, 2257, 2261, 2263, 3002, 3036, 3043, 3066, 4716, 5019, 5177, 5183, 5231, 5242, 5247, 5271, 5273, 5301, 5407, 5424, 5436, 5705, 5708, 5757, 5758, 5667, 5761, 5773, 5827, 5832, 5849, 5886, 5888, 5898, 5916, 5920, 5927, 5973, 6038, 6116, 6233, 6448, 6483, 6888, 7042, 7150, 7218, 9835, 15494, 15871, 15875, 18245, 20180, 22294
Cevdet: Belediye/5522, Sihhiye/89, 132, 208, 255, 551, 569, 644, 749, 1074, 1204, 1230
Topkapı Sarayı Müzesi Arşivi [Archives of Topkapi Palace, Istanbul]:
evrak 93/1–2, 2211/7, 2657/1–5, 11942/7–11, 13–16, 18, 25, 28, 30–33, 37, 41, 43–46, 48, 56, 60, 66, 67–69, 71, 73, 75, 78–82, 85, 87–90, 92, 96–98, 102–5, 112, 118, 122–25, 127–28, 131
defter 7017/1, 1781
Topkapı Sarayı Müzesi Kütüphanesi [Library of Topkapi Palace, Istanbul]: B. 408

Vakıflar Genel Müdürlüğü Arşivi [Archives of the General Directorate for Charitable Institutions, Ankara]:
defter 574, 575, 608/22, 608/23, 613, 990
dolap 1550
kasa 58

Manuscripts

"Book of Prayers." Wellcome Library for the History of Medicine, WMS. Turkish.25.

Dā'ūd al-Anṭākī. "Tadhkirat ūlā al-albāb wal-jamī' al-mu'jab al-a'jāb." Cambridge University Library, Add. 3510 (11).

Emir Çelebi, "Enmüzec-ül-tibb." British Library, OIOC. Or. 7282.

Ghazzī, Najm al-Dīn Muḥammad b. Muḥammad, al-. "Al-kawākib al-sā'ira fī a'yān al-mi'ā al-'āshira." Süleymaniye Library, H. Hüsnü Paşa 876.

Katip Çelebi. "Mizan al-hakk fi ikhtiyar al-ahakk." Cambridge University Library, Add. 442.

Ibn Kemāl Paşa, Shams al-Dīn Ahmad b. Süleyman. "Al-risāla fī al-tā'ūn wa al-wabā'." British Library, OIOC. Or. 9009.

Ibn Sallūm, Ṣāliḥ b. Naṣrallah. "Ghāyat al-bayān fī tadbīr badan al-insān." Cambridge University Library, P.27 Brown; Princeton University Library, Garret 1181H; New Series 998.

———. "Ghāyat al-itqān fī tadbīr badan al-insān." Cambridge University Library, Add. 3532.

"Kitab feraset-ül-yad." Wellcome Institute for the History of Medicine Library. Wms.Turkish.19.

Suyūṭī, Jalāl al-Dīn, al-. "Al-Manhaj al-sawī wal-manhal al-rawī f al-ṭibb al-nabawī." Wellcome Institute for the History of Medicine Library, Wms.Or.90.

Tashköprüzade, Ahmad b. Mustafa. "Al-shaqā'īq al-nu'māniyya." Süleymaniye Library, Esad Ef. 2308.

"Wonders of Art and Nature." British Library, Harl. 5500.

Zeyn al-Din al-Abidin b. Halil. "Shifa'-ı al-feva'id." Wellcome Institute for the History of Medicine Library, WMs.Turkish 15.

Printed Primary Sources

'Abd al-Ḥamīd, Muḥammad Muḥī al-Dīn. *Sharḥ Maqāmāt Badī' al-Zamān al-Hamādhānī*. Miṣr: Maktaba wa-Maṭa'at Muḥammad "Alī Ṣabīḥ, 1962/1381 A.H.

Albucasis. *Albucasis on Surgery and Instruments*. Trans. and ed. M. S. Spink and G. L. Lewis. London: Wellcome Institute of the History of Medicine, 1973.

Ali, Mustafa bin Ahmet. *Muṣṭafā 'Ālī's "Counsel for Sultans" of 1581*. Trans and ed. Andrea Tietze. 2 vols. Vienna: Verlag der Osterreichischen Akademie der Wissenschaften, 1979–82.

———. *Muṣṭafā 'Ālī's Description of Cairo of 1599*. Trans. and ed. Andreas Tietze. Vienna: Verlag der Osterreichischen Akademie der Wissenschaften, 1975.

'Asqalānī, Ibn Hajar, al-. *Fatḥ al-Bārī bi-Sharḥ al-Bukhārī*. 12 vols. Miṣr: Maktabat wa-Maṭba'at Muṣṭafā al-Bābī al-Ḥalabī, 1378H/1958.

Ata'i, Nev'izade. *Hada'iq al-Haqa'iq fi Takmilat al-Shaqa'iq*. 2 vols. İstanbul: Matbaa-i Amire, 1268H [1851].

Ayvanseray, Hafiz Hüseyn b. al-Haj Ismail. *Hadiqat-ül-Jamai'*. 2 vols. İstanbul: Matbaa-i Amire, 1281H [1865].

Barkan, Ömer Lutfi. "Edirne ve Civarındaki Bazı İmāret Tesislerinin Yıllık Muhasebe Bilānçoları." *Belgeler* 1, nos. 1–2 (1964): 235–377.

———. "Fatih Câmi ve İmareti Tesîslerini 1489–1490 Yıllarına âit Muhasebe Bilânçoları." *İstanbul Üniversitesi İktisat Fakültesi Mecmuası* 23, nos. 1–2 (1962–63): 297–341.

———. "İstanbul Saraylarına ait Muhasebe Defterleri." *Belgeler* 9, no. 13 (1979): 1–380.

Bassano, Luigi. *Costumi et i modi particolari della vita De'turchi, Roma 1545.* Monaco di Baviera: M. Huber, 1963.

Baydabā. *Kalīla wa Dimna.* Beirut: Dār al-Kutub al-'Āmiya, 1970.

Blount, Henry. *A Voyage into the Levant*. London, 1636.

Bon, Otaviano. *The Sultan's Seraglio: An Intimate Portrait of Life at the Ottoman Court*. London: Saqi Books, 1996.

Brookes, Douglas Scott. "Table of Delicacies Concerning the Rules of Social Gatherings: An Annotated Translation of Gelibolulu Mustafa Âli's *Mevâ'idü'n-Nefâ'is fi Kavâ'idi'l-Mecâlis*." PhD. diss., University of California, Berkeley, 1998.

Bryce, C. "Sketch of the State and Practice of Medicine at Constantinople." *Edinburgh Medical and Surgical Journal* 35 (1831): 1–12.

Bukhārī, Muḥammad b. Ismā'īl, al-. *Al-Jāmi' al-Ṣaḥīḥ*. 3 vols. [Cairo:] Dār wa-Maṭābi' al-Sha'b, 1378H [1958].

Busbecq, Ogier Ghislain de. *The Turkish Letters of Ogier Ghiselin de Busbecq*. Translated from the Latin of the Elzevir edition of 1633 by Edward Seymour Forster. Oxford: Clarendon Press, 1968.

Chronicle of the World Health Organization 1 (1947): 1–43.

Crone, Patricia, and Shmuel Moreh, trans. *The Book of Strangers: The Medieval Arabic Graffiti on the Theme of Nostalgia*. Princeton, NJ: M. Wiener Publishers, 2000.

Daniel, William. *A Journal or Account of William Daniel: His Late Expedition or Undertaking to go from London to Surrat in India . . .* London, 1702.

Dernschwam, Hans. *Tagebuch einer Reise nach der Konstantinopel und Kleinasien (1553–1555)*. Munich: Duncker & Humblot, 1932.

Düzdağ, M. Ertuğrul. *Şeyhülislâm Ebussu'ûd Efendi'nin Fatvalarına Göre Kanunī Devrinde Osmanlı Hayatı*. İstanbul: Şûle Yayınları, 1998. (Orig. pub. 1972.)

Evliya Çelebi. *The Intimate Life of an Ottoman Statesman: Melek Ahmed Paşa (1588–1662)*. Trans. and ed. R. Dankoff. Albany: State University of New York Press, 1991.

———. *Narrative of Travels in Europe, Asia, and Africa in the Seventeenth Century.* Trans. Ritter Joseph von Hammer. New York: Johnson Reprint Corp., 1968. (Photocopy of the London, 1834 ed.)

———. *Seyahatname.* 10 vols. İstanbul: Matbaa-i 'Amire, 1314 [1894–1938].

———. *The "Seyahatname" of Evliya Çelebi: Facsimile of Topkapı Sarayı Bağdat 304.* Cambridge, MA: Harvard University Press, 1993.

———. *Turkish Instruments of Music in the Seventeenth Century as Describes in the "Siyāḥat nāma" of Ewliyā Chelebi.* Trans. and ed. Henry George Farmer. Portland, ME: Longwood Press, 1976. (Orig. pub. 1937.)

Fatih Mehmet II Vakfiyeleri. Ankara: n.p., 1938.

Fisher, C. G., and A. Fisher. "Topkapi Sarayi in the Mid-Seventeenth Century: Bobovi's Description." *Archivum Ottomanicum* 10 (1985 [1987]): 5–81.

Ghazzī, Najm al-Dīn Muḥammad b. Muḥammad, al-. *Luṭf al-Samr wa-Qaṭf al-Thamr.* Dimashq: Wizārat al-Thaqāfa wal-Irshād al-Qawmī, 1981.

Gökbilgin, M. Tayyib. *XV-XVI Asırlarda Edirne ve Paşa Livāsi.* İstanbul: Üçler Basımevi, 1952.

Hill, Aaron. *A Full and Just Account of the Present State of the Ottoman Empire* . . . London, 1709.

Ibn Iyās, *Badā'i' al-Zuhūr fī Waqā'i' al-Duhūr.* Ed. Muḥammad Muṣṭafā. Al-Qāhira: Al-Hay'a al-Miṣriyya al-'Āmma lil-kitāb, 1403H/1982.

Ibn Māja, Abū 'Abdallah Muḥammad b. Yazīd. *Ṣaḥīḥ Sunan Ibn Māja.* 2 vols. Riyadh: Maktab al-Tarbiya al-'Arabī li-Duwal al-Khalīj, 1408H/1988.

Ibn Ridwan, Ali ibn Ali ibn Ja'far. *Medieval Islamic Medicine: Ibn Ridwan's Treatise "On the Prevention of Bodily Ills in Egypt."* Trans. Michael W. Dols; Arabic text edited by Adil S. Gamal. Berkeley and Los Angeles: University of California Press, 1984.

Kâhya, Esin. *Şemseddîn-I İtâkî'nin Resimli Anatomi Kitabı.* Ankara: Atatürk Kültür Merkezi Yayını, 1996.

Katip Çelebi [Hajji Khalifa]. *The Balance of the Truth.* Trans. G. L. Lewis. London: G. Allen and Unwin, 1957.

———. *Kashf al-Ẓunūn an Asāmī al-Kutūb wal-Funūn.* 2 vols. İstanbul: Wakālat al-Ma'arif, 1360–62 AH/1941–43.

Keppel, George. *Narrative of a Journey across the Balcan.* London, 1831.

Kürkçüoğlu, Kemāl Edīb, ed. *Süleymaniye Vakfiyesi.* Ankara: Kesimli Posta Matbaası, 1962.

Leo Africanus. *The History and Description of Africa and the Notable Things Therein Contained.* 3 vols. New York: B. Franklin, 1960. (Orig. pub. 1896.)

Lithgow, William. *The Total Discourse of the Rare Adventures and Painful Peregrinations of Long Nineteen Yeares Traveyles from Scotland to the Most Famous Kingdoms in Europe, Asia and Africa.* London, 1632.

Lokman Çelebi, Seyyid. *Kiyâfetü'l-İnsâniyye fî Şemâili'l-'Osmâniyye.* İstanbul: Historical Research Foundation, Istanbul Research Center, 1987.

Malki, Refa'el Mordekhai. *Ma'amarim bi-Refu'a le-Rabi Refa'el Mordekhai Malki.* Ed. Meir Benayahu. Jerusalem: Yad ha-Rav Nissim, 1986. (In Hebrew)

Maqrizī, Aḥmad b. 'Alī, al-. *Al-Mawā'iẓ wal-I'tibār fī Dhikr al-Khiṭaṭ wal-Athar.* 2 vols. Beirut: Dār Ṣādir, 196.

Meri, Josef W., trans. *A Lonely Wayfarer's Guide to Pilgrimage: 'Alī ibn Abī Bakr al-Harawī's "Kitāb al-Ishārāt ilā Ma'rifat al-Ziyārāt."* Princeton, NJ: Darwin Press, 2004.

Montagu, Mary Wortley. *The Complete Letters of Lady Mary Wortley Montagu.* Ed. R. Halsbad. 3 vols. Oxford: Clarendon Press, 1965–67.

Muḥibbī, Muḥammad Amīn b. Faḍlallah, al-. *Tarīkh Khulaṣat al-Athr fī A'yān al-Qarn al-Ḥādī Ashar.* 4 vols. Beirut: Maktabat Khayyāṭ, n.d.

Na'ima, Mustafa. *Tarih-i Naima: Rawdat al-Husayn fi Khulasat Akhbar al-Khafiqin.* 6 vols. İstanbul: Matbaa-i Amire, 1281H.

Nicolay, Nicolas, de. *The Navigations, Peregrinations, and Voyages, Made into Turkie by Nicolas de Nicolay. . . .* Trans. T. Washington. London, 1593 [1585].

Öztürk, Said. *Askeri Kassama ait Onyedinci Asır İstanbul Tereke Defterleri (Sosyo-Ekonomik Tahlil).* İstanbul: OSAV, 1995.

Peçevi, İbrahim. *Tarih-i Peçevi.* 2 vols. İstanbul: Matbaa-i Amire, 1283 [1867].

Rashed, Muhammad b. Mustafa. *Tarih-i Rashed.* 6 vols. İstanbul: Matbaa-i Amire, 1282H.

Ray, John, ed. *A Collection of Curious Travels . . .* London, 1693.

Refik, Ahmet Altınay. *İstanbul Hayatı.* 4 vols. İstanbul: Enderun Kitabevi, 1988. (Orig. pub. 1917–1932.)

Robson, James, trans. *Tracts on Listening to Music.* In *Theology, Ethics and Metaphysics: Royal Asiatic Society Classics of Islam,* ed. Hiroyuki Mashita. London: RoutledgeCurzon, 2003. (Orig. pub. London, 1938.)

Rycaut, Paul. *The History of the Turkish Empire from the Year 1623 to the Year 1677 . . .* London, 1680.

———. *The Present State of the Ottoman Empire . . .* London, 1668.

Sabuncuoğlu, Şerefeddin. *Cerrahiyyetü'l-H̱āniyye.* Trans. and ed. İlter Uzel. 2 vols. Ankara: Türk Tarih Kurumu, 1992.

Sandys, George. *A Relation of a Journey Begun an. Dom. 1610 Containing a Description of the Turkish Empire . . .* 6th ed.; London, 1670.

Schweigger, Salomon. *Ein Newe Reyssbeschreibung auss Teutschland nach Constantinopel und Jerusalem.* Graz: Akademische Druck-u. Verlagsanstalt, 1964.

Süreyya, Mehmet. *Sijill-i Osmānī.* 4 vols. İstanbul: Matbaa-i Amire, 1308 [1890].

Tavernier, Jean Baptiste. *A New Relation of the Inner-Part of the Grand Seignior's Seraglio.* London, 1677.

Thevenot, Jean. *The Travells of Monsieur de Thevenot into the Levant . . .* London, 1687.

Thomas, Tho. *An Account of the City of Prusa in Bythinia, and a Continuation of the Historical Observation Relating to Constantinople . . .* In *A Collection of Curious Travels and Voyages,* ed. John Ray. London, 1693.

Secondary Literature

Abdel Haleem, M. A. S. "Medical Ethics in Islam." In *Choices and Decisions in Health Care,* ed. Andrew Grubb, 1–20. Chichester: J. Wiley, 1993.

Aberth, John, ed. *The Black Death: The Great Mortality of 1348–1350: A Brief History with Documents.* Boston: Bedford/St. Martin's, 2005.

Abou-Lughod, Janet. "The Islamic City—Historic Myth, Islamic Essence, and Contemporary Relevance." *International Journal of Middle East Studies* 19 (1987): 155–76.

Adamson, Peter. *The Arabic Plotinus: A Philosophical Study of the Theology of Aristotle*. London: Duckworth, 2002.

Adıvar, Adnan Abdülhāk. *Osmanlı Türklerinde İlim*. 5. printing; İstanbul: Remzi Kitabevi, 1991.

Ahmad, A. D. Ibrāhīm Khalīl. "Al-Amrāḍ wa-al-Awbī'a wa-In'ikasātuhā 'alā Mujtama' al-Mawṣil ibbānā al-'Ahd al-'Uthmānī." *Arab Historical Review for Ottoman Studies/Al-Majalla al-Ta'rīkhiyya al-'Arabiyya lil-Dirāsāt al-'Uthmāniyya* 17–18 (1998): 19–26.

Agmon, Iris. *Family and Court: Legal Culture and Modernity in Late Ottoman Palestine*. Syracuse, NY: Syracuse University Press, 2005.

Ahsan, Muhammad Manazir. *Social Life under the Abbasids, 170–289 AH, 786–902 AD*. London: Longman, 1979.

Alshech, Eli. " 'Do Not Enter Houses Other than Your Own": The Evolution of the Notion of a Private Domestic Sphere in Early Sunnī Islamic Thought." *Islamic Law and Society* 11 (2004): 292–332.

Altıntaş, Ayten. "Fatih Darüşşifası Tıp Eğitim Yapılıyor Muydu?" *Tarih ve Toplum* 27, no. 161 (May 1997): 291–95.

Álvarez-Millán, Cristina. "Graeco-Roman Case Histories and Their Influence on Medieval Islamic Clinical Accounts." *Social History of Medicine* 12 (1999): 19–43.

———. "Practice versus Theory: Tenth-Century Case Histories from Islamic Middle East." *Social History of Medicine* 13 (2000): 293–306.

Ambraseys, N. N., and C. F. Finkel. *The Seismicity of Turkey and Adjacent Areas: A Historical Review, 1500–1800*. Istanbul: Eren, 1995.

And, Metin. *Istanbul in the 16th Century: The City, the Palace, Daily Life*. Istanbul: Akbank, 1994.

Arberry, Arthur J. *The Koran Interpreted*. London: G. Allen & Unwin, 1955.

Arjomand, Said Amir. "Philanthropy, the Law, and Public Policy in the Islamic World before the Modern Era." In *Philanthropy in the World's Traditions*, ed. Warren F. Ilchman, Stanley N. Katz, and Edward L. Queen II, 109–32. Bloomington: Indiana University Press, 1998.

Arslan, Hüseyin. *16yy. Osmanlı Toplumunda Yönetim, Nüfus, İskân, Göç ve Sürgün*. İstanbul: Kaknüs Yayınları, 2001.

Artan, Tülay. "Aspects of the Ottoman Elites' Food Consumption: Looking for 'Staples,' 'Luxuries' and 'Delicacies' in a Changing Century." In *Consumption Studies and the History of the Ottoman Empire, 1550–1922*, ed. Donald Quatert, 107–200. Albany: State University New York Press, 2000.

'Asalī, Kāmil Jamīl, al-. *Muqaddama fī Ta'rīkh al-Ṭibb fī al-Quds*. Amman: Al-Jāmi'a al-Urduniyya, 1994.

Ashtor, E. "The Diet of Salaried Classes in the Medieval Near East." *Journal of Asian History* 4 (1970): 1–24.

Atıl, Esin. *The Age of Sultan Süleyman the Magnificent*. Washington, DC: National Gallery of Art, 1987.

Aybash, Aḥmad, al-, and D. Qutayba al-Shihābī, eds. *Dimashq al-Shām fī Nuṣūṣ al-Raḥāllīn wal-Jughrāfiyyin wal-Buldāniyyin al-'Arab wal-Muslimīn min al-Qarn al-Thālith ilā al-Qarn al-Thālith 'Ashr lil-Hijra*. Vol. 2. Dimashq: Wizārat al-Thaqāfa, 1998.

Babinger, Franz. *Die Geschichtsschreiber des Osmanen und ihre Werke*. Leipzig: Otto Harrassowitz, 1927.

Baer, Gabriel. "Patrons and Clients in Ottoman Cairo." In *Mèmorial Ömer Lütfi Barkan*, 11–18. Paris: Adrien Maisonneuve, 1980.

Baldry, John. "The Ottoman Quarantine Station on Karaman Island, 1881–1914." *Studies in History of Medicine* 2 (1978): 3–138.

Barkai, Ron. "Between East and West: Jewish Doctor from Spain." In *Intercultural Contacts in the Medieval Mediterranean,* ed. Benjamin Arbel, 49–63. London: F. Cass, 1996.

Barnett, Charles. " 'Spiritual Medicine': Music and Healing in Islam and Its Influence in Western Medicine." In *Musical Healing in Cultural Contexts,* ed. Penelope Gouk, 85–91. Aldershot, UK: Ashgate, 2000.

Baykal, Ismail. "Yeni Sarayda 'Enderun Hastahanesi.' " *Türk Tıb Tarihi Arkivi* 17 (1940): 33–41.

Bayram, Sadi. "Sağlık Hizmetlerimiz ve Vakif Guraba Hastanesi." *Vakıflar Dergisi* 14 (1982): 101–18.

Beg, M. A. J. "Ghassāl." *Encyclopaedia of Islam,* 2nd ed., suppl.

Behrens-Abouseif, Doris. *Fath Allāh and Abū Zakariyya: Physicians under the Mamluks*. Cairo: Institut Francais d'Archeologie Orientale, 1987.

———. "Gardens in Islamic Egypt." *Der Islam* 69 (1992): 302–12.

———. "The Image of the Physician: Arab Biographies of the Post-Classical Age." *Der Islam* 66 (1989): 331–43.

Biesterfeldt, H. H. "Some Opinions on the Physician's Remuneration in Medieval Islam." *Bulletin of the History of Medicine* 58 (1984): 16–27.

Birnbaum, Eleazar. "The Questing Mind: Kātib Chelebi, 1609–1657." In *Corolla Torontonesis: Studies in Honour of Ronald Morton Smith,* ed. Emmet Robins and Stella Sandahl, 133–58. Toronto: TSAR, 1994.

———. "Vice Triumphant: The Spread of Coffee and Tobacco in Turkey." *Durham University Journal* 49, n.s. 18 (1956–57): 21–27.

Black, Deborah L. "Psychology: Soul and Intellect." In *The Cambridge Companion to Arabic Philosophy,* ed. Peter Adamson and Richard C. Taylor, 308–26. Cambridge: Cambridge University Press, 2005.

Bodrogligeti, A. J. E. "Ḳutadghu Bilig," *Encyclopeaedia of Islam,* 2nd ed.

Bonner, Michael, Mine Ener, and Amy Singer, eds. *Poverty and Charity in Middle Eastern Contexts.* Albany: State University New York Press, 2003.

Bos, Gerrit. "Ibn al-Jazzār on Medicine for the Poor and Destitute," *Journal of the American Oriental Society* 118 (1998): 365–75.

Braudel, Fernand. *Civilization and Capitalism 15th–18th Century.* Vol. 1: *The Structures of Everyday Life: The Limits of the Possible.* New York: Harper & Row, 1985.

Brodman, James William. *Charity and Welfare: Hospitals and the Poor in Medieval Catalonia.* Philadelphia: University of Pennsylvania Press, 1998.

Brody, Howard. "The Doctor as Therapeutic Agent: A Placebo Effect Research Agenda." In *The Placebo Effect*, ed. Anne Harrington, 77–92. Cambridge, MA: Harvard University Press, 1997.

Browne, Edward G. *A Hand-list of the Muhammadan Manuscripts including all those Written in the Arabic Character Preserved in the Library of the University of Cambridge*. Cambridge: Cambridge University Press, 1900.

———. *A Supplementary Hand-List of the Muhammadan Manuscripts including all those Written in the Arabic Character, Preserved in the Libraries of the University and Colleges of Cambridge*. Cambridge: Cambridge University Press, 1922.

Burelli, Augusto Romano. "Visions and Representation of Urban Space." *Enviromental Design* 5, nos. 5–6 (1987): 42–51.

Bürgel, Johann Cristoph. *The Feather of Simurgh: The "Licit Magic" of the Arts in Medieval Islam*. New York: New York University Press, 1988.

———. Psychosomatic Methods of Cures in the Islamic Middle Ages." *Humaniora Islamica* 1 (1973): 157–72.

———. "Secular and Religious Features of Medieval Medicine." In *Asian Medical Systems: A Comparative Survey*, ed. Charles Leslie, 44–62. Berkeley and Los Angeles: University of California Press, 1976.

Bynum, W. F., and Roy Porter, eds. *Medicine and the Five Senses*. Cambridge: Cambridge University Press, 1993.

Cameron, Euan, ed. *Early Modern Europe*. Oxford: Oxford University Press, 2001.

Cantay [Güreşsever], Gönül. *Anadolu Selçuklu ve Osmanlı Darüşşifaları*. Ankara: Atatürk Kültür Merkezi Yayını, 1992.

———. "Kitab al-Cerrahiyet al-Hāniye (İstanbul Tıp Tarihi Enstitüsü Nüshası) Minyatürler." In *I. Milletarası Türkoloji Kongresi. Tebliğler*, 3:771–85. 3 vols. İstanbul: n.p., 1979.

Carlino, Andrea. " 'Know Thyself': Anatomical Figures in Early Modern Europe," *Res* 27 (1995): 52–69.

Cerasi, Maurice. "The Deeper Structures of Ottoman Urban Housing Fabric: Conservation of Space and Forms through Basic Parameters." In *The Ottoman House: Papers from the Amasya Symposium, 24–27 September 1996*, ed. Stanley Ireland and William Bechhoefer, 9–15. London: British Institute of Archaeology at Ankara, 1998.

———. "The Formation of Ottoman House Types: A Comparative Study in Interaction with Neighboring Cultures." *Muqarnas* 15 (1998): 116–56.

———. "The Many Masters and Artisans of the Ottoman Town's Form and Culture: Chaos out of Order, Syncretism out of Separation—the Eighteenth and Nineteenth Centuries." Paper delivered at *Order in Anarchy: The Management of Urban Space and Society in the Islamic World*, the third annual international workshop of the Program for Middle East History at Ben-Gurion University of the Negev, Israel, April 1997.

———. "Open Space, Water and Trees in Ottoman Urban Culture in the XVIIIth–XIXth Centuries." *A.A.R.P. Environmental Design* 2 (1985): 36–49.

Cevdet, Mehmet. "Sivas Darüşşifası Vakfiyesi ve Tercümesi." *Vakıflar Dergisi* 1 (1938): 35–38.

Chabrier, Jean-Claude. "Musical Science." In *Encyclopedia of the History of Arabic Science,* ed. Roshdi Rashed, 2:581–613. 3 vols. London: Routledge, 1996.

Chaumont, E. "Tabann^{in}." *Encyclopeaedia of Islam,* 2nd ed., suppl.

Chaumont, E., and R. Shaham, "Yatīm." *Encyclopeaedia of Islam,* 2nd ed.

Chishti, Saadia Khawar. "*Fitra*: An Islamic Model for Human and the Environment." In *Islam and Ecology: A Bestowed Trust,* ed. Richard C. Foltz, Frederick M. Denny, and Azizan Baharuddin, 67–82. Cambridge, MA: Center for the Study of World Religions, Harvard Divinity School; distributed by Harvard University Press, 2003.

Cipolla, C. M. *Public Health and the Medical Profession in the Renaissance.* Cambridge: Cambridge University Press, 1976.

Clark, Emma. *The Art of the Islamic Garden.* Ramsbury, UK: Crowood Press, 2004.

Clinton, Jerome W. "Madness and Cure in the 1001 Nights." *Studia Islamica* 61 (1985): 107–25.

Cohen, Amnon. "Coffee and Coffeehouses in Jerusalem." In *Studies in the History of Muslim Peoples: Papers Presented at a Conference in Memory of David Ayalon, 9 June 1999,* 103–12 Jerusalem: Israel Academy of Sciences and Humanities, 2006. (In Hebrew)

———. *Economic Life in Ottoman Jerusalem.* Cambridge: Cambridge University Press, 1989.

———, Elisheva Simon-Pikali, and Ovadia Salama. *Jews in the Moslem Religious Court: Society, Economy and Commercial Organization in the XVIIIth Century; Documents from Ottoman Jerusalem.* Jerusalem: Yad Ben-Zvi, 1996. (In Hebrew)

———, Elisheva Ben-Shimon, and Eyal Ginio. *Jews in the Moslem Religious Court: Society, Economy and Commercial Organization in the XIXth Century; Documents from Ottoman Jerusalem.* Jerusalem: Yad Ben-Zvi, 2003. (In Hebrew)

———. *A World Within: Jewish Life as Reflected in Muslim Court Documents from the "Sijill" of Jerusalem (XVIth Century).* Philadelphia: Center for Judaic Studies, University of Pennsylvania, 1984.

Cohen, Amnon, and Elisheva Simon-Pikali. *Jews in the Moslem Religious Court: Society, Economy and Communal Organization in the XVI Century; Documents from Ottoman Jerusalem.* Jerusalem: Yad Ben-Zvi, 1993. (In Hebrew)

Cohen, Mark R. "The Foreign Jewish Poor in Medieval Egypt." In *Poverty and Charity in Middle Eastern Contexts,* ed. Michael Bonner, Mine Ener, and Amy Singer, 53–72. Albany: State University New York Press, 2003.

———. *Poverty and Charity in the Jewish Community of Medieval Egypt.* Princeton, NJ: Princeton University Press, 2005.

Conrad, Lawrence I. "Arabic Plague Chronologies and Treatises: Social and Historical Factors in the Formation of a Literary Genre." *Studia Islamica* 54 (1981): 51–93.

———. "The Arab-Islamic Medical Tradition." In *The Western Medical Tradition, 800 BC to AD 1800*, ed. Lawrence I. Conrad et al., 93–138. Cambridge: Cambridge University Press, 1995.

———. "Epidemic Diseases in Formal and Popular Thought in Early Islamic Society." In *Epidemics and Ideas: Essays on the Historical Perception of Pestilence*, ed. Terence Ranger and Paul Slack, 77–99. Cambridge: Cambridge University Press, 1992.

———. "Medicine—Traditional Practice." In *The Oxford Encyclopedia of the Modern Islamic World*, 3:85–88. 4 vols. New York: Oxford University Press, 1995.

———. "Medicine and Martyrdom: Some Discussions of Suffering and Divine Justice in Early Islamic Society." In *Religion, Health and Suffering*, ed. John R. Hinnells and Roy Porter, 212–36. London: Routledge, 1999.

———. "A Ninth-Century Muslim Scholar's Discussion of Contagion." In *Contagion: Perspectives from Pre-Modern Societies*, ed. Lawrence I. Conrad and Dominik Wujastyk, 163–77. Aldershot, UK: Ashgate, 2000.

———. "Scholarship and Social Context in the Near East." In *Knowledge and the Scholarly Medical Traditions*, ed. Don Bates, 81–101. Cambridge: Cambridge University Press, 1995.

———. "Tāʿūn and Wabāʾ: Conceptions of Plague and Pestilence in Early Islam." *Journal of the Economic and Social History of the Orient* 25 (1982): 268–307.

Crosby, Alfred W. "The Past and Present of Environmental History." *American Historical Review* 100 (1995): 1177–89.

Cunningham, Andrew. *The Anatomical Renaissance: The Resurrection of Anatomical Projects of the Ancients*. Aldershot, UK: Scolar Press, 1997.

Dankoff, Robert. *An Ottoman Mentality: The World of Evliya Çelebi*. Leiden: Brill, 2004.

Delcambre, A.-M. "Laḳīṭ," *Encyclopaedia of Islam*, 2nd ed..

Demirhan, Ayşegül. "The Evolution of Opium in the Islamic World and Anatolian Turks." *Studies in History of Medicine* 4 (1980): 73–97.

———. *Mısır Çarşısı Drogları*. İstanbul: Sermet Matbaası, 1975.

Dengler, Ian C. "Turkish Women in the Ottoman Empire: The Classical Age." In *Women in the Muslim World*, ed. Lois Beck and Nikki Keddie, 229–44. Cambridge, MA: Harvard University Press, 1978.

Deursaeh, Nurdeen. "Is Imbibing al-Khamr (Intoxicating Drink) for Medical Purposes Permissible by Islamic Law?" *Arab Law Quarterly* 18 (2003): 355–64.

Dickie, James (Yaqub Zaki). "Garden and Cemetery in Sinan's Istanbul." *Environmental Design* 5, nos. 5–6 (1987): 70–85.

Dikötter, Frank, Lars Laamann, and Zhou Xun. *Narcotic Culture: A History of Drugs in China*. Chicago: University of Chicago Press, 2004.

Dols, Michael W. *The Black Death in the Middle East*. Princeton, NJ: Princeton University Press, 1977.

———. "Insanity and Its Treatment in Islamic Society." *Medical History* 31 (1987): 1–14.

———. "Insanity in Byzantine and Islamic Medicine." *Symposium on Byzantine Medicine, Dumbarton Oaks Papers* 38 (1984): 136–48.

———. "Islam and Medicine." *History of Science* 26 (1988): 417–25.

———. "The Leper in Medieval Islamic Society." *Speculum* 58 (1983): 891–916.

———. "Leprosy in Medieval Arabic Medicine." *Journal of the History of Medicine and Allied Sciences* 34 (1979): 314–33.

———. *Majnūn: The Madman in Medieval Islamic Society*. Oxford: Clarendon Press, 1992.

———. "The Origins of the Islamic Hospital: Myth and Reality." *Bulletin of the History of Medicine* 61 (1987): 367–90.

———. "Plague in Early Islamic History." *Journal of the American Oriental Society* 94 (1974): 376–83.

———. "The Second Plague Pandemic and Its Recurrences in the Middle East: 1347–1894." *Journal of the Economic and Social History of the Orient* 22 (1979): 162–89.

Druart, Thérèse-Anne. "The Human Soul's Individuation and Its Survival after the Body's Death: Avicenna of the Causal Relation between Body and Soul." *Arabic Sciences and Philosophy* 10 (2000): 259–73.

Elgood, Cyril. *A Medical History of Persia and the Eastern Caliphate*. London: Cambridge University Press, 1951.

———. *Medicine in Persia*. New York: Hoeber, 1934.

———. *Safavid Medical Practice or the Practice of Medicine, Surgery and Gynaecology in Persia between 1500 A.D. and 1750 A.D.* London: Luzac, 1970.

Elling, Roy H. "The Hospital-Support Game in Urban Centers." In *The Hospital in Modern Society*, ed. Eliot Freidson, 73–111. New York: Free Press of Glencoe, 1963.

Ellis, Harold. *A History of Surgery*. London: Greenwich Medical Media, 2001.

Enderwitz, Susanne. "Homesickness and Love in Arabic Poetry." In *Myths, Historical Archetypes, and Symbolic Figures in Arabic Literature: Towards a New Hermeneutic Approach*, ed. A. Neuwirth, B. Embaló, S. Günther, and M. Jarrar, 59–70. Beirut: In Kommission bei Franz Steiner Verlag, 1999.

Ergun, Nılgün, and Özge İskender. "Gardens of the Topkapi Palace: An Example of Turkish Garden Art." *Studies in the History of Gardens and Designed Landscape* 23 (2003): 57–71.

Estes, J. Worth, and Laverne Kuhnke. "French Observations of Disease and Drug Use in Late Eighteenth-Century Cairo." *Journal of the History of Medicine and Allied Sciences* 39 (1984): 121–52.

Ettinghausen, Richard. Introduction to *The Islamic Garden*, ed. Elisabeth B. MacDougall and Richard Ettinghausen, 3–10. Washington, DC: Dumbarton Oaks, Trustees for Harvard University, 1976.

Eyuboğlu, İsmet Zeki. *Anadolu Halk İlaçları*. İstanbul: Hür Yayın ve Ticaret A.Ş., 1977.

Fahd, T. "Firāsa." *Encyclopaedia of Islam*, 2nd ed.

———. "Ḳiyāfa." *Encyclopaedia of Islam*, 2nd ed.

Fahmy, Khaled. "The Anatomy of Justice: Forensic Medicine and Criminal Law in Nineteenth-Century Egypt." *Islamic Law and Society* 6 (1999): 224–71.

———. "Law, Medicine and Society in Nineteenth-Century Egypt." *Egypte/Monde Arabe* 24 (1998): 17–51.

———. "Medicine and Power: Towards a Social History of Medicine in Nineteenth-Century Egypt." *New Frontiers in the Social History of the Middle East/Cairo Papers in Social Science* 23 (2000): 15–62.

———. "Women, Medicine, and Power in Nineteenth-Century Egypt." In *Remaking Women: Feminism and Modernity in the Middle East,* ed. Lila Abu-Lughod, 35–72. Princeton, NJ: Princeton University Press, 1998.

Farmer, Henry George. *A History of Arabian Music to the XIIIth Century*. London: Luzac, 1929.

Faroqhi, Suraiya. *Pilgrimage & Sultans: The Hajj under the Ottomans*. London: I. B. Tauris, 1994.

———. *Towns and Townsmen of Ottoman Anatolia: Trade, Crafts and Food Production in an Urban Setting, 1520–1650*. Cambridge: Cambridge University Press, 1984.

Feldman, Walter. *Music of the Ottoman Court: Makam, Composition and the Early Ottoman Instrumental Repertoire*. Berlin: VWB-Verlag fur Wissenschaft und Bildung, 1996.

Figueroa, Robert, and Sandra Harding, eds. *Science and Other Cultures: Issues in Philosophies of Science and Technology*. New York: Routledge, 2003.

Fleischer, Cornell H. *Bureaucrat and Intellectual in the Ottoman Empire: The Historian Mustafa Âli (1541–1600)*. Princeton, NJ: Princeton University Press, 1986.

Foltz, Richard C. *Animals in Islamic Tradition and Muslim Cultures*. Oxford: Oneworld, 2006.

Foster, George M., and Barbara G. Anderson. *Medical Anthropology*. New York: J. Wiley, 1978.

Foucault, Michel. *The Archaeology of Knowledge*. Trans. A. M. Sheridan Smith. New York: Pantheon Books, 1972.

———. *The Birth of the Clinic: An Archaeology of Medical Perception*. Trans. A. M. Sheridan. London: Tavistock Publications, 1976.

———. *Discipline and Punish: The Birth of the Prison*. Trans. A. M. Sheridan. New York: Pantheon Books, 1977.

———. *Madness and Civilization: A History of Insanity in the Age of Reason*. Trans. Richard Howard. London: Tavistock Publications, 1967.

Gallagher, Nancy. "Contagion and Quarantine in Tunis and Cairo, 1800–1870." *Maghreb Review* 7 (1982): 108–11.

———. *Egypt's Other Wars: Epidemics and the Politics of Public Health*. Syracuse, NY: Syracuse University Press, 1990.

———. *Medicine and Power in Tunisia, 1780–1900*. Cambridge: Cambridge University Press, 1983.

García Sánchez, Expiración. "Dietic Aspects of Food in al-Andalus." In *Patterns of Everyday Life,* ed. David Waines, 275–88. Aldershot, UK: Ashgate, 2002.

Geoffrey, E. "Al-Suyūṭī Abū al-Faḍl 'Abd al-Raḥmān b. Abū Bakr b. Muḥammad Djalāl al-Dīn," *Encyclopeaedia of Islam*, 2nd ed.

Georgeon, François. "Ottomans and Drinkers: The Consumption of Alcohol in the Nineteenth Century." In *Outside In: On the Margins of the Modern Middle East*, ed. Eugene Rogan, 7–30. London: I. B. Tauris, 2001.

Ghaly, Mohammad M. I. "Writings on Disability in Islam: The 16th-century Polemic on Ibn Fahd's al-Nukat al-Ziraf." *Arab Studies Journal* 14 (2006): 9–38.

Goitein, S. D. *A Mediterranean Society: The Jewish Communities of the Arab World as Portrayed in the Documents of the Cairo Geniza*. 5 vols. Berkeley and Los Angeles: University of California Press, 1967–88.

Gökyay, Orhan Şaık. "Kātib Çelebi." *Encyclopaedia of Islam*, 2nd ed.

Good, Byron J. and Mary-Jo Del Vecchio Good. "The Semantics of Medical Discourse." In *Sciences and Cultures: Anthropological and Historical Studies of the Sciences*, ed. Everett Mendelsohn and Yehuda Elkana, 177–212. Dordrecht: D. Reidel, 1981.

Goodwin, Godfrey. *A History of Ottoman Architecture*. London: Thames and Hudson, 1971.

———. "Sinan and City Planning." *Environmental Design* 5, nos. 5–6 (1987): 10–19.

Goodwin, Jason. *Lords of the Horizons*. London: Vintage, 1998.

Goody, Jack. *Cooking, Cuisine and Class*. Cambridge: Cambridge University Press, 1982.

Goubert, J. P. "Twenty Years On: Problems of Historical Methodology in the History of Health." In *Problems and Methods in the History of Medicine*, ed. Roy Porter and Andrew Wear, 40–56. London: Croom Helm, 1987.

Gouk, Penelope, ed. *Musical Healing in Cultural Contexts*. Aldershot, UK: Ashgate, 2000.

Grehan, James. "Smoking and 'Early Modern' Sociability: The Great Tobacco Debate in the Ottoman Middle East (Seventeenth to Eighteenth Centuries)." *American Historical Review* 111 (2006): 1352–77.

Green, Monica H. "Women's Medical Practice and Health Care in Medieval Europe." In *Sisters and Workers in the Middle Ages*, ed. J. M. Bennet, E. A. Clark, J. F. O'Barr, and B. A. Villen, 39–78. Chicago: Chicago University Press, 1989.

Grell, Ole Peter. "The Protestant Imperative of Christian Care and Neighbourly Love." In *Health Care and Poor Relief in Protestant Europe 1500–1700*, ed. Ole Peter Grell and Andrew Cunningham, 43–65. London: Routledge, 1997.

Grell, Ole Peter, and Andrew Cunningham. "The Reformation and Changes in Welfare Provision in Early Modern Northern Europe." In *Health Care and Poor Relief in Protestant Europe 1500–1700*, ed. Ole Peter Grell and Andrew Cunningham, 1–42. London: Routledge, 1997.

———. "The Counter-Reformation and Welfare Provision in Southern Europe." In *Health Care and Poor Relief in Counter-Reformation Europe*, ed. Ole Peter Grell and Andrew Cunningham, 1–17. London: Routledge, 1999.

———. "Health Care and Poor Relief in 18th and 19th Century Northern Europe." In *Health Care and Poor Relief in 18th and 19th Century Northern Europe,* ed. Ole Peter Grell, Andrew Cunningham, and Robert Jütte, 3–14. Aldershot, UK: Ashgate, 2002.

Grunebaum, Gustave E. von. "The Response to Nature in Arabic Poetry." *Journal of Near Eastern Studies* 4 (1945): 137–51.

Guo, Li. "Paradise Lost: Ibn Dāniyāl's Response to Baybars' Campaign against Vice in Cairo." *Journal of the American Oriental Society* 121 (2001): 219–35.

Gutas, Dimitri. "Philopnus and Avicenna on the Separability of the Intellect: A Case of Orthodox Christian-Muslim Agreement." *Greek Orthodox Theological Review* 31 (1986): 121–29.

Güvenç, Rahmi Oruç. "The Tradition of Turkish Music Therapy." In *Culture and Arts,* ed. Kemal Çiçek, 651–56. Vol. 4 of *The Great Ottoman-Turkish Civilization.* Ankara: Yeni Türkiye, 2000.

Hagen, Gottfried. *Ein Osmanischer Geograph bei der Arbeit Entstehung und Gedankenwelt von Kātib Čelebis Ǧihānnümā.* Berlin: Klaus Schwartz Verlag, 2003.

———. "Some Considerations on the Study of Ottoman Geographical Writing." *Archivum Ottomanicum* 18 (2000): 183–93.

Halıcı, Nevin. "Anadolu Mutfağinida Haşhaş." In *İkinci Milletarası Yemek Kongresi (3–10 Eylül 1988),* ed. Feyzi Halıcı, 170–80. Konya: Konya Kültür ve Turizm Vakfı Yayınları, 1989.

———. "Ottoman Cuisine." In *Culture and Arts,* ed. Kemal Çiçek, 93–103. Vol. 4 of *The Great Ottoman-Turkish Civilization.* Ankara: Yeni Türkiye, 2000.

Hamadeh, Shirine. "Splash and Spectacle: The Obsession with Fountains in Eighteenth-Century Istanbul." *Muqarnas* 19 (2002): 123–48.

Hamarneh, Sami K. *Catalogue of Arabic Manuscripts on Medicine and Pharmacy at the British Library.* Cairo: n.p., 1975.

———. "Development of Hospitals in Islam." *Journal of the History of Medicine and Allied Sciences* 17 (1962): 366–84.

———. *Drawings and Pharmacy in al-Zahrawi's 10th Century Surgical Treatise.* Washington, DC: Smithsonian Institution, 1961.

———. "Pharmacy in Medieval Islam and the History of Drug Addiction." *Medical History* 16 (1972): 226–37.

Hamarneh, Sami K., and Henri Amin Awad. "Glass Vessel Stamp Data for Materia Medica." In *Fustat Finds: Beads, Coins, Medical Instruments, Textiles, and Other Artifacts from the Awad Collection,* ed. Jere L. Bacharach, 167–75. Cairo: American University in Cairo Press, 2002.

Hamdy, Sherine F. "Blinding Ignorance: Medical Science Diseased Eyes, and Religious Practice in Egypt." *Arab Studies Journal* 13 (2005): 26–45.

Haq, S. Nomanul. "Islam." In *A Companion to Environmental Philosophy,* ed. Dale Jamieson, 111–29. Oxford: Blackwell, 2001.

———. "Islam and Ecology: Toward Retrieval and Reconstruction." *Daedalus* 130, no. 4 (Fall 2001): 141–78.

Harding, Sandra. *Is Science Multi-Cultural? Postcolonialisms, Feminisms, and Epistemologies*. Bloomington: Indiana University Press, 1998.
Hardwig, John. "What About the Family." *Hastings Center Report* 20, no. 2 (March/April 1990): 5–10.
Hattox, Ralph S. *Coffee and Coffeehouses: The Origins of a Social Beverage in the Medieval Near East*. Seattle: University of Washington Press, 1988.
Heine, P. "Nabīdh." *Encyclopaedia of Islam,* 2nd ed.
Heyd, Uriel. "Moses Hamon, Chief Jewish Physician to Sultan Suleyman the Magnificent," *Oriens,* 16 (1963): 152–70.
———. "Turkish Documents about Building Tiberias in the Sixteenth Century." *Sephunot* 10 (1966). (In Hebrew)
———. "An Unknown Turkish Treatise by a Jewish Physician under Suleyman the Magnificent." *Eretz Israel* 7 (1964): 48*–53*.
Horden, Peregrine. "A Discipline of Relevance: The Historiography of the Later Medieval Hospital." *Social History of Medicine* 1 (1988): 360–74.
———. "The Earliest Hospitals in Byzantium, Western Europe, and Islam." *Journal of Interdisciplinary History* 35 (2005): 361–89.
———. "The Millennium Bug: Health and Medicine around the Year 1000." *Social History of Medicine* 13 (2000): 201–19.
———. "Religion as Medicine: Music in Medieval Hospitals." In *Religion and Medicine in the Middle Ages,* ed. Peter Biller and Joseph Ziegler, 135–53. Woodsbridge, UK: York Medieval Press, 2001.
———. "Ritual and Public Health in the Early Medieval City." In *Body and City: Histories of Urban Public Health,* ed. Sally Sheard and Helen Power, 17–40. Aldershot, UK: Ashgate, 2000.
Horsburgh, C. Robert, Jr. "Healing by Design." *New England Journal of Medicine* 333 (1995): 735–40. (Subsequent correspondence between author and readers is in 334 (1996): 334–36.)
Hosain, Hidayet. "Al-Hudjwīrī," *Encyclopaedia of Islam,* 2nd ed.
Hourani, Albert. "How Should We Write the History of the Middle East?" *International Journal of Middle East Studies* 23 (1991): 125–35.
Hoyland, Robert. "Physiognomy in Islam." *Jerusalem Studies in Arabic and Islam* 30 (2005): 361–402.
Hughes, Jonathan. "The 'Matchbox on a Muffin': The Design of Hospitals in the Early NHS." *Medical History* 44 (2000): 21–56.
Hutton, Patrick H. "The History of Mentalities: The New Map of Cultural History." *History and Theory* 20 (1981): 237–59.
Ihsanoğlu, Ekmeleddin. *Science, Technology, and Learning in the Ottoman Empire: Western Influence, Local Institutions, and the Transfer of Knowledge*. Aldershot, UK: Ashgate, 2004.
———. "Türkçe Tibb-i Nebevī Yazmaları." *Tıp Tarihi Araştırmaları* 2 (1998): 34–39.
Inalcik, H. "Istanbul." *Encyclopaedia of Islam,* 2nd ed.
———. "Istanbul: An Islamic City." *Journal of Islamic Studies* 1 (1990): 1–23.

———. "Maṭbakh." *Encyclopaedia of Islam,* 2nd ed.
Inayatullah, Sh. "Contribution to the Historical Study of Hospitals in Medieval Islam." *Islamic Culture* 18 (1944): 1–14.
Ireland, Stanley, and William Bechhoefer, eds. *The Ottoman House: Papers from the Amasya Symposium, 24–27 September 1996.* London: British Institute of Archeology at Ankara, 1998.
'Īsā, Ahmad. *Ta'rīkh al-Bīmāristānāt fī al-Islām.* 2nd ed. Beirut: Dār al-Rā'īd al-'Arabī, 1401 [1981].
İzgi, Cevat. *Osmanlı Medreselerinde İlim.* 2 vols. İstanbul: İz Yayıncılık, 1997.
Jacquart, Danielle. "La physiognomonie à l'époque de Frédéric II: Le traité de Michel Scot." *Micrologus* 2 (1994): 19–37.
Jadon, Samira. "The Physicians of Syria during the Reign of Ṣalāḫ al-Dīn 570–598 A.H. 1174–1193 A.D." *Journal of the History of Medicine and Allied Science* 25 (1970): 323–40.
Jennings, Ronald. "The Society and Economy of Maçuka in the Ottoman Judicial Registers of Trabzon, 1560–1640." In *Continuity and Change in Late Byzantine and Early Ottoman Society,* ed. Anthony Bryer and Heath Lowry, 129–54. Birmingham: Centre for Byzantine Studies & Modern Greek, University of Birmingham, 1986.
Joralemon, Donald. *Exploring Medical Anthropology.* 2nd ed. Boston, MA: Allyn & Bacon, 2006.
Jordanova, Ludmilla. "The Art and Science of Seeing in Medicine: Physiognomy 1780–1820." In *Medicine and the Five Senses,* ed. W. F. Bynum and Roy Porter, 297–98 (notes). Cambridge: Cambridge University Press, 1993.
Juynboll, G. H. A. "Muslim b. al- Hadjdjādj," *Encyclopaedia of Islam,* 2nd ed.
Kafesçioğlu, Çiğdem. "The Ottoman Capital in the Making: The Reconstruction of Constantinople in the Fifteenth Century." PhD diss., Harvard University, 1996.
Kâhya, Esin. "One of the Samples of the Influences of Avicenna on the Ottoman Medicine, Shams al-Din Itaqi." *Belleten* 64, no. 4 (2000): 63–68.
——— and Aysegül D. Erdemir. *Bilimin Işığında Osmanlıdan Cumhuriyete Tıp ve Sağlık Kurumları.* Ankara: Türkiye Diyanet Vakfı Yayınları, 2000.
Karatay, Fehmi Edhem. *Topkapı Sarayı Müzesi Kütüphanesi Arapça Kataloğu.* Vol. 3. İstanbul: Topkapı Sarayı Müzesi, 1966.
Karmi, Ghada. "The Colonisation of Traditional Arabic Medicine." In *Patients and Practitioners: Lay Perceptions of Medicine in Pre-Industrial Society,* ed. Roy Porter, 315–39. Cambridge: Cambridge University Press, 1985.
Kassler, Jamie Croy. "Apollo and Dionysus: Music Theory and the Western Tradition of Epistemology." In *Music and Civilization: Essays in Honor of Paul Henry Lang,* ed. Edmond Strainchamps and Maria Rika Maniates, 457–71. New York: W. W. Norton, 1984.
———. "Man—A Musical Instrument: Models of the Brain and Mental Functions before the Computer." *History of Science* 22 (1984): 59–92.
Kedar, B.Z. "News from the Hospital." *'Et-mol* 5, no. 145 (July 1999): 6–9. (In Hebrew)

Khouri, Fuad I. *The Body in Islamic Culture.* London: Saqi Books, 2001.

Khoury, Dina Rizk. "Slippers at the Entrance or Behind Closed Doors: Domestic and Public Spaces for Mosuli Women." In *Women in the Ottoman Empire: Middle Eastern Women in the Early Modern Era,* ed. Madeline C. Zilfi, 105–27. Leiden: Brill, 1997.

King, Helen. "Introduction: What is Health?" In *Health in Antiquity,* ed. Helen King, 1–11. London: Routledge, 2005.

Kisacky, Jeane. "Restructuring Isolation: Hospital Architecture, Medicine, and Disease Prevention." *Bulletin of the History of Medicine* 79 (2005): 1–49.

Klein-Franke, Felix. "Health and Healing in Medieval Muslim Palestine." In *Health and Disease in the Holy Land,* ed. Manfred Wassermann and Samuel S. Kottek, 103–34. Lewiston, NY: E. Mellen Press, 1996.

———. "No Smoking in Paradise: The Habit of Tobacco Smoking Judged by Muslim law." *Le Muséon* 106 (1993): 155–83.

Kleinman, Arthur. "The Meaning Context of Illness and Care: Reflection on a Central Theme in the Anthropology of Medicine." In *Sciences and Cultures: Anthropological and Historical Studies of the Sciences,* ed. Everett Mendelsohn and Yehuda Elkana, 161–76. Dordrecht: D. Reidel, 1981.

Koenigsberger, H. G. *Early Modern Europe, 1500–1789.* London: Longman, 1987.

Kohlberg, E. "Vision and the Imams." In *Autour de Regard: Mélanges Gimaret,* ed. É. Chaumont, D. Aigle, M. A. Amir-Moezzi, and P. Lory, 125–57. Louvain: Peeters, 2003.

Konyalı, İbrahim Hakki. "Kanunī Sultan Süleyman'in Annesi Hafsa Sultan'ın Vakfiyyesi ve Manisa'daki Hayir Eserleri." *Vakıflar Dergisi* 8 (1969): 47–56.

Krawietz, Birgit. "Islamic Conception of the Evil Eye." *Medicine and Law* 21 (2002): 339–55.

Kudlick, Catherine J. "Disability History: Why We Need Another 'Other.' " *American Historical Review* 108 (2003): 763–93.

Kuhnke, LaVerne. *Lives at Risk: Public Health in Nineteenth Century Egypt.* Berkeley and Los Angeles: University of California Press, 1990.

Kuniholm, Peter Ian. "Dendochronologically Dated Ottoman Monuments." In *A Historical Archaeology of the Ottoman Empire,* ed. Uzi Baram and Lynda Carroll, 93–136. New York: Kluwer Academic/Plenum Publishers, 2000.

Kunt, I. Metin. *The Sultan's Servants: The Transformation of Ottoman Provincial Government, 1550–1650.* New York: Columbia University Press, 1983.

Kuran, Aptullah. *The Mosque in Early Ottoman Architecture.* Chicago: University of Chicago Press, 1968.

———. *Sinan: The Grand Old Master of Ottoman Architecture.* Washington, DC: Institute of Turkish Studies; Istanbul: Ada Press Publishers, 1985.

———. "A Spatial Study of Three Ottoman Capitals: Bursa, Edirne and Istanbul." *Muqarnas* 13 (1996): 114–31.

Landau-Tessaron, Ella. "Adoption, Paternity and False Genealogical Claims." *Bulletin of the School of Oriental and African Studies* 66 (2003): 169–92.

Lawrence, Christopher, and George Weisz, eds. *Greater than the Parts: Holism in Biomedicine, 1920–1950*. New York: Oxford University Press, 1998.

Leaman, Oliver. *Islamic Aesthetics: An Introduction*. Edinburgh: Edinburgh University Press, 2004.

Leeuwen, Marco H. D. van. "Histories of Risk and Welfare in Europe during the 18th and 19th Centuries." In *Health Care and Poor Relief in 18th and 19th Century Northern Europe*, ed. Ole Peter Grell, Andrew Cunningham, and Robert Jütte, 32–66. Aldershot, UK: Ashgate, 2002.

———. "Logic of Charity: Poor Relief in Pre-Industrial Europe." *Journal of Interdisciplinary History* 24 (1994): 589–613.

Leiser, Gary. "Medical Education in Islamic Lands from the Seventeenth to the Fourteenth Century." *Journal of History of Medicine and Allied Sciences* 38 (1983): 48–75.

Leiser, Gary, and Michael Dols, "Evliya Chelebi's Description of Medicine in Seventeenth-Century Egypt." *Sudhoff's Archiv* 71 (1987): 197–216; 72 (1988): 49–86.

Le Roy Ladurie, Emmanuel. "Presentation." *Annales: Economies, Sociétés, Civilizations* 29 (1974): 537.

Levanoni, Amalia. "Food and Cooking during the Mamluk Era: Social and Political Implications." *Mamlūk Studies Review* 9, no. 2 (2005): 201–22.

Levey, Martin. *Early Arabic Pharmacology*. Leiden: Brill, 1973.

Lewicka, Paulina B. "Restaurants, Inns and Taverns that Never Eere: Some Reflections on Public Consumption in Medieval Cairo." *Journal of the Economic and Social History of the Orient* 48 (2005): 40–91.

Lewis, Bernard. *The Jews of Islam*. Princeton, NJ: Princeton University Press, 1984.

———. *A Middle East Mosaic: Fragments of Life, Letters and History*. New York: Random House, 2000.

Lindemann, Mary, *Medicine and Society in Early Modern Europe*. Cambridge: Cambridge University Press, 1999.

Livingston, J. W. "Evliya Çelebi on Surgical Operation in Vienna." *Al-Abhāth* 23 (1970): 223–45.

Louis, A. L. "Ḥammām—Maghrib." *Encyclopaedia of Islam*, 2nd ed.

Luz, Nimrod. "Urban Residential Houses in Mamluk Syria: Forms, Characteristics and the Impact of Socio-Cultural Forces." In *The Mamluks in Egyptian and Syrian Politics and Society*, ed. Michael Winter and Amalia Levanoni, 339–55. Leiden: Brill, 2004.

Malti-Douglas, Fedwa. "Mentalités and Marginality: Blindness and Mamlûk Civilization." In *The Islamic World from Classical to Modern Times: Essays in Honor of Bernard Lewis*, ed. C. E. Bosworth, C. Issawi, R. Savory, and A. L. Udovitch, 211–37. Princeton, NJ: Darwin Press, 1989.

Mandler, Peter. "Poverty and Charity in the Nineteenth-Century Metropolis: An Introduction." In *The Uses of Charity: The Poor on Relief in the Nineteenth-Century Metropolis*, ed. Peter Mandler, 1–37. Philadelphia: University of Pennsylvania Press, 1990.

Marcus, Abraham. *The Middle East on the Eve of Modernity: Aleppo in the 18th Century*. New York: Columbia University Press, 1989.

———. "Privacy in Eighteenth-Century Aleppo: The Limits of Cultural Ideals." *International Journal of Middle East Studies* 18 (1986): 165–83.

Marcus, Clare Cooper, and Marni Barnes, eds. *Healing Gardens: Therapeutic Benefits and Design Recommendation*. New York: J. Wiley, 1999.

Marín, Manuela, and David Waines. "The Balanced Way: Food for Pleasure and Health in Medieval Islam." *Manuscripts of the Middle East* 4 (1989): 123–32.

Marmura, Michael. "Avicenna's 'Flying Man' in Context." *Monist* 69 (1986): 383–95.

Massée, H., D. B. MacDonald, D. N. Baratov, K. A. Nizami, and P. Voorhoeve. "Djīnn." *Encyclopaedia of Islam,* 2nd ed.

Mattson, Ingrid. "Status-Based Definitions of Need in Early Islamic *Zakat* and Maintenance Laws." In *Poverty and Charity in Middle Eastern Contexts,* ed. Michael Bonner, Mine Ener, and Amy Singer, 31–51. Albany: State University New York Press, 2003.

Mauss, Marcel. *The Gift: Forms and Functions of Exchange in Archaic Societies*. Trans. Ian Cunnison. London: Cohen & West, 1954.

McIntosh, Marjorie K. "Local Responses to the Poor in Late Medieval and Tudor England." *Continuity and Change* 3 (1988): 209–45.

Ménage, V. L. "Ḥadīdī." *Encyclopaedia of Islam,* 2nd ed.

Meyerhof, Max. *"The Book of the Ten Treatises on the Eye" Ascribed to Hunain ibn Is-haq (809–877 A.D.)*. Cairo: Govt. Press, 1928.

———. *Sarh Asma' al-Uqqar (Explication des nom de drogues): Un glossaire de matière medicale*. Le Caire: Impr. de l'Institut francais d'archeologie orientale, 1940.

———. *The Theologus Autodidactus of Ibn al-Nafis*. Oxford: Clarendon Press, 1968.

Meyerhof, Max, and Joseph Schacht. *The Medico-Philosophical Controversy between Ibn Butlan of Baghdad and Ibn Ridwan of Cairo: A Contribution to the History of Greek Learning among the Arabs*. Cairo: n.p., 1937.

———. "Ibn al-Nafīs." *Encyclopaedia of Islam,* 2nd ed.

Miller, Barnette. *Beyond the Sublime Porte*. New Haven, CT: Yale University Press, 1931.

Miller, Timothy S. *The Birth of the Hospital in the Byzantine Empire*. Rev. ed. Baltimore: Johns Hopkins University Press, 1997.

Mollat, Michel. *The Poor in the Middle Ages: An Essay in Social History*. New Haven, CT: Yale University Press, 1986.

Morrison, Robert G. "The Portrayal of Nature in a Medieval Qur'an Commentary." *Studia Islamica* 94 (2002): 115–37.

———. "Reasons for a Scientific Portrayal of Nature in Medieval Commentaries on the Qur'ān." *Arabica* 52 (2005): 182–203.

Müller, Kathrine. "*Al-ḥanīn ilā l-awṭān* in Early *Adab* Literature." In *Myths, Historical Archetypes, and Symbolic Figures in Arabic Literature: Towards a New Hermeneutic Approach,* ed. A. Neuwrith, B. Embaló, S. Günther, and M. Jarrar, 33–58. Beirut: In Kommission bei Franz Steiner Verlag, 1999.

Murphey, Rhoads. "Ottoman Medicine and Transculturalism from the 16th Century." *Bulletin of the History of Medicine* 66 (1992): 376–403.

———. *Ottoman Warfare 1500–1700.* New Brunswick, NJ: Rutgers University Press, 1999.

Murray, Stephen O. "Homosexuality among Slave Elites in Ottoman Turkey." In *Islamic Homosexualities: Culture, History, and Literature,* ed. Stephen O. Murray and Will Roscoe, 174–86. New York: New York University Press, 1997.

Naqvi, Ali Raza. "Adoption in Muslim Law." *Muslim Studies* 19 (1980): 283–302.

Necipoğlu, Gülru. *Architecture, Ceremonial, and Power: The Topkapı Palace in the Fifteenth and Sixteenth Centuries.* Cambridge, MA: MIT Press, 1991.

———. "Framing the Gaze in Ottoman, Safavid, and Mughal Palaces." *Ars Orientalis* 34 (1993): 303–42.

———. "From International Timurid to Ottoman: A Change of Taste in Sixteenth-Century Ceramic Tiles." *Muqarnas* 7 (1990): 136–70.

———. "A Ḳānūn for the State, a Canon for the Arts: Conceptualizing the Classical Synthesis of Ottoman Arts and Architecture." In *Soliman le Magnifique et son temps,* ed. Gilles Veinstein, 195–216. Paris: Documentation française, 1992.

———. "Plans and Models in 15th- and 16th-Century Ottoman Architectural Practice." *Journal of the Society of Architectural Historians* 45 (1986): 224–43.

———. "The Suburban Landscape of Sixteenth-Century Istanbul as a Mirror of Classical Ottoman Garden Culture." In *Gardens in the Time of the Great Muslim Empires,* ed. Attilio Petruccioli, 32–71. Leiden: Brill, 1997.

———. "The Süleymaniye Complex in Istanbul: An Interpretation." *Muqarnas* 7 (1996): 92–117.

Needham, Joseph. "Hygiene and Preventive Medicine." With Lu Gwei-Djen. *Journal of the History of Medicine and Allied Sciences* 17 (1962): 429–78.

Nelson, Hilde Lindemann, and James Lindemann Nelson. *The Patient in the Family: An Ethics of Medicine and Families.* New York: Routledge, 1995.

Nicholson, Reynold A., ed. *The Kashf al-Mahjūb: The Oldest Persian Treatise on Sufiism.* New ed. London: Printed for the Trustees of the "E. J. W. Gibb Memorial" and published by Luzac, 1976.

Nihat, M., and Baha Dörder. *Türk Tiatrosu Ansiklopedisi.* İstanbul: n.p., 1967.

Nutton, Vivian. *Ancient Medicine.* London: Routledge, 2004.

———. "God, Galen and the Depaganization of Ancient Medicine." In *Religion and Medicine in the Middle Ages,* ed. Peter Biller and Joseph Ziegler, 17–32. Woodsbridge, UK: York Medieval Press, 2001.

Opsomer-Halleux, Carmélia "The Medieval Garden and Its Role in Medicine." In *Medieval Gardens,* ed. Elisabeth B. MacDougall, 95–113. Washington, DC: Dumbarton Oaks Research Library and Collection, 1986.

Ormos, István. "The Theory of Humours in Islam (Avicenna)." *Quaderni di Studi Arabi* 5–6 (1987–88): 601–7.

Ortner, Sherry B. "Theory in Anthropology since the Sixties." *Comparative Studies in Society and History* 26 (1984): 126–66.

Özbek, Nadir. "Imperial Gifts and Sultanic Legitimation during the Late Ottoman Empire, 1876–1909." In *Poverty and Charity in Middle Eastern Contexts,* ed. Michael Bonner, Mine Ener, and Amy Singer, 203–20. Albany: State University New York Press, 2003.

———. "The Politics of Poor Relief in the Late Ottoman Empire, 1876–1914." *New Perspectives on Turkey* 21 (1999): 1–33.

Özçelik, Sadettin. "Bāsur Hastalığı ve Tedavisiyle İlgili 15. Yüzyılda ait bir Metin." *Yeni Tıp Tarihi Araştıtmaları* 4 (1998): 207–24.

Özçelikay, Gülbin, Eris Aşıl, Sevgi Şar, and Kenan Süveren. "A Study on Prescription Samples Prepared in Ottoman Empire Period [*sic*]." *Hamdard Medicus* 37 (1994): 28–35.

Özdemir, İbrahim. "Toward an Understanding of Environmental Ethics from a Qur'anic Perspective." In *Islam and Ecology: A Bestowed Trust,* ed. Richard C. Foltz, Frederick M. Denny, and Azizan Baharuddin, 3–37. Cambridge, MA: Center for the Study of World Religions, Harvard Divinity School; distributed by Harvard University Press, 2003.

Öztürk, O. M. "Folk Interpretation of Illness in Turkey and Its Psychological Significance." *Turkish Journal of Pediatrics* 7 (1965): 165–79.

———. "Folk Treatment of Mental Illness in Turkey." In *Magic, Faith and Healing,* ed. A. Kiev, 343–63. New York: Free Press of Glencoe, 1964.

Öztürk, O. M., and V. Volkan. "The Theory and Practice of Psychiatry in Turkey." In *Psychological Dimensions of Near Eastern Studies,* ed. L. C. Brown and N. Itzkowitz, 330–61. Princeton, NJ: Darwin Press, 1977.

Panzac, Daniel. *La peste dans l'Empire Ottoman 1700–1850.* Louvain: Peeters, 1985.

———. "La peste dans les possessions insulaires du grand seigneur (XVIIe–XIX siècles)." In *Insularités Ottomans,* ed. Nicolas Vatin and Gilles Veinstein, 223–40. Paris: Maisonneuve & Larose, 2004.

———. "Politique Sanitaire et Fixation des Frontièrs: L'example Ottoman (XVIIIe–XIXe siècles)." *Turcica* 31 (1999): 87–108.

Park, Katherine. "Healing the Poor: Hospitals and Medical Assistance in Renaissance Florence," In *Medicine and Charity before the Welfare State,* ed. Jonathan Barry and Colin Jones, 26–45. London: Routledge, 1991.

Park, Katherine, and John Henderson. " 'The First Hospital among Christians': The Opsedale di Santa Maria Nuova in Early Sixteenth-Century Florence." *Medical History* 35 (1991): 164–88.

Parker, Kenneth, ed. *Early Modern Tales of Orient: A Critical Anthology.* London: Routledge, 1999.

Peirce, Leslie. "The Family as Factions: Dynastic Politics in the Reign of Süleymân." In *Soliman le Magnifique et son temps,* ed. Gilles Veinstein, 105–16. Paris: Documentation française, 1992.

———. *The Imperial Harem: Women and Sovereignty in the Ottoman Empire.* New York: Oxford University Press, 1993.

———. *Morality Tales: Law and Gender in the Ottoman Court of Aintab*. Berkeley and Los Angeles: University of California Press, 2003.

Peirone, Federico. "Islam and Ecology in the Mediterranean Muslim *Kulturkreise*." *Hamdard Islamicus* 5, no. 2 (1981): 3–31.

Pelling, Margaret. "Healing the Sick Poor: Social Policy and Disability in Norwich, 1550–1640." *Medical History* 29 (1985): 115–37.

———. "Illness among the Poor in an Early Modern English Town: The Norwich Census of 1570." *Continuity and Change* 3 (1988): 273–90.

Perho, Iremli. *The Prophet's Medicine: A Creation of the Muslim Traditionalist Scholars*. Helsinki: Finnish Oriental Society, 1995.

Petruccioli, Attilio. "Nature in Islamic Urbanism: The Garden in Practice and in Metaphor." In *Islam and Ecology: A Bestowed Trust*, ed. Richard C. Foltz, Frederick M. Denny, and Azizan Baharuddin, 499–510. Cambridge, MA: Center for the Study of World Religions, Harvard Divinity School; distributed by Harvard University Press, 2003.

Pormann, Peter E. "The Physician and the Other: Images of the Charlatan in Medieval Islam." *Bulletin of the History of Medicine* 79 (2005): 189–227.

Pormann, Peter E., and Emilie Savage-Smith, *Medieval Islamic Medicine*. Edinburgh: Edinburgh University Press, 2007.

Porter, Roy. *The Greatest Benefit to Mankind*. London: Harper Collins, 1997.

———. "The Gift Relation: Philanthropy and Provincial Hospitals in Eighteenth-Century England." In *The Hospital in History*, ed. Lindsay Granshaw and Roy Porter, 149–78. London: Routledge, 1989.

———. "The Patient's View: Doing Medical History from Below." *Theory and Society* 14 (1985): 175–98.

Prawer, Joshua. "The Jewish Community in Jerusalem in the Crusader Period." In *The History of Jerusalem: Crusaders and Ayyubids (1099–1250)*, ed. Joshua Prawer and Haggai Ben-Shammai, 194–212. Jerusalem: Yad Ben-Zvi, 1991. (In Hebrew)

Prior, Lindsay. "The Architecture of the Hospital: A Study of Spatial Organization and Medical Knowledge." *British Journal of Sociology* 39 (1988): 86–94.

———. "The Local Space of Medical Discourse: Disease, Illness and Hospital Architecture." In *The Social Construction of Illness*, ed. Jens Lachmund and Gunner Stollberg, 67–84. Stuttgart: Robert Bosch Stiftung, 1992.

Pullan, Brian. "Support and Redeem: Charity and Poor Relief in Italian Cities from the Fourteenth to the Seventeenth Century." *Continuity and Change* 3 (1988): 177–208.

Qadi, Wadad, al-. "Expressions of Alienation in Early Arabic Literature." In *Myths, Historical Archetypes, and Symbolic Figures in Arabic Literature: Towards a New Hermeneutic Approach*, ed. A. Neuwrith, B. Embaló, S. Günther, and M. Jarrar, 3–31. Beirut: In Kommission bei Franz Steiner Verlag, 1999.

Quataert, Donald. "The Social History of Labor in the Ottoman Empire: 1800–1914." In *The Social History of Labor in the Middle East*, ed. Ellis Jay Goldberg, 19–36. Boulder, CO: Westview Press, 1996.

Rahman, Fazlur. *Health and Medicine in Islamic Tradition*. New York: ABC International Group, 1989.

Rawcliffe, Carole. "Hospital Nurses and Their Work." In *Daily Life in the Late Middle Ages,* ed. Richard Britnell, 53–64. Stroud: Sutton Pub., 1998.

———. "Medicine for the Soul: The Medieval English Hospital and the Quest for Spiritual Health." In *Religion, Health and Suffering,* ed. John R. Hinnells and Roy Porter, 316–38. London: Kegan Paul International, 1999.

Reindl-Kiel, Hedda. "The Chicken of Paradise: Official Meals in the Mid-Seventeeenth Century Ottoman Palace." In *The Illuminated Table, The Prosperous House: Food and Shelter in Ottoman Material Culture,* ed. Suraiya Faroqhi and Christoph K. Neumann, 59–88. Würzburg: Ergon in Kommission, 2003.

Rice, Eugene F. *The Foundations of Early Modern Europe, 1460–1559.* With Anthony Grafton. New York: W. W. Norton, 1994.

Risse, Guenter B. *Mending Bodies, Saving Souls*. New York: Oxford University Press, 1999.

Robson, J. "Al-Bukhārī, Muḥammad b. Isma'īl." *Encyclopaedia of Islam,* 2nd ed.

Rogers, J. Michael. "Innovation and Continuity in Islamic Urbanism." In *The Arab City: Its Characteristics and Islamic Cultural Heritage,* ed. Ismail Serageldin and Samir El-Sadek, 53–61. Riyadh: Arab Urban Development Institute, 1982.

———. "The Palace, Potions and the Public: Some Lists of Drugs in Mid–16th Century Ottoman Turkey." In *Studies in Ottoman History in Honour of Professor V. L. Mènage,* ed. Colin Heywood and Colin Imber, 273–95. Istanbul: Isis Press, 1994.

Rosen, George. *A History of Public Health*. New York: MD Publications, 1958.

———. *Madness in Society: Chapters in the Historical Sociology of Mental Illness*. Chicago: University of Chicago Press, 1968.

Rosenberg, Charles E. "Body and Mind in Nineteenth-Century Medicine: Some Clinical Origins of the Neurosis Construct." In *Explaining Epidemics and Other Studies in the History of Medicine,* 74–89. Cambridge: Cambridge University Press, 1992.

. *The Care of Strangers: The Rise of America's Hospital System*. New York: Basic Books, 1997.

———. *Explaining Epidemics and Other Studies in the History of Medicine*. Cambridge: Cambridge University Press, 1992.

Rosenthal, Franz. "The Defense of Medicine in the Medieval Muslim World." *Bulletin of the History of Medicine* 43 (1969): 519–32.

———. *The Herb: Hashish versus Medieval Muslim Society*. Leiden: Brill, 1971.

———. "The Physician in Medieval Muslim Society." *Bulletin of the History of Medicine* 52 (1978): 476–91.

———. "The Stranger in Medieval Islam." *Arabica* 44 (1997): 35–75.

Rosner, David. "Social Control and Social Service: The Changing Use of Space in Charity Hospitals." *Radical History Review* 21 (1979): 183–97.

Rubin, Miri. *Charity and Community in Medieval Cambridge*. Cambridge: Cambridge University Press, 1987.

———. "Development and Change in English Hospitals, 1100–1500." In *The Hospital in History*, ed. Lindsay Granshaw and Roy Porter, 41–59. London: Routledge, 1989.

Rubin, Uri. "Muḥammad the Exorcist: Aspects of Islamic-Jewish Polemics." *Jerusalem Studies in Islam* 30 (2005): 94–111.

Rugh, Andrea B. "Orphanages in Egypt: Contradiction or Affirmation in a Family-Oriented Society." In *Children in the Muslim Middle East*, ed. Elizabeth Warnock Fernea, 124–41. Austin: University of Texas Press, 1995.

Ruggles, D. Fairchild. *Gardens, Landscape, and Vision in the Palaces of Islamic Spain*. University Park: Pennsylvania State University Press, 2000.

———. "Humayun's Tomb and Garden." In *Gardens in the Time of the Great Muslim Empires*, ed. Attilio Petruccioli, 173–86. Leiden: Brill, 1997.

Russell, Gül A. " 'The Owl and the Pussycat': The Process of Cultural Transmission in Anatomical Illustration." In *Transfer of Modern Science and Technology to the Muslim World*, ed. Ekmeleddin Ihsanoğlu, 180–212. Istanbul: Research Centre for Islamic History, Art and Culture, 1992.

———. "Physicians at the Ottoman Court." *Medical History* 34 (1990): 243–67.

Sabra, Adam A. *Poverty and Charity in Medieval Islam: Mamluk Egypt, 1250–1517*. Cambridge: Cambridge University Press, 2000.

Sadan, J. "Khamr," *Encyclopaedia of Islam*, 2nd ed.

———. "Mashrūbāt," *Encyclopaedia of Islam*, 2nd ed.

Sahillioğlu, Halil. "Üsküdar'ın Mamure (Cedide) Mahallesi Fıtık Cerrahları." *Yeni Tıp Tarihi Araştıtmaları* 4 (1998): 59–66.

Sakaoğlu, Necdet. "Sources for Our Ancient Culinary Culture." In *The Illuminated Table, The Prosperous House: Food and Shelter in Ottoman Material Culture*, ed. Suraiya Faroqhi and Christoph K. Neumann, 34–49. Würzburg: Ergon in Kommission, 2003.

Saleh, Marlis J. "Al-Suyuti and His Works: Their Place in Islamic Scholarship from Mamluk Times to the Present." *Mamlūk Studies Review* 5 (2001): 73–89.

Saraçgil, Ayşe. "Generi voluttuari e region di stato: Politiche repressive del consumo di vino, caffè e tobacco nell'Impero Ottomano nei secc. XVI e XVII." *Turcica* 28 (1996): 163–94.

Sargutan, Erdal. "Selçuklular'da Tıb ve Tıb Kurulusları." *Vakıflar Dergisi* 11 (1976): 313–22.

Sarı, Nil (Akdeniz). "Educating the Ottoman Physician." *Yeni Tıp Tarihi Araştırmaları* 2 (1998): 40–64.

———. "Osmanlı Darüşşifalarına Tayin Edilecek Görevlilerde Aranan Nitlikler." *Yeni Tıp Tarihi Araştırmaları* 1 (1995): 11–54.

———. "Türk Tıp Tarihinde Yelemk ile Tıp Arasındaki İlişkiye ait Örnekler." In *İkinci Milletarası Yemek Kongresi (3–10 Eylül 1988)*, ed. Feyzi Halıcı, 392–402. Konya: Konya Kültür ve Turizm Vakfı Yayınları, 1989.

Sarı, Nil (Akdeniz), and Ali H. Bayat. "The Medical Organization at the Ottoman Court." *Studies in History of Medicine and Science* n.s., 16 (1999–2000): 37–51.

Sarı, Nil (Akdeniz), and M. Bedizel Zülfikar. "Islâm Tıbbından Osmanlı Tıbbına Kuşlarla Tedavi." In *Dördüncü Milletlerarası Yemek Kongresi, 3–6 Eylül 1992,* ed. Feyzi Halıcı, 259–71. Konya: Konya Kültür ve Turizm Vakfı Yayınları, 1993.

Savage-Smith, Emilie. "Al-Zahrāwī, Abū al-Ḳāsim Khalaf b. al-'Abbās," *Encyclopaedia of Islam,* 2nd ed.

———. "Attitudes toward Dissection in Medieval Islam." *Journal of the History of Medicine and Allied Sciences* 50 (1995): 67–110.

———. "Gleanings from an Arabist's Workshop: Current Trends in the Study of Medieval Islamic Science and Medicine." *Isis* 79 (1988): 246–66.

———. "Medicine." In *Encyclopedia of the History of Arabic Science,* ed. Roshdi Rashed, 3:903–61. 3 vols. London: Routledge, 1996.

———. "The Practice of Surgery in Islamic Lands: Myth and Reality," *Social History of Medicine,* 13 (2000): 307–21.

———. "Tashrīḥ," *Encyclopaedia of Islam,* 2nd ed.

Scalenghe, Sara. "The Deaf in Ottoman Syria, 16th–18th Centuries." *Arab Studies Journal* 13 (2005): 10–25.

Schacht, Joseph *An Introduction to Islamic Law.* Oxford: Clarendon Press, 1964.

Seçkin, Yasin Çağatay. "Gardens of the Ninteenth-Century Imperial Palaces in Istanbul." *Studies in the History of Gardens and Designed Landscape* 23 (2003): 72–86.

Sedgwick, Peter. "Michel Foucault: The Anti-History of Psychiatry." *Psychological Medicine* 11 (1981): 235–48.

Şehsuvaroğlu, Bedi N. *İstanbul'da 500 Yıllık Sağlık Hayatımız.* İstanbul: İstanbul Fetih Derneği Neşriyati, 1953.

———. Ayşegül Erdemir Demirhan, and Gönül Cantay Güreşsever. *Türk Tıp Tarihi.* Bursa: n.p., 1984.

Semerdjian, Elyse. "Sinful Professions: Illegal Occupations of Women in Ottoman Aleppo, Syria." *Hawwa* 1 (2003): 60–85.

Shah-Khan. "The Song of Creation: Sufi Themes on Nature." *Sufi* (London) 18 (Summer 1993): 27–30.

Shapiro, Arthur K., and Elaine Shapiro. "The Placebo Effect: Is It Much Ado about Nothing?." In *The Placebo Effect,* ed. Anne Harrington, 12–36. Cambridge, MA: Harvard University Press, 1997.

———. *The Powerful Placebo: From Ancient Priest to Modern Physician.* Baltimore: Johns Hopkins University Press, 1997.

Sheard, Sally, and Helen Power, eds. *Body and City: Histories of Urban Public Health.* Aldershot, UK: Ashgate, 2000.

Shefer, Miri. "Charity and Hospitals in the Ottoman Empire in the Early Modern Period." In *Poverty and Charity in Middle Eastern Contexts,* ed. Michael Bonner, Mine Ener, and Amy Singer, 121–43. Albany: State University New York Press, 2003.

———. "Hospitals in the Three Ottoman Capitals: Bursa, Edirne and Istanbul in the Sixteenth and Seventeenth Centuries," PhD diss., Tel Aviv University. Tel Aviv, 2001. (In Hebrew)

———. "Insanity and the Insane in the Ottoman Empire." In *Minorities, Foreigners and Marginals,* ed. Shulamit Volkov, 91–204. Jerusalem: Zalman Shazar Center, 2000. (In Hebrew)

———. "Medical and Professional Ethics in Sixteenth-Century Istanbul: Towards an Understanding of the Relationships between the Ottoman State and the Medical Guilds." *Medicine and Law* 21 (2002): 307–19.

———. "Old Patterns, New Meaning: The 1845 Hospital of Bezm-i 'Alem in Istanbul." *Dynamis* 25 (2005): 329–50.

Shehadi, Fadlou. *Philosophies of Music in Medieval Islam.* Leiden: Brill, 1995.

Shiloah, Amnon. "Jewish and Muslim Tradition of Music Therapy." In *Music as Medicine: The History of Music Therapy since Antiquity,* ed. Peregrine Horden, 69–83. Aldershot, UK: Ashgate, 2000.

———. "Musical Modes and the Medical Dimension: The Arabic Sources." In *Metaphor: A Musical Dimension,* ed. Jamie C. Kassler, 147–59. Sydney: Currency Press, 1991.

———. *Music in the World of Islam: A Socio-Cultural Study.* Detroit: Wayne State University Press, 1995.

———. *The Theory of Music in Arabic Writings (c.900—1900).* Munich: G. Henle, 1979.

Shoshan, Boaz. "The State and Madness in Medieval Islam." *International Journal of Middle East Studies* 35 (2003): 329–40.

Singer, Amy. *Constructing Ottoman Beneficence: An Imperial Soup Kitchen in Jerusalem.* Albany: State University New York Press, 2002.

———. "Serving Up Charity: The Ottoman Public Kitchen." *Journal of Interdisciplinary History* 35 (2005): 481–500.

Siraisi, Nancy G. "Some Current Trends in the Study of Renaissance Medicine." *Renaissance Quarterly* 37 (1984): 585–600.

Skilliter, Susan A. "Three Letters from Ottoman 'Sultana' Safiye to Queen Elizabeth I." In *Documents from Islamic Chanceries,* ed. S. M. Stern, 119–57. Oxford: B. Cassirer, 1965.

Slack, Paul. "Hospitals, Workhouses and the Relief of the Poor in Early Modern London." In *Health Care and Poor Relief in Protestant Europe 1500–1700,* ed. Ole Peter Grell and Andrew Cunningham, 234–51. London: Routledge, 1997.

Smuts, J. C. *Holism and Evolution.* London: Macmillan, 1926.

———. "Some Recent Scientific Advances in Their Bearing on Philosophy," in: *Our Changing World-View.* Johannesburg: University of the Witwatersrand Press, 1932.

Sohrweide, H. "Luḳmān b. Sayyid Ḥusayn." *Encyclopaedia of Islam,* 2nd ed.

Sonbol, Amira el-Azhary. "Adoption in Islamic Society: A Historical Survey." In *Children in the Muslim Middle East,* ed. Elizabeth Warnock Fernea, 45–67. Austin: University of Texas Press, 1995.

———. *The Creation of a Medical Profession in Egypt, 1800–1922*. Syracuse: Syracuse University Press, 1991.

Sontag, Susan. *Illness as Metaphor*. New York: Farrar, Straus and Giroux, 1978.

Stavroulakis, Nicholas. "The Flora of Ottoman Gardens: I. Trees." *Mediterranean Garden* 10 (1997): 7–16

———. "The Flora of Ottoman Gardens: II. Flowering Plants." *Mediterranean Garden* 11 (1997–98): 11–20.

Steinberg, Ted. "Down to Earth: Nature, Agency and Power in History." *American Historical Review* 107 (2002): 798–820.

Stillman, Norman A. "Charity and Social Service in Medieval Islam." *Societas* 5 (1975): 105–15.

———. "Khil'a." *Encyclopaedia of Islam*, 2nd ed.

Sujimon, M. S. "The Treatment of the Foundling (*al-laqīṭ*) according to the Ḥanafīs." *Islamic Law and Society* 9 (2002): 358–85.

Tannahill, Reay. *Food in History*. 2nd ed. Harmondsworth, UK: Penguin, 1988.

Tapper, Richard, and Nancy Tapper. " 'Eat This, It'll Do You a Power of Good': Food and Commensality among Durrani Pashtuns." *American Ethnologist* 13 (1986): 62–79.

Temkin, Owsei. "An Historical Analysis of the Concept of Infection." In *Studies in Intellectual History*, 123–47. Baltimore: Johns Hopkins University Press, 1953.

Terzioğlu, Arslan. "Evliya Çelebi's Beschreibung der Südosteuropäischen Hospitäler und Heilbäder des 17. Jahrhunderts und ihre Kulturgeschichtliche Bedeutung." *Revue des Études Sud-Est Européennes* 13 (1975): 429–42.

———. "15. ve 16. Yüzyılda Türk-İslam Hastane Yapıları ve Bunların Dünya Çapındaki Önemi." In *II. Ulusarası Türk-Islam Bilim ve Teknoloji Tarihi Kongresi (I.T.Ü 28 Nisan–2 Mayıs 1986)*, 155–97. Vol. 3. İstanbul: n.p., 1987.

———. *Die Hofspitäler und undere Gesundheitseinrichtungen der Osmanischen Palastbauten unter Berücksichtigung der Ursprungsfrage sowie Ihre Beziehungen zu den Abendländischen Hofspitälern*. Munich: Dr. Dr. Rudolf Trofenik, 1979.

Thompson, John A., and Grace Goldin. *The Hospital: A Social and Architectural History*. New Haven, CT: Yale University Press, 1975

Thompson, Mine F. "Turkey." In *Encyclopedia of Gardens: History and Design*, 3:1333–35. 3 vols. Chicago: Fitzroy Dearborn Publishers, 2001.

Tibi, Selma. *The Medicinal Use of Opium in Ninth-Century Baghdad*. Leiden: Brill, 2006.

Titley, Nora M. *Miniatures from Turkish Manuscripts: A Catalogue and Subject Index of Paintings in the British Library and British Museum*. London: Library, 1981.

Titley, Nora M., and Frances Wood. *Oriental Gardens: An Illustrated History*. San Francisco: Chronicle Books, 1992.

Toledano, Ehud. "The Emergence of Ottoman-Local Elites (1700–1800): A Framework for Research." In *Middle Eastern Politics and Ideas: A History*

from Within, ed. I. Pappe and M. Ma'oz, 145–62. London: Tauris Academic Studies, 1997.
Tolmacheva, Marina. "Female Piety and Patronage in the Medieval 'Hajj.' " In *Women in the Medieval Islamic World*, ed. Gavin R. G. Hambly, 161–79. New York: St. Martin's Press, 1998.
Tritton, A. S. "Djanāza." *Encyclopaedia of Islam*, 2nd ed.
———. "Ḥināṭa." *Encyclopaedia of Islam*, 2nd ed.
Ullmann, Manfred. *Islamic Medicine*. Edinburgh: Edinburgh University Press, 1978.
Uluçay, Çağatay. "Kanunī Sultan Süleyman ve Ailesi ile İlgili Bazi Notlar ve Vesikalar." In *Kanuni Armağanı*, 225–57. Ankara: Türk Tarih Kurumu, 1970.
[Uludağ], Osman Şevki. *Beş Büçük Asırlık Türk Ṭebābeti Ta'rihi*. İstanbul: Matbaa-i Amire, 1341H/1925.
———. "Haseki Darüşşifası." *Tıb Dünyası* 9 (1938): 3728–30.
Üngör, Ethem Ruhi. "The Turkish Music and Instruments in the Ottoman State." In *Culture and Arts*, ed. Kemal Çiçek, 535–47. Vol. 4 of *The Great Ottoman-Turkish Civilization*. Ankara: Yeni Türkiye, 2000.
Unschuld, Paul U. *Medicine in China: A History of Ideas*. Berkeley and Los Angeles: University of California Press, 1985.
Ünver, Ahmet Süheyl. "L'album d'Ahmed Ier." *Annali dell'Istituto Universitario Orientale di Napoli* 13 (1963): 127–62.
———. "Anadolu ve İstanbulda İmaretlerin Aşhane, Tabhane ve Misafirhanelerine ve Müessislerinin Ruhī Kemallerine dair." *İstanbul Üniversitesi Tıb Fakültesi Mecmuası* 4, no. 18 (1941): 2390–410.
———. "Büyük Selçuklu İmperatorluğu Zamaninda Vakıf Hastanelerin Bir Kismına Dair." *Vakıflar Dergisi* 1 (1938): 17–23.
———. "Eski Evlerimizde Mualece Dolapları, Sandıkları ve İhtiva Ettigi İlāçlara Ait Bir Misal." *Türk Tıp Tarihi Arkivi* 15 (1940): 120–24.
———. "Fatih Darüşşifası Plâni." *Türk Tıp Tarihi Arkivi*, 21–22 (1943): 23–28.
———. "Fatih Külliyesine ait Diğer Mühim bir Vakfiye." *Vakıflar Dergisi* 1 (1938): 39–45.
———. "Fatih Külliyesinin Ilk Vakfiyesine Göre Fatih Darüşşifası." *Türk Tıb Tarihi Arkivi* 17 (1940): 13–17.
———. "Four Medical Vignettes from Turkey." *International Record of Medicine* 171 (1958): 52–57.
———. "İstanbul'un Bazı Acı ve Tatlı Sularının Halkça Maruf Şifa Hassaları Hakkında." *Türk Tıp Tarihi Arkivi* 18 (1940): 90–96.
———. *İstanbul Üniversitesi Tarihi Baslangıç, Fatih Külliyesi ve Zamanı Hayatı*. İstanbul: n.p., 1946.
———. "İstanbul'un Zabtından Sonra Türklerde Tibbī Tekāmüle Bir Bakış." *Vakıflar Dergisi* 2 (1939): 71–81.
———. "Kanunī Süleyman'a İlkbaharda İlāç Yapılması." *Türk Tıp Tarihi Arkivi* 14, no. 4 (1939): 83–86.
———. "Türk Hamamları." *Türk Dünyası* 5 (1950): 198–203.

———. "XVinci Asırda Türkiyede Tecrubi Tababete ait İki Misal." *İstanbul Üniversitesi Tıp Fakültesi Mecmuası* 3 (1949): 1–4.

Uslu, Recep. "Musicians in the Ottoman Empire and Central Asia in the 15th Century According to an Unknown Work of Aydınlı Şemseddin Nahifi." In *Culture and Arts*, ed. Kemal Çiçek, 548–55. Vol. 4 of *The Great Ottoman-Turkish Civilization.* Ankara: Yeni Türkiye, 2000.

Veselý, Rudolf. "Neues zur Familie al-Qūṣūnī: Ein Beitrag zue Genealogie einer Ägyptischen Ärzte- und Gelehrtenfamilie." *Oriens* 33 (1992): 437–44.

Vogt-Göknil, Ulya. *Living Architecture: Ottoman.* Photography by Edward Widmer. London: Grosset & Dunlap, 1966.

Waines, David. "Abū Zayd al-Balkhī on the Nature of Forbidden Drink: A Medieval Islamic Controversy." In *La alimentación en las culturas islámicas*, ed. Manuela Marín and David Waines, 111–26. Madrid: Agenica Española de Cooperación Internacional, 1994.

Walsh, J. "ʿAṭāʾī." *Encyclopaedia of Islam*, 2nd ed.

Wear, Andrew. "Interfaces: Perceptions of Health and Illness in Early Modern England." In *Problems and Methods in the History of Medicine*, ed. Roy Porter and Andrew Wear, 230–55. New York: Croom Helm, 1987.

Wear, R. K. French, and I. M. Lonie, eds. *The Medical Renaissance of the Sixteenth Century.* Cambridge: Cambridge University Press, 1985.

Weiler, Ingomar. "Inverted *Kalokagathia.*" In *Representing the Body of the Slave*, ed. Thomas Wiedemann and Jane Gardner, 11–28. London: Frank Cass, 2002.

Weir, T. H., and A. Zysow. "Sadaḳa." *Encyclopaedia of Islam*, 2nd ed., s.v. "Sadaḳa," by T. H. Weir and A. Zysow.

West, Martin. *Ancient Greek Medicine.* Oxford: Oxford University Press, 1992.

———. "Music Therapy in Antiquity." In *Music as Medicine: The History of Music Therapy since Antiquity*, ed. Peregrine Horden, 51–68. Aldershot, UK: Ashgate, 2000.

Westcoat, James L. Jr. "From the Gardens of the Qur'an to the 'Gardens' of Lahore." In *Islam and Ecology: A Bestowed Trust*, ed. Richard C. Foltz, Frederick M. Denny, and Azizan Baharuddin, 511–26. Cambridge, MA: Center for the Study of World Religions, Harvard Divinity School; distributed by Harvard University Press, 2003.

Wilber, Ken. *The Marriage of Sense and Soul: Integrating Science and Religion.* Dublin: Gateway, 1998.

Winter, Michael. "Islamic Attitudes toward the Human Body." In *Religious Reflections on the Human Body*, ed. Jane Marie Law, 36–45. Bloomington: Indiana University Press, 1995.

White, George E. "Evil Spirits and the Evil Eye in Turkish Lore." *Moslem World* 9 (1919): 179–86.

Wright, O. "*Çargâh* in Turkish Classical Music versus Theory." *Bulletin of the School of Oriental and African Studies* 53 (1990): 224–44.

———. "On the Influence of a 'Timurid Music.' " *Oriente Moderno* n.s., 15 (1996): 665–81.

———. "Under the Influence? Preliminary Reflections on Arab Music during the Ottoman Period." In *The Balance of Truth: Essays in Honour of Professor Geoffrey Lewis*, ed. Çiğdem Balim-Harding and Colin Imber, 407–29. İstanbul: Isis Press, 2000.

———. *Words without Songs: A Musicological Study of an Early Ottoman Anthology and its Precursors*. London: School of Oriental and African Studies, University of London, 1992.

Yan, Yun-xiang. *The Flow of Gifts: Reciprocity and Social Networks in a Chinese Village*. Stanford, CA: Stanford University Press, 1996.

Yang, Mayfair Mei-Hui. *Gifts, Favors, and Banquets: The Art of Social Relationships in China*. Ithaca, NY: Cornell University Press, 1994.

Yazbak, Mahmoud. "Muslim Orphans and the *Sharīʿa* in Ottoman Palestine according to *Sijill* Records." *Journal of the Economic and Social History of the Orient* 44 (2001): 123–40.

Yürükoğlu, Nihad Nuri. *Manisa Bimarhanesi*. İstanbul: n.p., 1948.

Ze'evi, Dror. *An Ottoman Century: The District of Jerusalem in the 1600s*. Albany: State University New York Press, 1996.

———. "The Ottoman Century: The Sancak of Jerusalem in the 17th Century." PhD diss., Tel Aviv University, 1991. (In Hebrew)

———. *Producing Desire: Changing Sexual Discourse in the Ottoman Middle East, 1500–1900*. Berkeley and Los Angeles: University of California Press, 2006.

Ziegler, Joseph. "Religion and Medicine in the Middle Ages." In *Religion and Medicine in the Middle Ages*, ed. Peter Biller and Joseph Ziegler, 1–16. Rochester, NY: York Medieval Press, 2001.

Zysow, A. "Zakāt." *Encyclopaedia of Islam*, 2nd ed.

Internet

H-MedAnthro: An electronic forum for medical anthropologists, http://www.h-net.org/~medanthro.

Larson, Jean, and Mary Jo Kreitzer. "Healing by Design: Healing Gardens and Therapeutic Landscapes." *Implications* 2, no. 10 (a newsletter by InformeDesign, a Web site for design and human behavior research at the University of Minnesota), http://www.informedesign.umn.edu/_news/nov_v02-p.pdf.

Oxford English Dictionary: http://www.oed.com.

Ulrich, Roger S. "Health Benefits of Gardens in Hospitals." Paper for *Plants for People*, International Exhibition Floriade 2002, http://www.planterra.com/SymposiumUlrich.pdf.

Index